Assessing and Differentiating Reading & Writing Disorders

Multidimensional Model

LINDA J. LOMBARDINO, Ph.D.

Professor of Speech-Language Pathology
School of Special Education, School of Psychology,
and Early Childhood Studies
University of Florida

D1737615

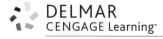

DELMAR
CENGAGE Learning™

Australia • Canada • Mexico • Singapore • Spain • United Kingdom • United States

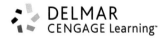
DELMAR
CENGAGE Learning™

Assessing and Differentiating Reading & Writing Disorders: Multidimensional Model
Linda J. Lombardino, Ph.D.

Director of Learning Solutions: Matthew Kane

Senior Acquisitions Editor: Sherry Dickinson

Associate Acquisitions Editor: Tom Stover

Managing Editor: Marah Bellegarde

Product Manager: Laura J. Wood

Editorial Assistant: Anthony Souza

Vice President, Marketing: Jennifer Baker

Marketing Director: Wendy E. Mapstone

Associate Marketing Manager: Jonathan Sheehan

Production Manager: Andrew Crouth

Senior Content Project Manager: Andrea Majot

Senior Art Director: David Arsenault

For product information and technology assistance, contact us at
Cengage Learning Customer & Sales Support, 1-800-354-9706
For permission to use material from this text or product,
submit all requests online at **www.cengage.com/permissions**.
Further permissions questions can be e-mailed to
permissionrequest@cengage.com

Library of Congress Control Number: 2011923837

ISBN-13: 978-1-1115-3989-4

ISBN-10: 1-1115-3989-8

Delmar
5 Maxwell Drive
Clifton Park, NY 12065-2919
USA

Cengage Learning is a leading provider of customized learning solutions with office locations around the globe, including Singapore, the United Kingdom, Australia, Mexico, Brazil, and Japan. Locate your local office at:
international.cengage.com/region

Cengage Learning products are represented in Canada by
Nelson Education, Ltd.

To learn more about Delmar, visit **www.cengage.com/delmar**

Purchase any of our products at your local college store or at our preferred online store **www.cengagebrain.com**

Notice to the Reader

Printed in the United States of America
1 2 3 4 5 6 7 14 13 12 11

Table of Contents

CHAPTER 3 • Application of the Multidimensional Assessment of Reading and Writing Disorders to the Diagnostic Process

CHAPTER 4 • Identifying and Classifying Children at Risk for Reading Deficits

CHAPTER 5 • Identifying and Classifying School-Age Children with Reading Disabilities

Preface

INTRODUCTION

This book is designed to provide practitioners with an integrated clinical and educational model called the *Multidimensional Model for Assessing Reading and Writing (MAR^{w}R)*. The MAR^{w}R is intended to provide a detailed roadmap needed to examine the multiple cognitive and language-based skill domains that support the acquisition of skilled reading. The fundamental tenets of this book are that (1) both broad and deep levels of knowledge about the cognitive processes that underlie reading and the component skills of reading must be understood to make a differential diagnosis of reading disorders; and (2) individual profiles of struggling readers' strengths and weaknesses are essential for determining the skills to be targeted in a comprehensive approach to intervention.

Because reading is by its very nature a dynamic and complex process, this book should appeal to a wide range of professionals in disciplines that include, but are not limited to: speech-language pathology, special education, school psychology, clinical psychology, and early childhood studies. The term "practitioner" is used throughout the book to represent the diversity of professionals from multiple disciplines who work with students who have reading and writing difficulties. The skills of the evaluator rather than the discipline that the evaluator represents will determine the sections of this book that are most relevant and useful to the individual practitioner.

CONCEPTUAL APPROACH

This book was designed to integrate the most recent cross-disciplinary scientific literature on factors that are strongly associated with understanding reading difficulties and evaluating reading strengths and weaknesses. After using this book, practitioners should be armed with the tools needed to conduct reading evaluations with greater depth and breadth, and to interpret assessment data with greater precision. Differentiated assessments should lead practitioners to (1) identify core weaknesses that underlie the struggling readers' difficulties, (2) provide diagnoses that have greater scientific validity, and (3) recommend specific reading intervention and accommodation plans.

In addition, this book is designed to provide practitioners with the knowledge necessary to understand the reading process and breakdowns in the process by answering the following questions:

- Which cognitive skills are most critical in supporting the acquisition of skilled reading (e.g., phonological memory, speed of word recognition)?

- How do cognitive processing skills and core component reading skills work together to support reading?

- What breakdowns can occur in any one or more of these processes and what reading skills are impacted?

- What are the optimal methods for evaluating component reading skills and underlying cognitive constructs?

- How can profiles of strengths and weaknesses be used to recognize learners who are at risk for future reading difficulties, to diagnose reading disabilities, to interpret assessment data, and to guide diagnosis and treatment?

ORGANIZATION OF TEXT

Each chapter addresses the assessment of reading in the context of the MAR^{w}R. Chapter 1, **Foundations for a Practitioner's Model of Reading Assessment**, is designed to provide practitioners with (a) an overview of issues related to components of reading, (b) connections between oral and written language, and (c) a historical perspective on the classifications of reading difficulties as the basis for establishing a foundation for the differential diagnosis of reading disability.

Chapter 2, **A Multidimensional Model for Assessing Reading and Writing**, is designed to (a) introduce practitioners to the 10 modules that compose MAR^{w}R, (b) provide practitioners with a cross-disciplinary perspective of the scientific literature that pertains to each of the 10 MAR^{w}R modules, and (c) describe developmental and graphic schemes for understanding how skills develop over time and how they interact with other skills to support reading and writing development.

Chapter 3, **Application of the Multidimensional Assessment of Reading and Writing Disorders to the Diagnostic Process**, is designed to (a) provide practitioners with a comprehensive selection of standardized tests and other procedures for gathering test data on the skills represented in the MAR^{w}R modules; (b) assist practitioners in interpreting the data in an effort to identify learners' core areas of weakness that impact their ability to advance as expected in the acquisition of skilled reading and in diagnosing the disabilities tied to these weaknesses; and (c) assist practitioners in developing informed intervention goals.

Chapter 4, **Identifying and Classifying Children at Risk for Reading Deficits**, aims to provide practitioners with (a) a framework for classifying profiles in young children with normal-range intellectual abilities who are showing difficulties in one or more domains of language during the preschool through first-grade years, placing them at risk for later reading difficulties; and (b) sample assessment protocols and diagnostic reports for three profiles of learners (spoken language and emergent literacy deficit, emergent literacy deficit, environmental disadvantage deficit) who are at risk for future reading disabilities.

Chapter 5, **Identifying and Classifying School-Age Learners with Reading Disorders**, is designed to provide practitioners with (a) a framework for classifying profiles in school-age children (dyslexia, mixed spoken and written language disability, comprehension deficit disorder) in the second semester of first grade and beyond who have normal-range intellectual abilities yet are showing difficulties in one or more domains of reading and who are failing to keep pace with their classroom peers; and (b) sample assessment protocols and diagnostic reports for three profiles of reading-impaired learners.

Finally, Chapter 6, **Counseling and Intervention,** is aimed at (a) equipping practitioners with tools and tips for diagnostic counseling, (b) reviewing critical factors and principles that need to be considered when transitioning from diagnosis to treatment, (c) outlining major component areas of reading that need to be addressed in treatment planning, and (d) providing practitioners with sample treatment plans for four of the reading profiles described in Chapters 4 and 5.

Linda J. Lombardino

About the Author

Linda J. Lombardino, Ph.D., CCC-SLP, has been a professor of speech-language pathology at the University of Florida for more than 30 years. Until recently, she resided in the Department of Communication Sciences and Disorders, where she taught graduate courses in spoken and written language disorders and established the University of Florida Reading Disabilities Diagnostics and Treatment Clinics. She has recently joined the School of Special Education, School Psychology, and Early Childhood Studies at the University of Florida, where she continues to teach in the areas of language and literacy. Her area of specialization is developmental dyslexia. She has published and presented numerous papers in this area and is a coauthor of *Assessment of Literacy and Language*.

Contributor Information

Rebecca Wiseheart, Ph.D., CCC-SLP, began her career teaching reading to middle school students with severe language and learning disabilities. Since 1993, she has worked almost exclusively with struggling readers in a variety of settings, including public and charter schools, juvenile detention centers, and in her own private practice. She received her undergraduate and graduate degrees from the University of Florida, where she also supervised students in the Reading Disabilities Diagnostic Clinic for many years. Her research, which has been presented at both national and international conferences, focuses on understanding the cognitive and linguistic processes involved in dyslexic reading.

Acknowledgments

I wish to thank many individuals who helped me along this journey, including:

The parents of hundreds of children with reading difficulties and the many university students who trusted me to help them find answers and solutions.

Kytja Voeller, who invited me to collaborate with a group of professionals studying learning disabilities many years ago.

Christiana Leonard, for her guidance in teaching me the neuroscience of reading disabilities and for many years of collaboration in research on the behavioral and neuroanatomical profiles of children with reading disabilities.

George Hynd, for introducing me to the importance of understanding brain-behavior relationships in children with dyslexia and for giving me the opportunity to study the language characteristics of these children many years ago.

Sally Ann Giess, for her insightful comments on many chapter drafts and for her constant encouragement to keep writing.

Laurie Mercado Gauger, for teaching many graduate students to conduct reading evaluations and for sharing diagnostic profiles to help many of us better understand the strengths of children with reading difficulties.

Shannon Brumfield, for her extraordinary dedication and skill in teaching graduate students to work with the children that our diagnostic team identified as having reading disabilities.

Sue Ann Eidson, for sharing with me her samples of writings by 3- and 4-year-old children.

Natalie Brugman, for sharing with me her data on school-based intensive instruction of high-risk children.

Andrea Buonaiuto, Pamela Carvajal, Alexandra Johnson, and Amanda Napolitano, for their well-integrated contributions to the section of Chapter 2 on the components of oral language.

Heeyoung Park, for organizing the bibliography for an early draft of this book and to both Heeyoung and Sunjung Kim for conducting literature searches over and over again!

R. Jane Lieberman, for her feedback on several iterations of these chapters and for her invaluable recommendations for the organizational structure of this book.

Rebecca Wiseheart and Lori Altmann, for their contributions to the development of the MAR^{w}R.

Sherry Dickinson, Laura Wood, Madhavi Prakashkumar, and Andrea Majot, my Delmar Cengage editors, for their extraordinary professionalism, assistance, and patience for a much longer period than any of us expected.

Professionals who reviewed this book and who provided me with extremely constructive and precise recommendations for both its organization and content.

Janet Ferguson, my personal "in-house" editor, who kept the multiple pieces of this book impeccably organized.

My mother, Rose Lombardino, and my sisters Diane Devosjoli and Susan Lombardino, for understanding so graciously the many times when I was not available to participate in family events.

And especially, Donald Beech, my partner in life, who did everything possible to support me while I was working on this book, including remedying my nearly daily computer glitches!

REVIEWERS

Heidi M. Harbers, Ph.D., CCC-SLP
Associate Professor
Illinois State University
Normal, Illinois

R. Malatesha Joshi, Ph.D.
Professor of Literacy Education, ESL, and Educational Psychology
Texas A & M University
College Station, Texas

Robert Kraemer, CCC-SLP, Ph.D.
Adjunct Faculty
University of Arizona
Tucson, Arizona

Michaela J. Ritter, CCC-SLP
Associate Chair
Department of Communication Sciences and Disorders, Baylor University
Waco, Texas

CHAPTER ONE

Foundations for a Practitioner's Model of Reading Assessment

THIS CHAPTER AIMS TO:

- Provide practitioners with a description of component skills that work both individually and synergistically In the evolution of becoming a skilled reader.
- Provide practitioners with an overview of issues related to components of reading, and connections between oral and written language.
- Provide practitioners with an understanding of core issues related to the discipline of learning disabilities.
- Provide practitioners with a historical perspective on the classifications of reading difficulties as the basis for introducing a multidimensional educational and clinical model for assessing and differentiating reading and writing disorders.

COMPONENT SKILLS OF READING

At the most fundamental level, reading refers to understanding or comprehending language that is written down (Ziegler & Goswami, 2005). As noted by Hannon and Daneman (2001), "because reading is a complex cognitive skill that draws on many component processes and resources, any of these component processes or resources has the potential for being a source of individual differences in reading ability" (p. 103). As defined by the National Reading Panel (2000), the primary component skills necessary for the acquisition and development of grade-level reading are phonological awareness, phonics, vocabulary, fluency, and reading comprehension.

- *Phonological awareness* is a broad term that refers to different levels of sensitivity to the sound structure of our language, from simple identification of similar segments in words such as rimes to the manipulation of individual sounds in words such as in tasks of sound deletion.

- *Phonics* refers to the ability to translate print into its spoken form by use of sound-letter mapping to determine a word's pronunciation.

- *Vocabulary* refers to the understanding of words and word meanings in both spoken and written language.

- *Fluency* refers to the ability to name rapidly familiar symbols such as letters or numbers, and to read words, phrases, sentences, and text with age-appropriate speed, accuracy, and expression.

- *Reading comprehension* refers to the ability to construct an accurate interpretation of the meaning of text.

In addition to these widely recognized skills, there are cognitive processes that involve memory and processing speed resources; such as the ability to *remember* the pronunciations of familiar words in print and to *retrieve quickly* the names for familiar symbols such as letters and digits that provide the foundation for developing word reading skills (Wagner et al., 1997). Individuals vary in their aptitude for the cognitive resources needed to support skilled reading. All of these skills contribute to the learner's ability to become a fluent reader. Meyer and Felton (1999) define fluent reading as "the ability to read connected text rapidly, smoothly, effortlessly, and automatically with little conscious attention to the mechanics of reading, such as decoding" (p. 284). Given adequate literacy socialization and adequate cognitive processing abilities, the component skills needed for reading, along with the cognitive processes that support them, should develop in a synchronistic manner such that the preliterate preschooler evolves into a fluent reader during the elementary school years. Unfortunately, however, as many as 36% of fourth-grade children are reading below basic levels (Perie, Grigg, & Donahue, 2005), the minimum level at which they understand what they are reading (Grigg, Donahue, & Dion, 2007).

To begin to unravel the nature of the struggling learner's difficulties, practitioners working as reading diagnosticians or interventionists need to possess an understanding of core domains of knowledge associated with learning to read (refer to Box 1-1). Knowledge in these areas provides practitioners with the fundamental tools needed to engage in a wide range of assessment and treatment practices with learners who are at risk for reading disorders or who have already begun to manifest reading deficits. These core domains of knowledge are discussed in detail throughout this book.

BOX 1-1   Core Domains of Knowledge for Practitioners

- Knowledge of component skills that work together to enable the development of skilled reading and writing (e.g., decoding, spelling)
- Knowledge of cognitive processes (e.g., working memory, processing speed) that underlie skilled reading and writing
- Knowledge of how cognitive processes and component reading skills work together to support reading
- Nature of breakdowns that can occur (1) at the level of cognitive processes that impact component skill development or (2) at the skill level alone
- Knowledge of how to evaluate both cognitive processes and component reading skills to understand root causes of reading and writing deficits
- Knowledge of how to interpret assessment data to arrive at a diagnosis and to prescribe specific, scientifically-based treatments for improving all component reading skills

© Cengage Learning 2012

Spoken Language and Written Language Connections

Learning to read is a dynamic process that spans many years and relies on the continuous interplay between prior knowledge and new information acquired through listening and reading. Reading acquisition begins long before the learner receives formal reading instruction. During the preschool years, the learner develops numerous skills that contribute to later success in learning to read (Adams, 1990; Scarborough, 1990; Scarborough & Dobrich, 1994; Bus, van Ijzendoorn, & Pellegrini, 1995; Van Kleeck & Schuele, 1987). These skills, represented by the term *emergent literacy* (Teale & Sulzby, 1986), refer to a wide range of behaviors that precede formal reading and writing instruction (e.g., paging through picture books and telling the story while looking at the pictures). In their seminal paper on relationships between early language and emergent literacy, Whitehurst and Lonigan (1998) presented a model of component reading skills and processes, *inside-out and outside-in,* to represent the interactions of two domains of knowledge that, when integrated, support fluent reading. Inside-out processes refer to children's understanding and knowledge of the correspondences between sound units (i.e., individual or groups of phonemes) and print units (i.e., individual or groups of graphemes) needed to pronounce or spell words. These skills are founded on children's knowledge of the alphabetic code needed to learn to read. Outside-in processes represent children's understanding of the language at a conceptual level. They require knowledge of word meanings, an understanding of how context impacts word meanings, and an appreciation for how language is used in different discourse environments (e.g., oral narrative storytelling, written expository text).

Some of the early skills identified in the emergent literacy research have obvious connections to reading, such as understanding that each word spoken can be represented in a printed form, whereas others, such as the amount of time taken to name familiar symbols on a page, have less obvious connections. Factors that influence reading encompass sociocultural values, cognitive processes, heritability, early literacy experiences, type and intensity of classroom instruction, and type and intensity of intervention (Neuman & Dickinson, 2002).

In both spoken and written language, the learner must possess an awareness that language can be segmented into units. However, the degree of conscious awareness of the segmental nature of language differs for spoken and written language. In spoken language, only an *implicit* awareness of the segmental nature of language is necessary for the learner to understand the acoustic boundaries that separate one word from the next word. In spoken language interactions, the word is perceived as a whole acoustic event because individual speech sounds are not physically separated into distinct units (Liberman, Cooper, Shankweiler, & Studdert-Kennedy, 1967; Liberman & Liberman, 1990). For example, in the spoken word "bat," it is physically impossible to say the initial sound /b/ in the word without making some form of a vowel sound; however, the listener does not need to

know this in order to speak or to understand the word. In contrast, an *explicit* awareness of sounds in words is necessary to read an alphabetic language because the learner must be able to segment words phoneme by phoneme in order to learn the sound-letter associations needed to pronounce words in print (Liberman, Shankweiler, Fischer, & Carter, 1974). Because reading requires a higher level of phonological sensitivity to the sounds of one's language than speaking, it does not develop with the same ease and spontaneity.

In order to read, the learner must be able to convert print on a page into meaningful language units by mapping the sounds of language onto their corresponding letters and letter sequences (Liberman et al., 1974). In addition to phonological awareness, several other oral language skills such as vocabulary and sentence structure knowledge are strongly associated with the development of reading (Scarborough, 2002). The nature of interactions between oral and printed language changes over the course of the learner's development (Deacon & Kirby, 2004; De Jong & van der Leij, 2002; Muter, Hulme, & Scarborough, 2004; Oakhill, Cain, & Bryant, 2003; Storch & Whitehurst, 2002; Torgesen, Wagner, Rashotte, Burgess, & Hecht, 1997).

During the preschool years, children learn thousands of root word meanings (Biemiller, 2006; Biemiller & Slonim, 2001), an accomplishment that greatly enhances their early word identification. At the same time, the learner should be developing an awareness that printed symbols convey meaning. By the end of kindergarten, the learner should be able to convert print on a page into meaningful language units by mapping the sounds of language onto their corresponding letters and letter sequences (Liberman, Mattingly, & Shankweiler, 1980). From first through third grade, educators teach children how to read by instructing them in the core component skills of decoding, word recognition, and the beginning of text comprehension. During this same period, the learner should be quite proficient at producing oral language narratives (Applebee, 1978; Westby, 1991). As early as the end of third grade, the learner should have acquired the foundational skills needed to become a skilled reader (Chall, 1983). Beyond third grade, the focus of reading instruction shifts to how to learn from reading, with an emphasis on acquiring information from text. At this juncture, the learner should be well on the way to becoming a skilled reader (Adams, 1990; Chall, 1983, 1996). Learners' knowledge of the morphophonemic structure of words (i.e., ways that pronunciations and meanings of words change when combined with specific sounds) provides them with the raw material to transition from reading narrative texts in the early grades to reading expository texts in third grade and beyond. By the late elementary and middle grades, discourse skills such as the ability to draw inferences and to understand story structures are associated with text-level comprehension (Oakhill & Cain, 2007a). In narrative texts, vocabulary tends to be more familiar, whereas expository texts introduce new words, many of which are derived from already learned words (Deane, Sheehan, Sabatini, Futagi, &

Kostin, 2006). The production and comprehension of expository text becomes critical for academic success during this period of development (Nippold, 2007; Paul, 2006; Nelson, Bahr, & Van Meter, 2004).

There are several stage models of reading acquisition (Chall, 1979; Frith, 1985; Ehri, 1995), some of which focus on word-level reading and others that depict a broader developmental picture of reading milestones. In this chapter, an adaptation of Chall's (1967, 1983) framework is shown in Table 1-1 because it differentiates the developmental landmarks of *learning to read* from *reading to learn* and describes general growth sequences in reading from preschool through college. Chall (1979, 1983) notes that her stages were based on assumptions about stage-level processes that underlie Piaget's stages of cognitive ability; therefore we can assume that the stages are hierarchical and invariant in sequence—each stage is both dependent on and an extension of the previous stage. In the early stages of development (0–2), the emphasis is on decoding skills, and in the later stages (3–5), the emphasis is on comprehension. For example, learners in Stage 0 span a large developmental period, with the youngest learners acquiring the spoken language foundations for literacy and the oldest developing phonological and print awareness. By the end of Stage 0, learners begin to understand the alphabetic principle—that letters represent sounds in printed words. Beginning in Stage 2, learners shift their emphasis from decoding to constructing meaning from text, and by the end of Stage 5, they have become

TABLE 1-1 Developmental Stages of Reading

	Stage	Age/Grade	Developing Skills
Learning to read	Stage 0: Prereading/Emergent Reading	Age: 5–6 Grade: Preschool–Kindergarten	• Making great gains in the semantic, syntactic aspects of spoken language and in producing well-structured stories • Understanding the concept of words as individual units in the stream of speech and that words can be segmented into parts (e.g., "cup/cake") • Becoming aware of the phonological similarities and differences in words (as in sound onsets and rimes) • Learning some letter names, especially letters in one's name • Beginning to understand the alphabetic principle
	Stage 1: Initial Reading or Decoding "Glued to Print"	Age: 6–7 Grade: 1–2	• Focusing on the printed code with little attention given to meaning • Learning the alphabetic principle and applying it to decode words • Recognizing words that occur frequently in print • Learning to apply phonological knowledge to spell words (i.e., invented spelling)
	Stage 2: Confirmation "Ungluing from Print"	Age: 7–8 Grade: 2–3	• Consolidating what has been learned by gaining greater automaticity in decoding words and in recognizing familiar words • Beginning to integrate print with meaning based on word knowledge and context • Becoming a fluent reader as words are recognized more quickly and attention begins to shift from form to meaning of text
Reading to learn	Stage 3: Reading for Learning the New from One Viewpoint	Age: 8–14 Grade: 4–8	• Shifting focus from an emphasis on the codes for reading to emphasis on the meaning of text • Learning from listening and watching begins to shift to learning from reading • Using prior knowledge to comprehend new information becomes important
	Stage 4: Multiple Viewpoints	Age: 14–18 Grade: High School	• Using layers of knowledge to understand and analyze others' perspectives • Taking opportunities to read a wide range of materials that assist in critically responding to others' ideas
	Stage 5: Construction and Reconstruction	Age: 18 and Above Grade: College	• Understanding how to read selectively to obtain information needed for understanding abstract concepts • Constructing knowledge to analyze, synthesize, and hypothesize

Adapted from Jeanne Chall (1967, 1983).

sophisticated comprehenders of text, with the ability to analyze, synthesize, and judge complex texts. Models of this nature provide the practitioner with a framework for identifying where learners fall along a developmental continuum and selecting content, instructional strategies, and programs to meet their developmental needs.

Relationships between Strengths and Weaknesses in Oral Language Skills and Reading Skills

The developmental skills most closely associated with reading ability involve language processes that are viewed along a continuum of processing complexity. Reading skills such as decoding, which require accessing sound-letter associations but do not require knowledge of word meanings, are considered *low-level processing* skills. In contrast, language skills such as word and text-level comprehension, which require accessing meaning, are considered *higher-level processing* skills (Hannon & Daneman, 2001). Bishop and Snowling (2004) recommended a two-dimensional model of reading. The first dimension consists of assessing strengths and weaknesses of *phonological skills* (low level language skills, e.g., segmenting, blending at the word level). The second dimension consists of assessing strengths and weaknesses in *nonphonological skills* (high-level language skills, e.g., multiple word meanings, listening comprehension). As shown in Table 1-2, this type of profiling yields different combinations of language strengths and weaknesses, thereby providing the practitioner with the initial junction for differentiating oral language strengths and

TABLE 1-2 Profile of Strengths and Weaknesses in the Phonological and Nonphonological Domains of Oral Language

Nonphonological Skill Strengths/Weaknesses	Phonological Skill Strengths/Weaknesses
−	−
+	−
−	+

© Cengage Learning 2012

weaknesses. Learners who show strengths in nonphonological skills such as listening comprehension and vocabulary but depressed phonological skills on tasks such as decoding and rapid word recognition exhibit a *more specific type of reading deficit* than learners who exhibit depressed phonological and nonphonological skills. Comparing and contrasting strengths and weaknesses across these two dimensions has advanced the field of reading disabilities by distinguishing the language profiles of children who show deficits in their reading abilities.

Profiling the learner's strengths and weaknesses based on the simple dimensions of nonphonological and phonological language skills helps the practitioner understand how isolated deficits in specific language systems can result in different types of reading profiles. The *type* of deficient processes along with the *number* of deficient processes will determine the nature and severity of the reading disability. For example, during the act of reading text, if the sound or phonological system alone is deficient, the learner may have difficulty decoding words and perhaps remembering the pronunciations of familiar words, but should be able to rely on knowledge of other dimensions of language (knowledge of word meanings in the context of text) to compensate for this deficit when attempting to comprehend text. On the other hand, if the semantic and syntactic systems are deficient while the phonological system is intact, the learner will be able to pronounce words but will have difficulty with comprehending text. If both the phonological system and the semantic and syntactic systems are deficient, the learner will have difficulty with decoding words and with text comprehension. These relationships are shown in Figure 1–1.

A PERSPECTIVE ON READING DIFFICULTIES

The terms *reading difficulty*, *reading deficit*, *reading disorder*, *reading disability*, and *struggling reader* are often used interchangeably to refer to a heterogeneous group of learners. In this book, the term *struggling reader* is used generically to refer to any learner who is having difficulty developing age- or grade-appropriate reading skills. The term *reading disability* is used to refer to reading difficulties that are consistent with a diagnosis of learning disability. Learning disabilities are assumed to result, at least in part, from neurobiological and neurocognitive factors that

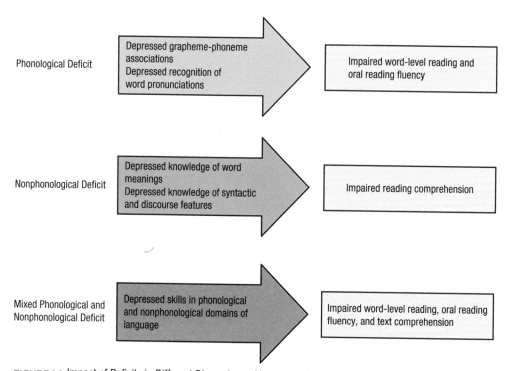

FIGURE 1-1 Impact of Deficits in Different Dimensions of Language Processing on Reading

© Cengage Learning 2012

interfere with the learner's efficient use of specific cognitive processes that are needed to develop reading at a typical rate (e.g., memory, processing speed).

At the most fundamental levels of causation, a reading deficit may be the result of environmental impoverishment, biological processing weaknesses, or a combination of these two factors. The degree to which environment and biology contribute to the root cause (or causes) of a reading deficit is often difficult to disentangle because each factor may contribute to similar deficits in reading, such as poor decoding or poor comprehension. For example, one learner may have difficulty decoding words because that learner was never taught the skill; another learner may have difficulty with this same skill because of a phonological processing weakness that impedes his ability to remember the pronunciations of familiar words in print, in spite of adequate instruction and opportunities for repetition. Vellutino and Fletcher (2005) emphasize the importance of making the distinction between learners' deficient reading behaviors (i.e., decoding deficit, comprehension deficit) and the root causes of their reading deficits (i.e., lack of knowledge due to poor instruction versus difficulty acquiring a skill in spite of adequate instruction).

Stanovich (2000) and Spear-Swerling and Sternberg (1996) underscore the pervasive impact of the environment in serving as both a causal factor and a contributory factor to reading success or failure. For example, a child who enters school from a disadvantaged environment, with little to

no literacy background and no intrinsic learning difficulties, can advance in his development of reading skills if given the adequate instruction needed to learn to read and the support to develop a positive attitude toward reading for learning and for pleasure. A less desirable outcome could arise for a child who has had adequate exposure to print prior to entering school yet fails to develop decoding skills at the rate of his peers because of a weakness in remembering phonological codes for sound-letter correspondences. If this child fails to receive adequate assistance and continues to struggle with word reading, he is likely to avoid reading as a source of information and pleasure. Early difficulties in learning to read words can affect motivation to read, resulting in dramatically reduced exposure to more advanced vocabulary and other language concepts learned through print (Stanovich, 1986; Spear-Swerling & Sternberg, 1996). Stanovich (1986) addressed individual differences in the reading-related skills of deficient readers by underscoring the cascading manner in which a deficit in one area of learning leads to deficits in other areas. He adopted the term *Matthew Effect*, in reference to a biblical parable ("the rich will get richer and the poor will get poorer"), to describe the downward spiral faced by many learners whose unsuccessful initial experiences with literacy result in a greater degree and range of reading deficits than would be predicted from the learner's general learning capabilities. Diminished exposure to written language can lead to deficiencies in a range of conceptual areas, especially vocabulary knowledge, that can impact the learner's ability to comprehend text (Cunningham & Stanovich, 1998; Echols, West, Stanovich, & Zehr, 1996). Multiple factors can affect the learner's degree of success with learning to read. These factors are shown in Box 1-2.

Learning Disabilities

Learning disability is a term used to represent a heterogeneous group of learners who have academic difficulties in one or more specific academic domains (Fletcher, Lyon, Fuchs, & Barnes, 2007). These difficulties are unexpected given the learners' sociocultural opportunities and overall intellectual functioning, and are assumed to be associated with neurobiologically and neurocognitively based processing deficits (Torgesen, 2004; Fletcher et al., 2007). The diagnosis of a learning disability (LD) occurs after children enter elementary school and have met school districts' performance criteria for this classification which is determined largely by performance on psycho-educational tests. (Fletcher, Morris, & Lyon, 2003). Children who are classified as having LD can present with a range of learning histories. For example, some children are identified as having speech or language disorders prior to entering school; others have no history of speech or language problems yet struggle in kindergarten with learning the precursors to reading, such as letter naming and sound segmentation; and others are not identified with learning difficulties until around the fourth grade, when reading or mathematics deficits become evident.

Federal guidelines for the designation of LD exclude sensory deficits, severe emotional problems, inadequate instruction, linguistic

---

BOX 1-2 **Environmental Factors and Biological Factors Associated with Literacy Acquisition**

Environmental Factors

- Poverty
- Maternal education
- Exposure to enriched oral language
- Exposure to literacy artifacts
- Engagement in joint activities, conversations, and narrative activities
- Engagement in sound-play activities such as rhyming
- Instruction in skills necessary for word decoding, including segmenting and blending and segmenting sounds in words, and sound-letter associations
- Instruction in print concepts such as matching words in speech to words in print
- Type of reading instruction
- Motivation to read

Biological Factors

- Cognitive processing skills such as ability to discriminate between sounds, isolate sounds in words, recall words' pronunciations, recall sound-letter associations, retrieve familiar words from memory, retrieve familiar letters and letter patterns for spelling (assuming adequate exposure to oral and written language)
- Family history of learning disability

Environmental and Biological Factors

- Age/grade at which spoken language and reading deficits are identified and remediated
- Type and intensity of remediation

diversity, and low intelligence as primary causes of learning disabilities and underscore the role of processing deficits (e.g., memory) as the root cause (United States Office of Education, 1977). The designation of LD is given to children who are exhibiting low achievement in one or more academic areas in comparison to their overall aptitude (typically defined as IQ) or their performance in other academic areas (Fletcher, Morris, & Lyon, 2003).

Learning disabilities manifest in a variety of ways and are often classified broadly into one of four categories: (1) language disability, (2) reading disability, (3) written language disability, or (4) mathematics disability. Specific types of behaviors that interfere with learning, such as inattention and hyperactivity, frequently co-occur with learning disabilities (Willcutt & Pennington, 2000). Understandably, the validity of using the discrepancy model to determine which learners qualify for LD services has been disputed strongly by many practitioners and researchers because (1) only learners who show an aptitude-achievement discrepancy qualify to receive LD services, leaving struggling learners without supplemental or alternative services; (2) correlations between IQ and reading are generally lower in LD learners than in typical learners; and (3) no differences have been shown between nondiscrepant struggling learners and discrepant struggling learners in their response to intervention (Fletcher et al., 1994; Fletcher, Coulter, Reschly, & Vaughn, 2004; Siegel, 2003). Because there are no standard operational criteria for identifying a learning disability, practitioners and researchers are left to adopt their own standards (Siegel & Lipka, 2008). Across educational institutions, the criteria used to define a discrepancy between IQ and achievement can range from one to two standard deviations (Perlmutter & Parus, 1983).

The IQ-achievement discrepancy model results in unfortunate consequences for many learners who have reading disabilities yet do not show the IQ-achievement gap required for the diagnosis of an LD (Aaron, 1997). By the time the required discrepancy manifests, often these learners have lost years of opportunity for special instruction, have fallen further behind in their reading skills and face social-emotional difficulties as a result of their academic failures (Aaron, Joshi, & Quatroche, 2008; Elbaum & Vaughn, 2003; Fletcher et al., 2004; Vaughn, Wanzek, Woodruff, & Linan-Thompson, 2007). In recent years, educational and research prevention and early identification initiatives have been instituted in response to the inadequacies inherent in the discrepancy model.

Further, a disturbingly high proportion of children from disadvantaged backgrounds enter school unprepared to begin reading instruction and consequently fail to achieve reading skills at the level of their peers because they are not provided classroom instruction in the foundational emergent literacy skills that elevate their knowledge to a level that is closer to being commensurate with their more advantaged peers. (Vaughn, Wanzek, Woodruff et al., 2007). Children from impoverished environments compose the largest group of learners who are at risk for reading failure in the United States (Vernon-Feagans, Hammer, Miccio, & Manlove, 2002). Although children from all social classes have difficulty learning to read (Snow, Burns, & Griffin, 1998; Vasilyeva & Waterfall, 2011), those who live in poverty and have minimal exposure to a rich and diverse vocabulary (Hart & Risely, 1995), literacy artifacts (i.e., printed materials), and literacy events within their home environments (e.g., shared reading time with an adult) are particularly vulnerable to future reading deficits (van Kleeck & Schuele, 1987). Low-income status and low quality of child care are two key environmental factors associated with risk for later reading difficulties (Dickinson & Sprague, 2002). Without systematic instruction in the classroom to help advance children's deficient foundational literacy skills, they often fail to acquire reading skills commensurate with their peers. Inadequate opportunities with spoken language or orthographic symbols (e.g., print) can result in weak phonological, semantic, and syntactic representations, thereby decreasing the expected rate of reading skill acquisition (Stanovich, 2000).

Research on English Language Learners

Furthermore, young children from disadvantaged backgrounds with the added burden of needing to learn a second language to succeed in school are at particular risk (National Reading Panel, 2000; Snow, Burns, & Griffin, 1998; Tabors & Snow, 2002). These children, commonly referred to as English language learners (ELLs) are at particularly high risk for reading difficulties when they are expected to learn to read in English before they are proficient in speaking English (August & Hakuta, 1997; Oller & Eilers, 2002; Ganske, Monroe, & Strickland, 2003). In their longitudinal study of Spanish-speaking children who had been exposed to English for varying amounts of time, Hammer, Scarpino, and Davison (2011) studied the language and literacy development of two groups of Spanish-speaking children in Head Start programs from preschool through first grade. One group of children was exposed to English at home before entering preschool, and the other group did not communicate in English until entering Head Start. During the preschool years, children who had longer exposure to English had stronger language skills in English and those who had less exposure to English had stronger language skills in Spanish. The authors stated that "over the 2-year period in Head Start, children made great advances in their English abilities. And once in elementary school, they caught up to their monolingual peers. They simply needed time to catch up" (p. 124). These data underscore the importance of immersing ELLs in English-speaking educational settings as early as possible.

Naturally, children identified as ELLs are a very heterogeneous group in that they represent a wide range of exposure to English and a broad continuum of sociocultural opportunities (Artiles & Ortiz, 2002). About 30% of children in Head Start are bilingual and nearly 85% of these children come from homes where Spanish is the dominant language (Hammer, Scarpino, & Davison, 2011). Latino children are at very high risk for reading deficits because of the high rate of poverty in this cultural group (National Center for Educational Statistics, 2009). These children often have difficulties in a range of skills, such as vocabulary and discourse patterns, necessary for reading comprehension (August, Francis, Hsu, & Snow, 2006). Artiles and Ortiz (2002) point out that ELLs are disproportionately represented in the group of children who show poor academic achievement. Samson and Lesaux (2009) found that ELLs appear to be underrepresented in special education in kindergarten and first grade but overrepresented in later grades. The reliability and validity of language and literacy test results for ELLs remains a major issue in the often difficult task of differentiating whether bilingualism alone or bilingualism in conjunction with a learning disability is the cause of ELLs' reading deficits (Abedi, 2008).

Educational Initiatives

As a result of the reauthorization of the Individuals with Disabilities Education Improvement Act of 2004 (IDEA, 2004), public schools are not required to use the IQ-achievement discrepancy model for diagnosing LD. Nationwide, many public schools have instituted a response-to-intervention (RTI) model to ensure that all children with learning difficulties have access to early identification and intervention (Fuchs & Fuchs, 2001; Wright & Wright, 2007). The IDEA 2004 legislation allows educators to use students' responsiveness to intervention to determine the nature and intensity of the intervention needed rather than relying on other standards, such as students' performance on a battery of tests, to determine if they qualify for additional instructional services. The motivation for this new instructional approach has been to prevent severe learning difficulties by identifying weaknesses as early as possible in

the elementary grades and by implementing a multitiered model of instruction (Fuchs & Fuchs, 2001). This multitiered model for reading instruction is typically depicted by a triangle that represents three levels of instruction (refer to Figure 6–1 and Chapter 6 for more complete information). In most educational settings, the RTI model represents three sequentially ordered stages of reading intervention. Tier 1 refers to the core classroom reading instruction, Tier 2 refers to supplemental small-group instruction and Tier 3 denotes an intensive very small group or individualized instruction that is highly differentiated to meet students' specific learning needs (Vaughn, Wanzek, & Fletcher, 2007). Approximately 70%–80% of students will meet the benchmarks for proficiency at Tier 1 instruction, 15%–20% will require Tier 2 intervention, and another 5%–10% will require Tier 3 intervention (Marchand-Martella, Ruby, & Martella, 2007). Because this model is a conceptual framework designed to be descriptive rather than prescriptive (Stewart, Benner, Martella, & Marchand-Martella, 2007), the way in which it is implemented varies across school districts and states. While RTI is being used widely across the country, discrepancy models continue to be used; federal guidelines permit the use of either RTI or the discrepancy model to diagnose LD (U.S. Department of Education, 2006).

Research on Differentiating Types of Reading Disabilities

The vast majority of learners with LD have reading disabilities (Lerner, 1989; Lyon, 1995). However, the designation of a reading disability does not differentiate the different types of profiles that have been most commonly identified in the reading disabilities literature. In discussing the need to distinguish among types of readers' disorders, Fletcher (2009) stated that "this distinction is important because the neuropsychological and neurobiological correlates will vary depending on the nature of the reading problems" (p. 502). As a result of the lack of scientifically based criteria for determining the nature of learning disabilities, many researchers use methods for identifying *intraindividual differences in the learner's strengths and weaknesses* to determine the nature of the learner's reading disabilities (Joshi & Aaron, 2008; Fletcher et al., 2004; Fletcher et al., 2003; Fletcher et al., 2007; Siegel, 2003; Siegel & Lipka, 2008; Stanovich, 1991). The intraindividual approach is based on the tenet that reading difficulties are not all alike and that an analysis of the learner's component skills of reading is *essential* for determining the nature of reading deficits and the optimal instructional intervention practices (Aaron & Joshi; 1992; Aaron, Joshi, & Williams, 1999; Carver, 2000). Researchers have studied both component skills of reading and cognitive processes associated with reading in an attempt to determine if specific strengths and weaknesses across these areas can be used to classify types of reading profiles (Joshi & Aaron, 2008; Bishop & Snowling, 2004; Berninger, 2008; Catts, Adlof, & Weismer, 2006; Catts, Hogan, & Fey, 2003; Puranik & Lombardino, 2006; Vellutino, Fletcher,

Snowling, & Scanlon, 2004; Stanovich, 1988b; Oakhill et al., 2003).

Practitioners who work with struggling readers need an assessment model supported by a developmental, multidimensional, and scientifically based framework that allows for the profiling of individual learners' strengths and deficits in the component skill areas of reading and in the cognitive processes that support reading. As the first step in this direction, Gough and Tunmer (1986) proposed a basic yet elegant formulaic model called the *Simple View of Reading* that depicts the inextricable link between spoken and written language. In this model, reading is the product of word decoding and listening comprehension. This formula is represented by the mathematical equation $R = D \times C$, in which R represents reading, D represents word decoding, and C represents listening comprehension. The significance of this model lies in its (a) ability to capture the necessity of establishing linkages between the explicit knowledge of letter-sound associations and implicit knowledge of language comprehension and (b) capacity to show how breakdowns in the reading process manifest when a disruption occurs in one or both of these component skills.

This simple view of reading provides a foundation for unraveling the complex interactions between word reading and listening comprehension (Stuart, Stainthorp, & Snowling, 2008). Scientific evidence shows that different relationships across these skill sets represent different types of reading problems (Aaron, Joshi, & Williams, 1999; Bishop & Snowling, 2004; Carver & Clark,

1998; Oakhill et al., 2003; Snowling & Hayiou-Thomas, 2006; Vellutino & Fletcher, 2005). For example, one group of struggling readers exhibits depressed word-level decoding skills with good listening comprehension, a profile that reflects a primary deficit in the phonological dimension of language, whereas another group of struggling readers exhibits deficits that extend beyond the phonological domain into other areas of language such as semantic knowledge (Aaron, Joshi, & Williams, 1999; Aaron, Joshi, & Quatroche, 2008; Bishop, 2008; Bishop & Snowling, 2004; Berninger, 2008; Carver & Clark, 1998; Catts & Kamhi, 2005). This simple formula spawned the development of more comprehensive and detailed diagnostic and treatment approaches designed to assist practitioners in identifying specific areas of deficits in individual readers and in informing intervention goals.

Carver (1997, 2000) developed a diagnostic model of reading called the *Rauding Diagnostic System*, a process based on the tenet that *listening comprehension* and *reading comprehension* represent the same fundamental language processes, and that reading disabilities can be more precisely identified and understood when the construct of comprehension is examined in both spoken and written language. Carver (2000) coined the term *rauding* by combining two words, reading and listening (auding) and defined the process of rauding as the ability to read at a grade-appropriate rate with a high level of comprehension.

The *Rauding Model* is a causal model of reading depicted in a four-level, tiered framework. Levels (i.e., echelons) in the model are organized relative to their proximity to the construct of reading achievement. Each level directly impacts the development of skills at the next proximal level to reading achievement. At top of the rauding model, level 4 factors include aptitude for spoken language, phonological decoding, and processing speed along with learning opportunities. These aptitude and learning factors have the most direct effect on level 3 behaviors, which include phonological decoding, vocabulary, and rapid word-retrieval skills. Following the same causal trajectory, level 3 skills have the most direct impact on level 2 behaviors, which include reading rate (i.e., speed) and reading accuracy (i.e., knowledge of words' meanings in text). Finally, reading rate and reading accuracy have a direct effect on level 1, reading achievement. Reading achievement, referred to by Carver as "rauding efficiency," represents the culmination of all experiences, processes, and skills in the upper echelons of the model.

Joshi and Aaron (2008) and Aaron, Joshi, Boulware-Gooden, and Bentum (2008) developed the *Componential Model of Reading* for diagnosing and treating reading disability. Their model is comprised of three domains: cognitive, psychological, and ecological. The component skills of reading, word recognition, and comprehension fall within the cognitive domain. Factors such as motivation, learning styles, and teacher expectations fall within the psychological domain, and factors such as sociocultural influences, classroom environment, dialect, and English as a second language fall within the ecological domain. Each domain represents an area of potential strength or weakness.

Finally, Fletcher et al. (2007) present a framework for representing core factors that must be considered when examining areas of variability in children who have LD. Their model depicts the influences of environmental, behavioral/psychosocial, cognitive, and neurobiological factors on specific skill deficits. Unidirectional and bidirectional interactions between these component domains are also shown. In this model, achievement deficits are necessary for a diagnosis of LD but are not sufficient for determining the nature of the learning disability.

SUMMARY OF THE FOUNDATIONS OF LITERACY

Reading relies on the integration of multiple domains of oral and written language knowledge (Hoover & Gough, 1990; Foorman, Francis, Shaywitz, Shaywitz, & Fletcher, 1997). Learners bring their own particular neurobiological makeup to the tasks of processing and connecting components of oral and written language. These biological skills are shaped by home and academic environments. The combination of these two powerful influences, biology and environment, determines the extent to which learners become proficient in their oral and written language skills. Fletcher and Lyon (2008) posit that "dyslexia results from an interaction of neurobiological factors that make the brain at risk and environmental factors that moderate this risk"

(p. 30). This same position aptly characterizes all learning disabilities.

The links between oral and written language are irrefutable and have been addressed in many resources on reading development and reading disabilities (Catts & Kamhi, 2003; Neuman & Dickinson, 2002; Dickinson & Neuman, 2006; Snowling & Hulme, 2005). While the profiles of persons with reading deficits are varied in nature, clinical and experimental data provide descriptions of commonly occurring patterns of strengths and weaknesses that allow practitioners to make decisions regarding the classification of reading disability types. Sample profiles and assessment procedures described in later chapters should help practitioners (1) *better identify* the strengths and weaknesses of learners who are at risk for reading deficits or (2) identify those who are already manifesting reading deficits and *more precisely target* core reading deficit areas in treatment.

The need to determine the specific nature of a learner's difficulty in acquiring reading skills is central to our understanding of how to advance the skills of struggling readers most efficiently and comprehensively. It is patently clear that difficulties with reading can arise from any number of factors, and that these factors must be understood as thoroughly as possible for practitioners to determine the appropriate course of intervention.

A new clinical framework is presented in the next chapter and serves as a blueprint for describing reading disabilities throughout this book. The *Multidimensional*

Model for Assessing Reading and Writing (MAR^wR) was inspired and influenced by several factors—the author's many years of evaluating and treating children with reading difficulties, the component models described above, and recent scientific advances in understanding predictable associations between component skills of reading and specific cognitive processes (e.g., working memory, processing speed). MAR^wR was developed as a guide for practioners across applied disciplines who participate in the assessment and diagnosis of reading deficits. This model is designed to assist practitioners in using scientific data and reading assessment profiles to understand the nature of learners' strengths and weakness and to inform treatment practices.

CHAPTER TWO

A Multidimensional Model for Assessing Reading and Writing

THIS CHAPTER AIMS TO:

- Introduce practitioners to the 10 modules that compose the Multidimensional Model for Assessing Reading and Writing (MAR^{W}R), a blueprint for the identification and the differential diagnosis of reading disability.
- Provide practitioners with a multidisciplinary perspective from the scientific literature that pertains to each of the 10 MAR^{W}R modules.
- Provide practitioners with visual schemes for developing a general understanding of how a range of pre-literacy skills develop over time and interact with other skills to support reading and writing development.

OVERVIEW OF THE MULTIDIMENSIONAL ASSESSMENT READING AND WRITING MODEL

The MAR^{w}R model was designed to guide practitioners in (1) developing profiles of literacy-related strengths and weaknesses for learners who are *at risk* for reading deficits or for learners who are *failing to achieve* expected levels of reading skill, (2) creating differential assessment blueprints that highlight the specific reading component strengths and weaknesses in the learner's profile, (3) using diagnostic categories for classifying the learner's type of reading deficit, and (4) designing evidence-based instruction for strengthening skills that lie at the root of the struggling reader's difficulties.

As shown in Figure 2-1, the MAR^{w}R model is organized into 10 modules that represent the range of domains shown to be associated with the development of reading in the scientific literature. The 10 modules that make up the MAR^{w}R are (1) environmental factors; (2) neurobiological and neurocognitive factors; (3) spoken language knowledge; (4) phonological knowledge; (5) print knowledge; (6) graphophonemic integration; (7) word-level reading; (8) word-level spelling; (9) text-level reading; and (10) text-level writing.

Within each module there are specific skills, processes, or external events that have been studied relative to their contribution to reading development. Research across several disciplines (e.g., psychology, education, speech-language pathology, neuroscience)

has been integrated to formulate these modules and their components. The modules in the MAR^{w}R model have been arranged to reflect a general causal trajectory of the specific processes, skills, and events that contribute to reading achievement. For example, factors associated with the first two modules have the most direct effect on the development of skills in the spoken language, phonological, and print knowledge modules. The spoken language knowledge module extends from the earliest preliteracy skills throughout the development of skilled reading. This was done to convey that the various component skills of spoken language influence the development of reading over the course of literacy development from the earliest stages of preliteracy knowledge to the attainment of skilled reading. The arrow, shown in Figure 2-1, demonstrates this hierarchical arrangement.

Definitions and scientific support are provided below for each of the MAR^{w}R modules. In later chapters, the MAR^{w}R framework is used to describe four types of emergent literacy profiles for preschool children who are at risk for reading difficulties and four types of literacy profiles for school-age children who have dyslexia and other types of reading disabilities.

ENVIRONMENTAL FACTORS MODULE

Definitions and Scientific Support

Environmental factors refer to difficulties that result from extrinsic influences that impede the learner's development. These factors

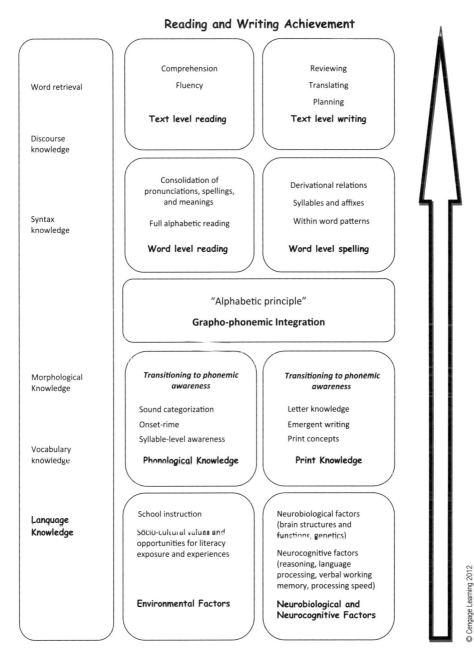

FIGURE 2-1 Multidimensional Model for Assessing Reading and Writing

are most commonly associated with a lack of exposure to language and literacy experiences in the home, at school, or across environments needed to support the learner's development of foundational reading skills (e.g., vocabulary, decoding), higher-level cognitive experiences (e.g., infcrential abilities), and general world knowledge. Worldwide, the majority of people who do not read, do not do so because of environmental factors (Olson, 2002).

Informal shared book-reading activities between parents and their children play an important role in later reading development because these activities facilitate preschoolers' knowledge of concepts of print and story structure language (Justice & Ezell, 2001, 2002; McCabe & Rollins, 1994). However, often more *direct* teaching strategies are needed to help children develop print-related skills such as letter identification and letter-sound correspondences (Evans, Williamson, & Pursoo, 2008; Sénéchal, LeFevre, Thomas, & Daley, 1998). Children who are faced with challenges in transitioning from relying solely on spoken language to learning the code of written language during their early school experiences are less likely to enjoy reading and more likely to avoid opportunities to read (Stanovich, 1986). The majority of children who are poor readers at the end of first grade remain depressed in their reading abilities throughout school (Juel, 2006; Torgesen & Burgess, 1998).

NEUROBIOLOGICAL AND NEUROCOGNITIVE FACTORS MODULE

Definitions and Scientific Support

Neurobiological Factors

Neurobiological factors refer to any difficulties that originate from deficits in neural processing. These factors are often referred to as intrinsic influences because they result from neurobiological or neurocognitive differences or dysfunctions in the learner. Learning disabilities have long been associated with neurobiological dysfunctions, but until recently these associations were based on inferences (e.g., "soft" neurological signs such as depressed language development) (Fletcher, Lyon, Fuchs, & Barnes, 2007; Reid, Fawcett, Manis, & Seigel, 2008). Studies within the last decade have shown that brain activation patterns during the processing of printed words are quite different in individuals who have dyslexia, a specific type of reading disability and the most common learning disability (Fletcher et al., 2007), than in individuals who are skilled at reading (Pugh et al., 2000; Shaywitz, 2003).

The study of the biological basis of reading disorders has been largely limited to the study of children who are diagnosed with dyslexia (Fletcher et al., 2007). Although a range of different types of neurobiological and neurocognitive investigations of brain regions have shown differences in the temporal-parietal-occipital brain regions of dyslexic learners when compared to learners without dyslexia (Shaywitz, Gruen, & Shaywitz, 2008), these imaging techniques are not yet available for use as diagnostic tools. Instead, practitioners must rely, in large part, on behavioral measures to examine specific types of cognitive processing that aid in the differential diagnosis of learning disabilities.

Over the last 10 years a substantial body of evidence has been accumulating steadily across academic disciplines and research methodologies to support a neurobiological basis for dyslexia (Habib, 2000; Lenhard, Lenhard, & Breitenbach, 2005; Shaywitz, Mody, & Shaywitz, 2006; Shaywitz & Shaywitz, 2007). Evidence comes from studies that examine (a) rapid temporal auditory processing (Gaab, Chang, Lee, Buechler, & Raschle, 2009); (b) visual attention span (Bosse, Tainturier, & Valdois, 2007) and atypical eye movement (Eden, Stein, Wood, & Wood, 1994; Prado, Dubois, & Valdois, 2007); (c) size and structure of brain anatomy, measured by magnetic resonance imaging (MRI) (Gauger, Lombardino, & Leonard, 1997; Leonard, Eckert, Given, Berninger, & Eden, 2006; Leonard, in press); (d) brain activity during reading and reading-related tasks, measured by functional magnetic resonance imaging (fMRI) (Landi, Frost, Mencl, Sandak, & Pugh, in press; Shaywitz et al., 2003); and (e) genetic influences on reading ability (Olson & Gayan, 2001; Keenan, Betjemann, Wadsworth, DeFries, & Olson, 2006; Olson, 2004; Pennington & Olson, 2005).

Leonard and colleagues (Leonard et al., 1996; Leonard et al., 2002; Eckert, Lombardino, & Leonard, 2001; Leonard et al., 2006; Leonard & Eckert, 2008; Leonard, Lombardino, Giess, & King, 2005) have examined a number of anatomical structures in the brains of normally developing children and in children who have developmental language disorders. Their data suggest that (1) asymmetry of the planum temporal is correlated with aspects of verbal ability and cognition; (2) individuals with multiple language and reading deficits are more likely to have small, symmetrical plana compared to reading-impaired individuals with phonological deficits but good overall verbal abilities who have a leftward asymmetry of the plana (Leonard et al., 2002); (3) an anatomical risk factor (ARF) index that combines a number of anatomical features, such as cerebral volume, cerebral asymmetry, and planum asymmetry, is sensitive to deficits in different components of reading; (4) a positive ARF index is associated with low cerebral volumes and symmetrical plana and globally impaired spoken language and reading (i.e., language learning disability); and (5) a negative ARF index is associated with high cerebral volumes and large leftward asymmetry of the plana and preserved reading comprehension (i.e., dyslexia). In a more recent study, Leonard et al. (2011) showed that adequate processing speed appears to serve as a protective factor in normal readers who show a negative ARF index. These data are consistent with a multiple-factors deficit model in that it appears that the direction of the ARF index predicts the type of the cognitive profile in individuals with reading disabilities.

The most compelling argument for using a modular framework to understand the neurobiological basis of reading disabilities comes from recent advances in brain imaging. Pugh et al. (2001) developed a model of the neural pathways involved in reading. The locations of these pathways in the brain and the connections between them are based partly on radiologic images of localized brain lesions that disrupt reading functions in adults and on functional images conducted on normal and dyslexic adults and children. These researchers identified three circuits as the primary regions of interest during reading, two posterior areas and one anterior area in the left hemisphere. The *temporoparietal area* is associated with integrating print, phonological, and lexical information during word reading; the *occipitotemporal area* is associated with rapid word identification; and the *inferior-frontal area*, the region around Broca's area, is associated with articulatory gestures. According to Shaywitz (2003), "as they read, good readers activate highly interconnected neural systems that encompass regions in the back and front of the left side of the brain" (p. 78). Figure 2-2 depicts these key reading areas in the brain.

Changes in neural activity within these reading circuits occurs with changes in age and reading skill level (Gaab et al., 2009; Schlaggar et al., 2002; Schlaggar & McCandliss, 2007; Shaywitz et al., 2004). Both children and adults with dyslexia show a disruption in the posterior neural circuits during word-processing tasks (Rumsey et al., 1997; Pugh et al., 2000; Shaywitz, 2003). This disruption is represented by a lower level of neural activity in these areas than found in typical readers.

In a recent review of the development of neural systems for reading, Schlaggar and McCandliss (2007) proposed an *interactive specialization* (IS) *framework* for understanding reading development. The basic tenet of

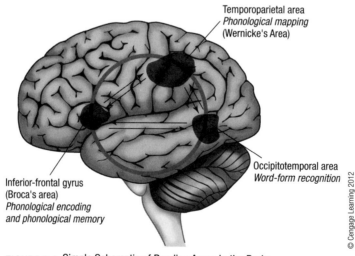

Temporoparietal area
Phonological mapping
(Wernicke's Area)

Occipitotemporal area
Word-form recognition

© Cengage Learning 2012

Inferior-frontal gyrus
(Broca's area)
*Phonological encoding
and phonological memory*

FIGURE 2-2 Simple Schematic of Reading Areas in the Brain

their framework is that the integration of extant circuits in the brain such as phonological and visual processing with cultural experiences (e.g., learning to map sounds onto letters) may allow for the development of novel circuitry in the brain that functions to support the relatively new cognitive skill of reading.

Reviews of treatment studies on both children and adults with reading disabilities have cited improved brain processing efficiency on functional magnetic resonance images following treatment (Shaywitz, Lyon, & Shaywitz, 2006; Richards et al., 2006; Simos et al., 2006).

Genetic Factors

The influence of family history on the activation of the brain centers related to reading is consistent with many years of genetic research in reading by Richard Olson, and colleagues (Byrne, Wadsworth, Corley, Samuelsson, Quain, DeFries, Willcutt, & Olson, 2005; Castles, Datta, Gayán, & Olson, 1999; Friend, DeFries, Wadsworth, & Olson, 2006, 2007; Gayán & Olson, 2001; Olson, 2002, 2006, 2007; Olson, Gillis, Rack, DeFries, & Fulker, 1991; Rack, Snowling, & Olson, 1992; Rack & Olson, 1993; Wadsworth, Olson, Pennington, & DeFries, 2000). The estimated heritability of reading disability is greater than 50% (Pennington & Olson, 2005). Olson (2004) reported that skills related to word reading such as phoneme decoding and phonological awareness are highly heritable, suggesting that word reading may be constrained by genetically influenced traits for learning phonological skills.

Keenan, Betjeman, Wadsworth, DeFries, and Olson (2006) found that word reading and listening comprehension account for independent genetic influences on reading comprehension, underscoring the modular nature of the component skills that underpin reading. In a recent investigation of neural premarkers of dyslexia in prereaders, Gaab, Chang, Buechler, and Raschle (2009) reported differences between prereaders with a positive family history for dyslexia and those with a negative family history for both structural measures of gray matter volume and brain activity in the auditory regions.

Neurocognitive Factors

A number of areas of cognitive processing have proven to be very useful in the differential diagnosis of reading disabilities. Neurocognitive factors refer to processing skills that subserve higher cortical functions such as speaking, listening, reading, and writing. These areas include but are probably not limited to: (1) reasoning ability, (2) language processing, (3) verbal working memory, and (4) processing speed. *Reasoning ability* refers to the ability to engage in abstract thinking by drawing inferences, understanding relationships between concepts and deciphering rules. *Language processing* refers to the ability to translate incoming speech into meaningful units that can be comprehended in the context in which they occur *and* to the ability to formulate semantically and syntactically accurate responses to fulfill a wide range of communicative functions (e.g., commenting, answering a question, inquiring, instructing, teasing, etc). The processing of phonological units has been the most widely studied language domain in the area of early reading readiness. *Verbal working memory aptitude* refers to the ability to listen to information, temporarily store and manipulate it, and then retrieve it. *Processing speed* refers to the ability to recognize, sort, and process information quickly.

These four domains have been included in the MAR^wR model because they target processes that have been associated with the different psycho-educational profiles of individuals with disabilities (Fletcher et al., 2007; Mody & Silliman, 2008; Stone, Silliman, Ehren, & Apel, 2006; Pennington, 2009). The assessment of these neurocognitive domains in conjunction with the evaluation of component skills in the areas of spoken language, phonological awareness, reading, and writing provide the practitioner with a more complete profile of the learner's strengths and weaknesses. A profile that includes information from these two global domains (i.e., components of reading and specific cognitive processes) will inform the practioner on (a) the nature of the learner's language learning deficit and (b) the optimal approach(es) for instruction and academic accommodations, when necessary.

Reading ability has long been associated with general intellectual and language abilities. However, in the last two decades, a substantial body of evidence has emerged to show more circumscribed associations between the reading skills of individuals who have obvious and unexpected reading disabilities and their cognitive processing abilities. These associations have

been studied most extensively in the areas of (1) language processing of phonological units (Stanovich, 1988a, 1988b; Wagner & Torgesen, 1987; Liberman & Liberman, 1990; Shankweiler & Liberman, 1989); (2) verbal working memory (Berninger, 2008; Swanson, Zheng, & Jerman, 2009; Pennington, 2009); and (3) processing speed (Laasonen, Lahti-Nuuttila, & Virsu, 2002; Ramus, 2003; Wolf & Bowers, 1999; Wolff, 2000; Stoodley & Stein, 2006).

Cognitive processes in the MAR^wR model are subsumed within the neurobiological and neurocognitive factors module because generalized strengths or weaknesses in these global areas (e.g., language processing at the phonological level; verbal working memory) appear to underlie the deficits in specific skills (e.g., decoding, language comprehension) that directly affect reading ability. The placement of these four cognitive processes within the neurobiological and neurocognitive factors module does not imply that facilities in these processes cannot be altered by environmental experiences; however, the degree to which aptitude in these core cognitive processes can be altered is not well understood. Specific cognitive skills in the phonological realm of language have proven to be most useful in identifying the key deficits that characterize children with dyslexia (Catts & Kamhi, 2005; Stanovich, 1988a, 2000; Siegel, 2003a; Vellutino & Fletcher, 2005).

Reasoning Abilities

Traditionally, intelligence has been viewed as a unitary factor composed of two types of reasoning, fluid intelligence (Gf) and crystallized intelligence (Gc) (Catell & Horn, 1978). Fluid intelligence represents the ability to perform tasks that require reasoning, holding information in memory, attending to details, and solving problems. In contrast, crystallized intelligence represents the ability to remember and apply acquired knowledge, such as defining the meaning of words or applying mathematical equations to solve problems.

Recent literature supports that fluid and crystallized intelligence can be disassociated to some degree and should be viewed independently (Blair, 2006), especially when profiling learners who have academic difficulties. The most commonly used test of intelligence, the *Wechsler Test of Intelligence–IV* (WISC-IV), attempts to separate fluid and crystallized abilities. The WISC-IV is composed of four core indices of cognitive skills: (1) verbal comprehensive index (crystallized intelligence), (2) perceptual reasoning index (fluid intelligence), (3) working memory index, and (4) processing speed index. On the *Woodcock-Johnson Test of Cognitive Ability–III* (WJ III COG), another widely used test of psycho-educational abilities, fluid and crystallized abilities are tested under the three constructs of (1) verbal ability, (3) thinking ability, and (3) cognitive efficiency.

While differing perspectives abound regarding the contribution of different types of intelligence to the traditional construct of general intelligence, children with learning disabilities show strengths on some tasks of cognition and weakness on others (Pennington, 2009). Their uneven, and often largely discrepant, performance on different types of tasks is consistent with Blair's suggestion that different types of cognitive skills should be examined independently of others. For example, it is well documented that children who have dyslexia show strengths in verbal comprehension and reasoning and weaknesses in phonological processing and verbal working memory (Shaywitz, 2003).

Language Processing

Language processing is a global construct that refers to (a) the ability to translate sounds heard in speech into meaningful units of information and comprehend them within the context in which they occur and to (2) the ability to generate meanings through the use of one's knowledge of semantics (word meanings), syntax (word forms), and pragmatics (word functions) (Aram & Nation, 1982).

Verbal comprehension aptitude is the most commonly assessed domain of language processing and is typically evaluated by measuring the learner's facility with surface word meanings (i.e., general vocabulary) and deep word meanings (e.g., antonyms, synonyms, analogies). This verbal comprehension construct is most frequently tested on comprehensive psycho-educational batteries such as the *WISC-IV* (Wechsler, 2003) and *WJ COG III* (Woodcock, McGrew, & Mather, 2001b). Weaknesses in verbal comprehension have been linked to reading difficulties in many studies (Berninger, 2008; Carver, 2000; Catts, Fey, Zhang, & Tomblin, 2001; Catts, Adlof, & Weismer, 2006; Cain & Oakhill, 2007a).

Dyslexia is the most frequently studied reading disability (Fletcher et al., 2007). For the past two decades, the *phonological deficit hypothesis* (PDH) (Vellutino & Fletcher, 2005) has been the predominant theory for explaining this specific learning disability. The PDH posits that phonological representations for sounds are weakly represented (sometimes referred to as "fuzzy representations") or underspecified in persons who have dyslexia (Shaywitz, 2003). These weak phonological representations account for the primary deficits that have been observed for decades in the reading skills of learners who have dyslexia; these deficits include depressed word reading, nonsense word reading, reading fluency, and spelling in spite of adequate language comprehension. As noted previously, the fact that different processes that contribute to reading (e.g., decoding, comprehension) can be dissociated suggests that the biological architecture of the brain that impacts reading skills may be modular in nature. For example, the neural network that allows for associations between letters and their corresponding sounds could be inefficient while the neural network needed to map sounds to meaning may be adequate (Cossu, 1999). In order for skilled reading to occur, information processing of print must proceed accurately and efficiently, with all neural networks working in concert.

Working Memory Processes

Working memory is a dynamic process that requires the ability to store information tem-porarily while engaging in other cognitive tasks (i.e., immediate recall and manipulation of information) (Baddeley, 1986). In contrast, short-term memory involves only the temporary storage of information without the added cognitive tasks of manipulating information (e.g., immediate verbatim recall) (Savage, Lavers, & Pillay, 2007), and long-term memory involves the storage and recall of information over a long period of time (recall over long periods of time) Atkinson & Shiffrin, 1968.

Baddeley's (1986) multicomponent working memory model is the most widely used framework for distinguishing between components of the temporary storage systems of memory, and it is the most frequently used model for discussing memory deficits in children with learning disabilities. In Baddeley's (2000) revised version of his model, shown in Figure 2-3, information in long-term memory represents knowledge that is "crystallized" and information in working memory represents knowledge that is "fluid." As noted earlier, crystallized intelligence refers to knowledge acquired through experiences and fluid intelligence refers to the ability to quickly perceive, understand, and manipulate information. Using Baddeley's model, deficits in "phonological" working memory represent fluid reasoning and are most closely linked to reading disability (Baddeley, 1986; Wagner & Torgesen, 1987; Swanson, 1994; Swanson & Ashbaker, 2000; Swanson & Berninger, 1995).

In this model, the "central executive" component functions as an "attentional-control" system that helps to direct the

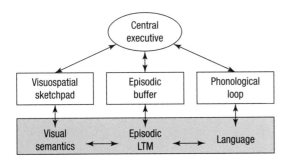

□ Fluid intelligence
▪ Crystallized intelligence

FIGURE 2-3 Baddeley's (2000) Revised Model of Working Memory

Reprinted from the *Journal of Communication Disorders*, Volume 36, Issue 3, by Alan Baddeley, Working memory and language: An overview, p. 20. Copyright 2000, with permission from Elsevier.

stream of information flowing between three "slave" storage systems: the phonological loop component, the visuospatial sketchpad component, and the episodic buffer (Baddeley, 2000).

The central executive system communicates bidirectionally with the verbal phonological loop system and the nonverbal visuospatial sketchpad system. The phonological loop serves as a short-term storage system for sounds and has the capacity to access verbal semantic information from long-term memory. In the same way, the visuospatial sketchpad serves as a short-term memory system for visual forms and has the capacity to access visual semantic information from long-term storage. The episodic buffer facilitates the processing of information by integrating verbal (e.g., sounds) and visual (e.g., letters) units with semantic information stored in long-term memory (Baddeley, 2003).

Pickering and Gathercole (2001) developed the *Working Memory Test Battery for Children* (WMTB-C) with tasks for assessing four components of working memory:

Phonological loop skills are measured on short-term memory tasks such as the immediate recall of series of digits or nonwords. Central executive *verbal working memory* is measured on more complex tasks such as listening to a series of sentences and then recalling the last word in each sentence. *Visuospatial sketchpad* skills are measured on short-term visual memory tasks such as immediate recall of the sequences in which blocks are touched. *Visuospatial central executive working memory* is measured by more complex procedures such as maze memory tasks.

Tasks of this nature appear to be useful in differentiating children's visual and verbal strengths and weaknesses. For example, deficits in both the phonological loop and in verbal working memory have been found in learners diagnosed with specific language impairment (Gathercole, Hitch, Service, & Martin, 1997; Gathercole, Tiffany, Briscoe, Thorn, and the ALSPAC team, 2005; Ellis-Weismer, Evans, & Hesketh, 1999; Hoffman & Gillam, 2004) and in learners diagnosed with reading disability (Siegel & Ryan, 1989; Stone & Brady, 1995; Swanson & Siegel, 2001; Swanson, 1993; de Jong, 1998; Gathercole, Alloway, Willis, & Adams, 2006; Vellutino, Scanlon, & Spearing, 1995). In a longitudinal study of children with poor phonological short-term memory who were tested at 5 and at 8 years of age, Gathercole et al. (2005) found that central executive verbal working memory deficits rather than phonological short-term memory deficits were associated with a general language learning deficit that extended beyond reading. These findings suggest *that perhaps different types of memory weaknesses reflect different types of language-based developmental disorders.* In their critique of studies on the role of working memory in developmental reading problems, Savage, Lavers, and Pillay (2007) state that "the clearest evidence on comprehension using groups carefully matched for nonsense word decoding skill tends to suggest that poor comprehenders do not necessarily experience domain-general working memory problems, and that poor decoders can often have only phonological loop deficits" (p. 215).

Berninger (2008) cites evidence from brain imaging research that words may be stored in memory in three different formats: phonological codes, morphological codes, and orthographic codes. Dyslexia appears to be strongly associated with inefficiencies in verbal working memory that involve mapping from one word form to another (e.g., mapping phonological units, or sounds, onto orthographic units, or spellings).

Speed of Processing

As noted above, interactions among neural circuits in the anterior and posterior portions of the brain are needed for reading. Breznitz (2006) notes that speed of processing (SOP) across brain circuits, such as in slow rate of reading, is a central and universal characteristic of individuals who have dyslexia and possibly of those who have more broadly based language disabilities.

Numerous studies have shown that children with reading disabilities are characteristically slower than their peers on tasks of rapid automatized naming (Bowers & Swanson, 1991; Denckla & Cutting, 1999; Denckla & Rudel, 1976; Wolff, Michel, & Ovrut, 1990). Breznitz (2006) summarized a range of studies that examined auditory and visual processing in elementary school and university dyslexic and nondyslexic students using reaction-time measures and online processing from event-related potentials (ERPs). She found that dyslexics at both ages were significantly slower than their nondyslexic peers and that the differences in speed of performance between the dyslexic and nondyslexic students increased with the complexity of the tasks. As a result of her findings, Breznitz (2008) has proposed the *asynchrony theory* to explain the root cause of the phonological deficits that characterize individuals who have dyslexia. She states:

> The complex process of word decoding can be compared to a concert which includes many instruments. The conductor must orchestrate the different musicians, to synchronize the instruments and make the output harmonious. Reading similarly requires one specific "harmonized" output. This process is also based on the activation of different brain entities (instruments) which are located in different areas of the brain (orchestra), and which process information in a different manner (sounds) (p. 25).

Thus, Breznitz posits that accurate decoding requires synchronistic activation between brain circuits and that it is a lack of synchrony at this level of decoding that leads to the phonological deficits that characterize dyslexia.

Although working memory and processing speed are not yet considered core differential diagnostic markers of dyslexia (Pennington, 2009), many learners with dyslexia show weaknesses in working memory (Berninger, 2008; Swanson, Zheng, & Jerman, 2009; Pennington, 2009) and in processing speed (Berninger, Abbott, Billingsley, & Nagy, 2001; Laasonen, Lahti-Nuuttila, & Virsu, 2002; Ramus, 2003; Wolf & Bowers, 1999; Wolff, Michel, & Ovrut, 1990; Stoodley & Stein, 2006; Park, Lombardino, & Altmann, 2010; Pennington, 2009) while showing strengths in verbal comprehension and reasoning (Fletcher & Lyon, 2008; Shaywitz, 2003; Shaywitz, Morris, & Shaywitz, 2008; Park, Kim, & Lombardino, 2010; Pennington, 2009).

The most frequently used tests of cognitive abilities, the Wechsler Intelligence Test for Children–IV (WISC-IV: Wechsler, 2003) and the Woodcock-Johnson Tests of Cognitive Ability-III (WJ III COG Woodcock, McGrew, & Mather, 2001b), allow for the examination of skills in four cognitive domains that have been shown to assist in distinguishing types of reading difficulties.

The Interaction of Biology and Environment

Reading development is influenced by both biological and environmental factors (Eckert, Lombardino, & Leonard, 2001). Children who live in poverty are at greater risk for prolonged health problems than middle-class children because of higher rates of prematurity, poor nutrition, prolonged illness such as chronic otitis media, and other factors that can impact their performance in learning to read (Vernon-Feagans, Hammer, Miccio, & Manlove, 2002). Regardless of whether the learner's initial difficulty with reading is rooted in biological or environmental influences, the manner in which the environment responds to the learner's difficulties is a *key factor* in determining the degree to which she will continue to advance in reading. Stanovich (2000) and Spear-Swerling and Sternberg (1996) underscore that the environment can serve as both a causal factor and a contributory factor to reading success or failure. For example, a child who enters school from a disadvantaged environment with little to no literacy background can advance in her development of reading skills if given adequate instruction and the support for learning to read both for both academic success and for pleasure. A less desirable outcome could arise for a child who has had adequate exposure to print prior to entering school yet fails to develop decoding skills because of an inability to learn the phonological codes for sound-letter correspondences with the efficiency of her peers. If this child fails to receive adequate assistance and continues to struggle with word reading, she is likely to avoid reading as a source of information and pleasure. Diminished exposure to written language can lead to deficiencies in a range of conceptual areas that can impact the learner's ability to comprehend text

(Cunningham & Stanovich, 1998; Echols, West, Stanovich, & Zehr, 1996).

Data from the University of Colorado's Learning Disabilities Research Center (CLDRC; Olson, 2006) support the interaction between genetic and environmental influences (G × E interactions) on reading disability. At this center, large numbers of identical and fraternal twins have been studied systematically for many years. When Friend, DeFries, and Olson (2008) examined G × E interactions in a large sample of twin pairs in which at least one twin had a reading disability and a comparison group of twin pairs with no history of reading disability, they found a heritability factor for reading disability of 0.61. They also found a stronger genetic influence in struggling readers with good environmental supports for reading (based on parents' education) than for struggling readers with who have fewer environmental supports. These data underscore the importance of considering both biological and environmental factors when evaluating and treating learners with reading deficits.

LANGUAGE KNOWLEDGE MODULE

Definitions and Scientific Support

Language knowledge refers to a wide range of verbal skills that contribute to reading acquisition and development. These skills include knowledge of meanings conveyed through words (i.e., vocabulary); word segments such as root words, prefixes, and suffixes (i.e., morphology); and text structures (e.g., story grammars, discourse structures).

The emergence of literacy is dependent on a range of spoken language skills. Spoken language plays both a direct and an indirect role in the development of literacy from the preschool years through at least third grade. These spoken language skills are not limited to vocabulary but extend to a broader range of language skills that include phonological, semantic, and syntactic knowledge (NICHD Early Child Care Research Network, 2005). Research supports that the components of language skills across the domains of phonology, semantics, syntax, and pragmatics impact reading achievement at varying stages of reading development. As noted in Chapter 1, a reciprocal relationship between spoken language and reading comprehension exists throughout the life span. This ongoing relationship is represented by the extension of the language knowledge module from the bottom to the top of the MAR^wR model of reading (Figure 2-1).

Vocabulary Knowledge

Vocabulary refers to knowledge of word meanings. It is central to learning one's native language, to learning additional languages, and to the normal acquisition of reading and writing (Coyne, Simmons, & Kame'enui, 2004; Biemiller, 2005; Biemiller & Slonim, 2001; Sénéchal, Ouellette, & Rodney, 2006; Stahl & Nagy, 2006). Spoken vocabulary size, as measured by standardized vocabulary tests, appears to be most directly related to word decoding and word recognition, whereas depth of word knowledge, as measured by tasks such as defining words and using figurative language, appears to be most directly related to reading comprehension (Tennenbaum, Torgesen, & Wagner, 2006; Ouellette, 2006). While vocabulary knowledge is a good predictor of later reading comprehension (Cutting & Scarborough, 2006; Cunningham & Stanovich, 1997; de Jong & ven der Leij, 2002; Seigneuric & Ehrlich, 2005), reading also provides a powerful vehicle for the expansion of vocabulary (Nagy & Scott, 2000).

During the preschool period, children learn thousands of root word meanings (Biemiller, 2006; Bicmiller & Slonim, 2001), an accomplishment that greatly enhances their early word identification. After examining data from studies on vocabulary-reading test score relationships, McGuinness (2005) concluded that receptive vocabulary appears to impact reading acquisition only when vocabulary scores are very depressed and that about 90% of school children have sufficiently adequate vocabularies to support learning to read. Children's understanding of word meanings in kindergarten predicts their reading comprehension as early as first and second grade (Roth, Speece, & Cooper, 2002) and is more strongly predictive of reading comprehension in middle school (de Jong & van der Leij, 2002; Seigneuric & Ehrlich, 2005). Vocabulary knowledge in the primary grades is predictive of reading comprehension in the middle grades and beyond (Cunningham & Stanovich, 1997; Scarborough, 1998; Sénéchal, Ouellette, & Rodney, 2006). This predictive relationship underscores the link between knowledge of word meanings and later text-reading fluency and comprehension. Learners acquire about 20,000 vocabulary words between grades 3 and 5, showing a steep growth in their knowledge of word meanings while moving into the middle school grades. When addressing the vocabulary needs of elementary and middle school children, it is important to distinguish between their spoken vocabulary size and their depth of word knowledge (Anglin, 1993; Perfetti, 1985).

Morphological Knowledge

Morphology refers to the smallest units of meaning in words. Morphemes link sounds to meaning just as phonemes link sounds to letters. Morphological knowledge is an important aspect of language and literacy development for children. Having knowledge of morphemes and their structure involves having morphological awareness (Carlisle, 2003). Morphological awareness refers to the awareness that words are made up of morphemes and an understanding of how to manipulate these morphemes (Carlisle, 2003; Nagy, Berninger, Abbott, Vaughan, & Vermeulen, 2003). Morphological awareness plays a key role in language acquisition and has a direct impact on literacy development, including vocabulary, phonology, and orthography; it is a core skill for expanding vocabulary. Children must have knowledge of the five types of morphologically based words that they encounter while reading: (1) root words, (2) inflected words, (3) derived words, (4) literal combinations, and (5) idioms (Anglin, 1993).

Beyond second grade, children learn approximately 1,000 root words each year, and this rapid vocabulary development provides them with the foundation for acquiring many new word meanings from print without being taught the words directly (Biemiller & Boote, 2006; Biemiller & Slonim, 2001). When entering the middle grades, learners acquire the meaning of new words by using their knowledge of morphological structures (e.g., prefixes, suffixes) to determine words' pronunciations and meanings. Morphological knowledge is foundational to vocabulary growth for printed words.

As learners are exposed to more and more words in print, they become more efficient at reading words quickly because they attend to segments of words that are larger than the phoneme, such as common prefixes (e.g., non-) and common suffixes (e.g., -tion). For example, once learners become familiar with the suffix -ment, as in the word *government*, they learn to associate this spelling pattern (i.e., four-letter orthographic unit) with its pronunciation. When they see the same pattern in a novel word, such as *supplement*, they are able to quickly process the letter sequence pattern -ment as a sound unit or chunk. Similarly, when they need to generate this pattern for spelling,

they are able to associate the pronunciation segment (sound sequence pattern) with its orthographic image (letter sequence pattern). Thus, as beginning readers become more proficient at holding the pronunciations for larger segments of printed words in memory, they are able to read unfamiliar words with greater fluency and spell unfamiliar words with greater accuracy.

Morphological knowledge contributes to both word-level and text-level comprehension (Anglin, 1993; Carlisle, 2000; Deacon & Kirby, 2004; Kirby, Desrochers, Roth, & Lai, 2008; Nagy, Berninger, & Abbott, 2006). Learners' knowledge of the morphemic structure of words provides them with the raw material to transition from reading narrative texts in the early grades to reading expository texts in third grade and beyond. In narrative texts, vocabulary tends to be familiar, whereas expository texts introduce new words, many of which are derived from already learned words (Deane, Sheehan, Sabatini, Futagi, & Kostin, 2006).

Syntactic Knowledge

Syntax refers to the rules that govern the grammatical structures of sentences. Syntactic skills can be viewed from two perspectives: syntactic knowledge and syntactic awareness (Cain & Oakhill, 2007a). In the context of reading, syntactic knowledge refers to the implicit knowledge needed to comprehend meaning from different syntactic constructions (e.g., passive-vs. active-voice constructions). Syntactic awareness, also known as grammatical awareness, is a metalinguistic skill and refers to one's ability to use explicit knowledge of syntax to reflect on and to manipulate grammatical forms in language (Bowey, 1986a, 1986b; Cain, 2007). Tasks of syntactic awareness vary in the degree to which they tax language knowledge and memory ability. For example, some syntactic awareness tasks require learners to make a judgment about the grammatical accuracy of a sentence while others require learners to correct some dimension of grammar such as ordering scrambled words into an accurate sentence or repairing a sentence that contains a grammatical error.

Bowey (1996) found that syntactic awareness and ability to monitor the grammaticality of sentences presented orally was related to reading skill and that the ability to identify these grammatical errors was directly related to children's reading comprehension skill. Similarly, Nation and Snowling (2000) found that poor comprehenders performed significantly poorer than their normal peers on a word-order correction tests.

In a well controlled study of syntactic awareness and reading ability, Cain (2007) examined the predictive power of performance on two types of syntactic awareness tasks (word-order correction and grammatical correction) on word reading and reading comprehension. Overall, she found that the two types of task were not equivalent; word-order correction was more dependent on memory skills while grammatical error correction was more dependent on grammatical knowledge. Most importantly, Cain's findings strongly support

that the link between syntactic awareness and reading comprehension "is indirect and arises from variance shared with vocabulary, grammatical knowledge, and memory" (p. 691).

Not surprisingly, verbal working memory weaknesses are believed to constrain higher-level language skills such as syntactic processing (Smith, Macaruso, Shankweiler, & Crain, 1989), resulting in impaired reading comprehension. Nation and Snowling (2000) noted that a subgroup of children, called poor comprehenders, showed depressed reading comprehension along with more general language processing deficits in spite of good word recognition. They concluded that a weakness in verbal working memory contributed to the poor comprehender's language processing limitations.

In their studies of children with dyslexia, Rispens, Roeleven, and Koster (2004) found that 8-year-old dyslexic children made significantly more errors than a control group in their production of subject-verb agreement in spontaneous speech and in their judgments of the grammatical accuracy of sentences. In a longitudinal study of preschoolers with a familial history of reading disability, Scarborough (2002) found that children's productive syntax between 30 and 48 months of age predicted their future reading abilities. However, although many children identified with spoken language impairments during their preschool years showed deficits in reading in the elementary grades, syntactic deficits were not always found in the preschool children who were diagnosed at school age with a reading disability (Bishop & Snowling, 2004).

Using the Bishop and Snowling (2004) two-dimensional model for classifying strengths and weaknesses in children's non-phonological (i.e., semantics, syntax) and phonological language skills (i.e., decoding), Snowling and Hayiou-Thomas (2006) identified three core deficit profiles: (a) phonological *and* nonphonological language deficits that characterize children who have specific language impairment, (b) phonological skill deficits *alone* that characterize children who have dyslexia, and (c) nonphonological skill deficits *alone* that characterize children who are poor comprehenders. Because profiles of strengths and weaknesses in reading-related skills vary, evaluations must be designed to tease apart the multiple types and levels of skills that can impact reading achievement.

Discourse Knowledge

Discourse refers to "a variety of spoken and written events" (Brinton & Fujiki, 1989, p. 2) that are organized into sentences and larger units to communicate a cohesive message.

Many skills are needed to successfully engage in discourse, ranging from the ability to choose the correct vocabulary words to express one's message coherently to the ability to actively engage in a conversation about abstract ideas. To be successful in discourse, children need to hold information in memory, make inferences, take into account the listeners' and the speakers' perspectives, and use language across different genres (e.g.,

conversational, narrative, or procedural discourse) (Fey, 1986; Johnston, 1982; Ripich & Griffith, 1988).

The roots of conversational discourse develop before children are familiar with literacy concepts and appear to prepare the way for the development of narrative discourse and other forms of literate language (Brinton & Fujiki, 1989; Hudson & Shapiro, 1991; Paris & Paris, 2003; Roth, Speece, & Cooper, 2002; Snow, 1983; Snow & Dickinson, 1990). The earliest roots of narrative development lie within a child's experience with listening to and participating in narrative exchanges (Boudreau, 2008, p. 103).

Narrative discourse appears to function as a bridge between oral language and literacy (Westby, 1984, 1991; Roth, Speece, & Cooper, 2002; Stadler & Ward, 2005). Narratives are accounts of daily events, scripts, or stories, and serve a range of functions such as sharing ideas, conveying information, entertaining, and socializing. Children's ability to comprehend and produce narratives prior to learning to read is an important indicator of their readiness to read beyond the level of word decoding (Paris & Paris, 2003), and is one index for predicting their future reading ability and overall academic success (McCabe & Rollins, 1994).

Learning to interpret and create narratives is challenging for all children, but this skill is especially challenging for children who have language learning difficulties (Johnson, 1995). Numerous studies have shown that narrative language is an area of vulnerability in children with language impairments (Boudreau & Hedberg, 1999; Gillam & Johnston, 1992; Scott & Windsor, 2000; Ripich & Griffith, 1988). Because the production of narratives and other types of discourse skills place demands on the cognitive and linguistic systems, deficiencies in these systems can impact the learner's use of language in social contexts and in the achievement of academic goals (Boudreau, 2008).

Stages of development (Applebee, 1978; Stadler & Ward, 2005) along with story grammar schemes (Stein & Glenn, 1979) are often used as developmental indices for examining children's narratives. Narrative skills emerge at around 20 to 24 months as children begin to talk about objects in the past and the future, referred to as *temporally displaced talk* (Nelson, 2010). In the first stage of narrative development, children's stories have no central theme (Applebee, 1978), and consist of assigning labels to actions and events (Stadler & Ward, 2005). At approximately 3 years of age, children enter the second stage of narrative development (Applebee, 1978), in which they use narrative schemes that include a central theme along with a setting. Neither a plot nor temporal events are present, but they label characters and describe characters' actions. This is also called the stage of "listing" (Stadler & Ward, 2005) because the events of the character are often literally presented as a list with no regard to time. At around 4 years of age, children begin to transition into the third stage of narrative development,

referred to as "primitive narratives" (Applebee, 1978), or "connecting" structures (Stadler & Ward, 2005). They can describe an initiating event, an action, and a consequence that revolves around a central person, object, or event, but temporal sequencing is still irrelevant and stories do not yet have resolutions. In the fourth stage, narrative scripts evolve into more completely sequenced and complex structures called narrative schemas (Paris & Paris, 2003). At this stage, children are capable of expressing cause-and-effect relationships in the context of an initiating event, an action, a consequence, and a vague plan (Applebee, 1978). Although children's story plots may still be weak in stage 4, their ability to sequence events is clearly evident in their more advanced use of language to coordinate ideas in a story. The "true narrative" is the final stage of development that occurs in normally developing children between 5 and 7 years of age (Applebee, 1978). Children at this stage can describe motivations behind characters' actions, provide a logical temporal sequence of actions and events for the reader to follow, and provide a resolution to the story. They are capable of taking into account the listener's perspective by providing the details needed to comprehend a story. Knowledge of the narrative structure facilitates both listening (Davies, Shanks, & Davies, 2004) and reading (Garner & Bochna, 2004; Paris & Paris, 2003) comprehension because it provides the learner with a framework for binding and knitting together individual sentences to create a cohesive story (Johnston, 2008).

Word Retrieval

Word retrieval refers to the ability to quickly access familiar words when speaking. For many years, word-retrieval deficits have been associated with the spoken and written language of learners who have language learning disabilities (German, 1984; Johnson & Myklebust, 1967; Wiig & Semel, 1984). The terms *lexical access*, *word retrieval*, and *word-finding* have been used interchangeably across disciplines; however, word finding has had the greatest longevity in characterizing the speech production of children with language learning disabilities. German and Newman (2007) state that word finding refers to "the mental activity of selecting or retrieving known words from the lexicon in order to express what you want to say or write. A word-finding difficulty is a disruption in this mental activity, resulting in problems generating words to express one's thoughts" (p. 399).

Word retrieval, or word finding, is critical to *fluent speaking and reading*. Word-finding deficits manifest both in spontaneous conversations and on tasks in which the rapid recall of familiar names from both open and closed sets of pictured stimuli are presented. Rapid word retrieval is typically assessed in a picture-naming format. Numerous studies on reading-impaired children have shown that they are slower and less accurate than their peers when naming pictures (German & Newman, 2007; Nation, Marshal, & Snowling, 2001; Nation,

Clarke, Marshall, & Durand, 2004; Nation, 2005a; Snowling, van Wagtendonk, & Stafford,1988; Swan & Goswami, 1997; Wolf & Goodglass, 1986). The task of Rapid Automatized Naming (RAN; Denckla & Rudel, 1972, 1974, 1976) is the most widely used measure of rapid serial naming and has continued to serve as a task that helps to distinguish good readers from poor readers from childhood through adulthood (Wolf, Bally, & Morris, 1986; Bowers & Wolf, 1993; Felton, Naylor, & Wood, 1990).

PHONOLOGICAL KNOWLEDGE MODULE

Definitions and Scientific Support

Phonology refers to the sound system of the language. Phonological knowledge, in the context of reading acquisition, refers to a broad range of skills that encompass *phonological awareness*, a sensitivity to the sound structure of words; *phonemic awareness*, a more advanced form of phonological awareness that allows one to consciously manipulate sounds in words; *phonological memory*, the ability to hold phonological units, such as nonsense words, in memory; and *phonological access*, the ability to automatically retrieve the pronunciations of familiar words (Wagner & Torgesen, 1987). This segment of the MAR^wR model addresses only the component skill of phonological awareness.

Phonological awareness refers to a continuum of skills that reflect different levels of sensitivity to the sounds in spoken words (Stahl & Murray, 1994). These skills develop over the span of several years from preschool through the early elementary school years. Stanovich (1992) described these levels on a continuum from *shallow to deep*, whereas Ball (1993) used the terms *emerging*, *simple*, and *complex* to represent the range of skills that represent this phonological construct. The developmental progression of phonological awareness is dependent on the size of the phonological unit; awareness of whole words precedes awareness of syllables and awareness of syllables precedes awareness of individual phonemes (Goswami & Bryant, 1990; Goswami, 2002; Lonigan, Burgess, Anthony, & Barker, 1998; Yopp, 1992).

At the *word level of awareness*, the learner is capable of identifying the number of words in a short sentence (e.g., See the cat.) but does not yet attempt to segment within a word. At the *syllable level of awareness*, learners understand how to segment spoken words into their component syllables. Learners who can count or tap out the number of syllables in compound words such as "base ... ball" and multisyllabic words such as "kit ... ten" or "el ... e ... phant" have acquired syllable-level phonological awareness. At the *intrasyllable level of awareness*, often called onset-rime awareness, learners can segment syllables into beginning and ending sounds. For example, in the word *bat*, /a/ is referred to as the *peak*, the part of the syllable that car-

ries the most vocal energy; /b/ is referred to as the *onset*, the part of the syllable that comes before the peak; and /t/ is referred to as the *coda*, the part of the syllable that comes after the peak. The onset consists of /b/ and the rime is represented by the peak plus the coda /a t/ (Morais, 2003). At this level, learners should be able to recognize similar sound units when asked to determine if two words start with the same sound (e.g., mop, mice) or to identify a word that does not begin with the same sound as the others (e. g., cup, cat, mop). Further, learners should be able to determine if words rime (e.g., sip, tip) and to identify a word in a group that does not rime (e.g., pit, mat, pat). In Figure 2-1, a crisscrossed line with an arrow is used to indicate the point at which the learner transitions to the phonemic level of sound awareness.

At the phonemic level of awareness, the learner is capable of identifying and manipulating individual sounds in words. Two of the most common phonemic manipulations are referred to as *segmenting* and *blending* phonemes. Segmenting represents the ability to parse individual sounds in words (e.g., counting the number of sounds in a word) and blending represents the ability to combine individual sounds into a whole unit (e.g., listening to individual sounds that make up a word then identifying the word).

Naturally, levels of complexity exist within the phonemic level of awareness. At about the time that learners come to understand that words are composed of individual sounds, they also come to understand that specific orthographic symbols (e.g., letters) correspond to specific phonemes (i.e., sounds). When this occurs, the learner has acquired the *alphabetic principle,* enabling him to segment and blend sounds (phonemes) and their corresponding letters (graphemes) for both word reading and spelling. As they continue to develop their sensitivity to and memory for phonological and orthographic patterns, they advance in their ability to manipulate sounds within words. Learners in second and third grades, for example, should be able to delete a sound in a consonant cluster or digraph (e.g., say the word "stand," now say it without the /t/), a process commonly referred to as elision (Rosner, 1979).

The construct of phonological awareness can be conceptualized by two types of operations: cognitive task complexity and linguistic complexity (Lonigan, 2006; Stahl & Murray, 1994). An understanding of how these operations impact the developmental progression of phonological skills is central to the assessment and treatment of learners who are delayed in their acquisition of these skills. Stahl and Murray (1994) examined the performance of kindergarten and first-grade children on four phonemic awareness tasks (blending, segmentation, phoneme isolation, and deletion) at four levels of linguistic complexity (onset-rime, vowel codas, cluster onsets, cluster codas). They found that both ways of defining phonological awareness (i.e., by type of

task, by level of linguistic complexity) yield a single common factor, but noted that linguistic complexity appears to be a better way to conceptualize phonological awareness. Their developmental hierarchy of tasks ranging from easiest to most difficult is shown below:

- Phoneme isolation (e.g., tell me the sound you hear in the beginning of the word *fat*)

- Phoneme blending (e.g., tell me what word I am saying when you hear one sound at a time, as in *m ... a ... p*)

- Phoneme deletion (e.g., say *meat*, now say it again, but don't say /m/)

- Phoneme segmentation (e.g., I will say a word such as *fish* and you tell me all the sounds that you hear in the word, like *f..i..sh*)

Many studies have shown that phonological awareness is strongly related to success in learning to read and spell (Adams, 1990; Blachman, 1997; Goswami & Bryant, 1990) and that phonological awareness improves as children become more proficient readers (Perfetti, Beck, Bell, & Hughes, 1987). Research on the precise relationships between phonological awareness skills and reading shows that learners can segment words into syllables and perform riming tasks prior to learning to read, but their ability to segment words into phonemes is acquired at about the same time they learn to read (Wagner & Torgesen, 1987; Liberman, Shankweiler, Fisher, & Carter, 1974). Along with letter identification, phonological awareness is one of the strongest predictors of reading achievement (Adams, 1990; Scarborough, 2002).

Tasks at the highest levels of phoneme manipulation require complex sound transpositions; examples include spoonerisms, Pig Latin, or other tasks that entail systematic changes in sound positions within and across words. To create spoonerisms, learners must be able to transpose the first sounds in two consecutive words, as in changing *John Lennon* to *Lohn Jennon*. To speak Pig Latin, learners must be able to place the first consonant in the word at the end of the word followed by the /ay/ sound, as in changing *dog* to *ogday*. Although it is likely that accomplished readers are more proficient at advanced phoneme manipulation tasks, proficiency at this high level of phonemic manipulation is not necessary to learn to read.

PRINT KNOWLEDGE MODULE

Definitions and Scientific Support

Print knowledge represents a wide range of print concepts that the learner must understand prior to reading. This knowledge can be categorized in three general areas: (1) *print concepts*: recognizing and understanding book conventions (e. g., cover, title page, front of book, a page), print mechanics (e.g., left to right, first line, last line), and letter discrimination (one letter, first letter, last letter); (2) *concept of word*: matching spoken words to print during reading; and (3) *letter orientation/discrimination*: matching symbols such as letters and numbers to one another (Clay, 1979; Henderson & Beers, 1980; Morris, 1981).

Performance on assessments of print knowledge predicts future reading achievement and relates strongly to more traditional measures of reading readiness (Adams, 1990). Furthermore, visual matching is one of the best discriminators of good and poor readers in grades 1 and 2 and of persistent good and poor readers in grades 6 and 7 (Badian, 1994, 1998).

Print Awareness

Print awareness skills are most often learned during joint reading activities in which preschoolers are actively engaged in book reading with adults (Scarborough & Dobrich, 1994; Bus, van Ijzendoorn, & Pellegrini, 1995). Storybook interactions between parents and their children have been shown to benefit children's spoken language skills (Frijters, Barron, & Brunello, 2000; Sénéchal & LeFevre, 2002). More direct teaching or instructional activities with adults that draw children's attention to concepts of print facilitate knowledge of letters and letter-sound associations (Evans, Williamson, & Pursoo, 2008; Ezell & Justice, 2000; Stephenson, Parrila, Georgiou, & Kirby, 2008).

Emergent Writing

Prior to learning that letters represent sounds in words, learners represent their preliterate knowledge in drawings, scribbling, and letter-like formations (Sulzby, Teale, & Kamberelis, 1989; Temple et al., 1992). Emergent writing refers to the learner's intention to use printed marks on paper to communicate ideas. These printed forms demonstrate that the learner understands that written information conveys ideas in a manner similar to spoken language. The skills that learners need to tell a narrative provide the foundation for their ability to convey a story using marks on paper. Children's attempts to convey their ideas in print can change dramatically during the course of one year. Emergent writing often begins as pictorial representations and evolves into forms that are more representative of print. Figure 2-4 shows a sample of a 42-month-old child's attempt to describe her grandmother's home through drawings. Figure 2-5 shows the same child's attempts to convey the same story in print at 56 months of age.

Once learners understand that printed words represent spoken words, they often begin to produce prephonological spellings. Traditionally, it was assumed that these spellings showed no direct sound-letter relationships with the words that they represented (e.g., *rvp* used to spell *fish*) and had been characterized as random spellings. Recently, however, Pollo, Treiman, and Kessler (2008a, 2008b) have shown that the prephonological spellings of prereaders are (a) not random, (b) influenced by the native language of the learners, and (c) predict spellings one year later. Hence, prephonological spellings appear to be a precursor to

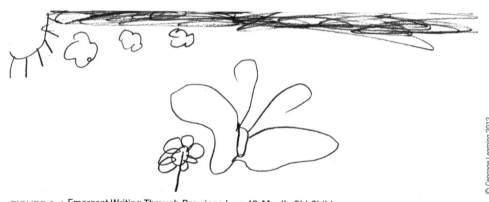

FIGURE 2-4 Emergent Writing Through Drawings by a 42-Month-Old Child

© Cengage Learning 2012

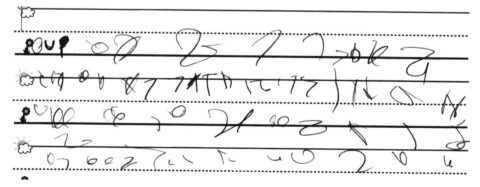

FIGURE 2-5 Emergent Writing by the Same Child on the Same Topic at 56 Months of Age

© Cengage Learning 2012

invented spellings, underscoring the importance of examining children's ability to "create" words in print prior to entering school. Furthermore, in a large scale study of emergent literacy skills in preschoolers between 4 and 5 years of age, Puranik, Lonigan, and Kim (2011) found that letter-writing ability made a significant and unique contribution to spelling skill when both name-writing and letter-writing skills were considered together.

Letter Knowledge

Letter knowledge has been shown consistently to serve as a good predictor of reading (Badian, 1982; Chall, 1983; Ehri, 1983; Gibson & Levin, 1975). Prereaders' ability to name letters is a strong predictor of their later phonemic awareness skills and their reading both in early and in later grades (Badian, 1994, 1995). In a recent study of longitudinal predictors of reading across several languages varying in orthographic consistency, Georgiou et al., (2010) reported that letter knowledge was the strongest predictor in each language. Walsh, Price, and Gillingham (1988) reported that letter-naming speed in kindergarten children is a very strong predictor of later reading but that speed loses it predictive value by second grade when typically developing children surpass a "threshold speed" for letter naming.

Ehri's (1992) research suggests that letter naming is a bridge to reading because several letter names (such as jay for the letter *J*; el for *L*) contain the sounds that correspond to the letters, thereby providing the learner with access to a connection between the printed symbol (e.g., J) and its phonological representation. Data from Badian (1995) and

Blaiklock (2004) suggest that the relationship between phonological awareness and later reading is mediated by children's letter knowledge. Hence, it appears that knowledge of letter names facilitates the awareness of individual phonemes and the awareness of individual phonemes facilitates word-level reading. Again, in Figure 2-1 an arrow is used to indicate that letter knowledge facilitates the transition to phonemic awareness.

GRAPHOPHONEMIC INTEGRATION MODULE

Definition and Scientific Support

The graphophonemic integration module represents the integration of phonemic awareness and letter knowledge (Ehri & Soffer, 1999; O'Connor, 2007). This level of knowledge is typically called the alphabetic principle because the learner understands that letters in print represent sounds in words. Understanding the alphabetic principle, that is, knowing that sounds can map onto letters and letters represent sounds, is necessary when decoding and blending sounds in words for reading and translating sounds into letters to generate spellings (Ehri, 1991; Liberman & Liberman, 1990).

Mapping Sound and Letter Units

Children's knowledge of the alphabetic principle is often first evident in their invented spellings (Gentry, 2000). Their ability to segment words along with identifying the names and sounds of letters prepares them to break through the alphabetic code of their writing system (Ehri & Roberts, 2006). Grapheme-phoneme mapping knowledge provides the "glue" that connects spellings to their pronunciations in memory (Ehri & Rosenthal, 2007). In fact, Al Otaiba et al. (2010) found that a one-minute letter-sound fluency task given in the spring of kindergarten was the best predictor of end-of-the-year kindergarten spelling achievement. An alphabetic script is, first and foremost (although not solely), a phonemic code or "blueprint"—a graphic dissection of the segmental structure of spoken words. Phonemic awareness and letter knowledge have been labeled *corequisites* (Share, 2005) or *codeterminants* (Bowey, 2005) to alphabetic literacy. Ehri and Soffer's (1999) term *graphophonemic awareness* aptly captures the inseparability of the two in learning to read and write in an alphabetic language such as English.

Invented Spelling

Invented spelling is a more advanced dimension of emergent writing. Learners' invented spellings emerge when they begin to apply their knowledge of how sounds heard represent letters in print, prior to learning conventional spellings. Invented spellings provide a window into the learner's level of phonemic awareness and knowledge of the alphabetic principle (Burns & Richgels, 1989; Gentry, 1982, 2000; Invernizzi, 1992; Morris, 1983; Morris, Nelson, & Perney, 1986; Read, 1971; Richgels, 2002; Treiman, 1993). For example, when prereaders spell "bk" for *back*, they demonstrate partial alphabetic knowledge of how sounds map onto letters (Ehri, 2005).

However, this level of phonemic awareness does not ensure that the learner will be able to segment and blend letters into the words that they represent. Although the ability to segment and blend sounds is a necessary skill in learning to develop the full alphabetic knowledge needed to decode words in alphabetic languages (Adams, 1990; Nation & Hulme, 1997; Spector, 1995), instruction in invented spelling has been shown to improve word reading (Tangel & Blachman, 1992, 1995; O'Connor & Jenkins, 1995).

In summary, preschool children who are not yet reading should be able to detect and manipulate larger linguistic segments such as words and syllables, and learners who are beginning to read should be able to blend and segment individual sounds in words (Wagner, Torgesen, & Rashotte, 1994). Explicit sensitivity to individual sounds in words and knowledge of how these sounds can be blended and segmented are necessary skills for learning to read, but they are not sufficient skills for reading. To apply phonemic knowledge to reading, learners must acquire the *alphabetic principle*, that is, "the understanding that letters in written words stand for sounds in spoken words" (Stahl & Murray, 1994, p. 232). The alphabetic principle is the basis for translating phonemes (sounds) in spoken language to their corresponding graphemes (letters) in written language (Adams, 1990; Adams, 2002; Moats, 2000). This principle is the foundation for word-level reading and must be taught explicitly (National Institute of Child Health and Human Development, National Reading Panel, 2000). Phoneme-level knowledge, along with knowledge of the alphabetic principle, create the perfect blend of skills needed to transition into decoding, a skill that is essential for the development of skilled word-level reading. Figure 2-6 shows the general developmental relationships among emergent literacy skills discussed in this section of the book.

A stable bidirectional relationship exists between phonological awareness and reading-related skills from preschool through second grade (Burgess & Lonigan, 1998; Perfetti, Beck, Bell, & Hughes, 1987; Wagner, Torgesen, & Rashotte, 1994). This means that phonological awareness enhances reading acquisition and is advanced by learning to read (Treiman, 1998; Figure 2-6). Although the importance of the units may differ depending on the native language of the learner (i.e., the

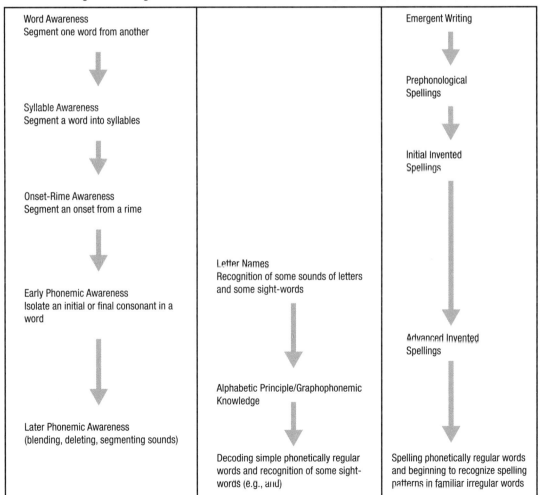

FIGURE 2-6 Approximate Parallel Development of Phonological and Phonological-Orthographic Skills

rime unit is more prominent in some languages than others), all children develop an awareness of larger phonological units before smaller units (Ziegler & Goswami, 2005).

WORD-LEVEL READING MODULE

Definitions and Scientific Support

At the rudimentary stages of sight-word reading, preschool children often learn to recognize their names in print (Treiman & Broderick, 1998) along with common environmental logos, long before they begin formal reading instruction. Children learn to make connections between visual cues from words themselves or from the contexts surrounding words and their pronunciations (Ehri & Wilce, 1987; Gough, Juel, & Griffith, 1992). Word-level knowledge should represent both the accuracy of the learner's knowledge of the *pronunciation* of words in print and the accuracy of the learner's knowledge of the *meaning* of these words.

The development of word recognition is dependent on sensitivity to sound segments of words at the phonemic level (i.e., mapping sounds onto letters), knowledge of the alphabetic principle (i.e., associating letters with their corresponding sounds), and decoding to arrive at the pronunciations of real words (e.g., "great") and nonsense words (e.g., "fut"). Thus, sight-words acquired without knowledge of sound-letter associations cannot support reading beyond a rudimentary level (Ehri, 1995). Decoding is the core skill required for learning to read in all languages that are based on an alphabetic

system. Learners' decoding skills are typically measured by tasks that require them to sound out phonetically predictable nonsense words, that is, words that comply with the spelling rules of one's language, such as "rane" or "lig" in the English language. Sight-word recognition occurs when learners can automatically access the pronunciation of a word along with its meaning. For most words, sight-word recognition is a direct result of having learned the sound segments of words and then storing pronunciations in memory where they can be retrieved readily upon seeing the words in print. Repeated exposure to a word's spelling strengthens the learner's association between the word's spelling and pronunciation.

Ehri and Roberts (2006) discussed three strategies that readers use to identify unfamiliar words: (1) use a decoding strategy to "sound out" or "map" sounds onto letters and then blend the sounds together to create words; (2) draw analogies between the letter patterns in the words with the pronunciations of the same letter patterns in familiar words (e.g., if the learner is familiar with the printed form and pronunciation of the word *train*, that learner is likely to use this knowledge to arrive at the accurate pronunciation of a novel word such as *gain*); and (3) predict the pronunciation and meaning of an unfamiliar word by using contextual cues surrounding the word along with any clues gleaned from the word's spelling.

A learner's knowledge of individual word meanings is assessed most stringently with words that are lexically ambiguous (Perfetti & Hart, 2001). Lexical ambiguities occur in words that have (1) the *same* phonology and spelling but *differ* in meaning (homonyms, e.g., *fly*, as in the action; *fly*, as in the insect); (2) words that have the *same* phonology but *differ* in spelling and in meaning (homophones, e.g., *threw* and *through*); and (3) words that have the *same* spellings but *differ* in phonology and in meaning (homographs, e.g., *bass*, as in the fish, and *bass*, as in the instrument). The rapid comprehension of potentially ambiguous words in print requires strong links between the words' phonology (sounds), orthography (spelling), and semantic (meaning) representations (Perfetti, 2007; Perfetti & Hart, 2001).

True sight-word reading is a direct growth of having learned the sound segments of words and then storing their pronunciations in memory so that they can be retrieved readily upon seeing the words in print. Repeated exposure to a word's spelling strengthens the learner's association between the word's spelling and its pronunciation. A large store of sight-words in memory occurs when words' phonological, orthographic, and semantic elements become consolidated after repeated exposure (Ehri & Roberts, 2006). Automatic recognition is essential for skilled reading because it allows the reader to attend to the meaning of text rather than the identification of individual words (LaBerge & Samuels, 1974). This integrative and systematic process that links words' spellings, pronunciations, and meanings represents the core of Ehri's (1992) amalgamation model of word-level reading.

Stages of Word-Level Reading

Based on her observation of children's early word-reading strategies, Ehri (1995, 2005) developed a three-phase framework for explaining the evolution of word-level reading that serves as a useful paradigm for describing stages of word-reading development. A summary of these phases is shown in Table 2-1. In *the prealphabetic* phase, learners recognize words by using visual word patterns rather than letter-sound connections to identify a word that they have learned. For example, they may recognize the word *ball* because of the two vertical letters at the end of the word, or they may recognize environmental print because of cues that occur on a sign, such as a girl with red hair and pigtails to represent Wendy's fast-food restaurant. In the *partial alphabetic* phase, learners use their limited knowledge of letter names and letter-sound connections to read words. For example, they may read *bell* as *ball* or may spell *ball* as "bl," reflecting partial knowledge of grapheme-phoneme relationships. Finally, in the *full alphabetic* phase, learners have acquired knowledge of most letter-sound associations. They are able to sound out and spell decodable words such as *bat* and *dig*. They develop the ability to quickly retrieve the pronunciations for these words when they see them in print because every time they see the same words, they strengthen their memories for the associations between the word's orthography (how it looks in print) and its pronunciation.

Consistent with preceding discussions in this chapter but emphasizing a neurobiological perspective, Shaywitz (2003)

TABLE 2-1 Ehri's Three-Phase Model of Word-Level Reading

Phase I: Prealphabetic Stage of Word Reading (Visual-Cue Stage) Preschool*

Key characteristic:
- Learners recognize words by connecting salient visual cues within or around the word with words' pronunciations or meanings (aka visual-cue reading)

Primary Indicators:
- Recognizing a word only when it occurs in a specific context
- Not recognizing when letters in a word are replaced or letters are rearranged (e.g., Pepsi spelled as Zepsi)
- Unable to identify letters in own printed name even if name is recognized

Examples:
- Relying on contextual cues such as familiar logos (e.g., McDonald's golden arches) to recognize a McDonald's sign
- Relying on the shape and color of a stop sign to recognize the word *stop*
- Relying on a meaningful pattern, such as the two "eyes" in the word *bee* or the circle at the end of Pogo's name, to recognize words in print

"Because the visual cues forming connections are not unique to individual words, children mistake visually similar words for one another" (Ehri, 1992, p. 125).

Transition from Prealphabetic to Partial Alphabetic Stage

Learners begin to use knowledge of a few letter names to form connections between letters and corresponding sounds at the beginning or end of words (e.g, child uses the letter *l* to represent the sounds in *ball* when attempting to spell it).

Phase 2: Partial Alphabetic Stage of Word Reading (Phonetic-Cue Stage) Kindergarten*

Key characteristic:
- Learners recognize words by connecting letters with sounds

Primary Indicators:
- Knowing the names of most letters in the alphabet
- Showing the ability to segment the initial sound in a word from the remainder of the word
- Using knowledge of letter names and ability to partially segment words (phonemic awareness) to make systematic connections between letters and their corresponding sounds, especially at the beginning and end of words. Knowing letter names gives access to phonetic cues that can be used to attempt reading words

Examples:
- Spelling flower as "FLR" by using letter names to guide spelling
- Misreading simple words such as *for* for *from* and *like* for *lake* while indicating the use of phonetic cues as a strategy for reading

"It is important to note that sight word reading during the partial alphabetic phase is an imperfect process that occurs among beginners who lack full knowledge of the alphabetic system and phonemic segmentation skill" (Ehri, 2005, p. 145).

Transition from Partial Alphabetic Stage to Full Alphabetic Stage

Learners use both visual and phonetic cues to read novel words.

Phase 3: Full Alphabetic Stage of Word-Reading (Alphabetic Coding Stage) First–Second Grade

Key characteristic:
- Learner can integrate knowledge of phonemic segmentation with knowledge of letter-sound associations to decode words
- Learner is able to quickly identify familiar words by retrieving spellings and pronunciations stored in memory

Primary Indicators:
- Segmenting and blending unfamiliar, phonetically regular words to arrive at accurate pronunciations of words in print

At this level, children are "able to form connections between all of the graphemes in spellings and the phonemes in pronunciations to remember how to read words" (Ehri, 2005, p. 148).

Adapted from Ehri (1992, 1995, 2005).
*Period of development indicated by grades is an approximation.

---

notes that practice in reading a word correctly allows the learner to develop a neural representation of the word and that eventually the learner's "internal representation of the word reflects its precise pronunciation, meaning, and spelling" (p. 189). This neural consolidation of a word's sounds, spelling, and meaning into whole word units allows the learner to read individual words accurately and quickly.

WORD-LEVEL SPELLING MODULE

Definitions and Scientific Support

Spelling is a linguistic skill and spelling disability is a linguistic problem (Moats, 1995). Learning the spelling patterns for words not only facilitates the learner's ability to acquire and retain words' pronunciations but also enhances the learner's knowledge of word meanings (Ehri & Rosenthal, 2007). Cassar and Treiman (2004) underscore the necessity of the learner's ability to integrate phonological

and orthographic knowledge to become a skilled speller. They noted that "typical errors of young spellers reveal their developing phonological skills. As children gain experience with printed words, their orthographic and morphological knowledge begins to have a larger influence on their spelling choices" (p. 630). Because children with reading and spelling disabilities show the same pattern of spelling errors as their younger typical-learning peers, we know that using a developmental framework for evaluating spelling is the most productive approach for determining instructional initiatives (Stanovich, Siegel, & Gottardo, 1997; Cassar, Treiman, Moats, Pollo, & Kessler, 2005).

Stages of Spelling Development

Several developmental and stage-oriented frameworks are available for analyzing spelling patterns. The early work of Henderson (1981) and the later work of Bear, Invernizzi, Templeton, and Johnston (2004); Ganske

(2000); and Masterson, Apel, and Wasowicz (2003) have provided descriptive and prescriptive paradigms for evaluating the spelling errors of struggling spellers at various stages of orthographic development (Apel, Masterson, & Niessen, 2004). Bear et al's. (2004) stage-based scheme for describing

spellings in emergent writing to spellings at advanced levels of derivational knowledge, is shown in Table 2-2.

Spelling deficits are common among children who have reading difficulties (Berninger et al., 2000; Moats, 1995), and are pervasive in the written language of children

TABLE 2-2 Developmental Stages of Spelling

Stages and Approximate Grades	Characteristics of Spelling Arranged Developmentally within Stages
Stage 1: Emergent Writing (preschool)	• Scribbling patterns • Letter and number symbols arranged horizontally • Beginning sound-letter associations as in prephonological spellings
Stage 2: Letter-Naming-Alphabetic Spelling (K–1st grade)	• Initial invented spelling using primarily consonant sounds (e.g., "b," or "bl" for *ball*) • Invented spelling with vowel sound marked (e.g., "bol" or "bal" for *ball*); invented spellings that mark less phonemically salient sounds such as nasal sounds (m, n, ing) in front of other consonant sounds (e.g., "chomp" for *jump*) • Correct alphabetic spellings
Stage 3: Within-Word Pattern Spelling (2nd–3rd grade)	• Knowledge of all initial and final consonants, consonant blends (e.g., *street*), and digraphs (e.g., ra*in*) • Correct spelling of *r* in most single syllable words (e.g., *third*) • Correct use of silent rule in single syllable words (e.g., fram*e*)
Stage 4: Syllables and Affixes Spelling (3rd–5th grade)	• Beginning to use consonant doubling rule (e.g., ho*pp*ing) • Learning to spell multisyllabic words by using prefixes and suffixes and by linking forms (-s,- ed) to number (e.g., present*s*) and tense (e.g., record*ed*) • Learning syllabication rules and relationships between syllable segments and meaning (e.g.,pro/gress, in/for/mal)
Stage 5: Derivational Relations Spelling (5th grade–college)	• Ability to spell most words correctly • Knowledge of the role of prefixes, suffixes, and root (Latin and Greek) words (e.g., in/struct/ive) in making connections between meaning segments and corresponding spellings (e.g., form, inform, information, informal, informant; trans-, transit, transfer, transport, transportation)

Adapted from Bear et al., (2004).

who have dyslexia (Berninger & Wolf, 2009; Frith, 1980; Snowling, 2000). Spelling deficits in individuals with dyslexia often persist into adulthood and are a hallmark of dyslexia in adults, even those who have succeeded in becoming quite skilled in reading (Bruck, 1993; Snowling, 2000). The severity and persistence of spelling deficits are key factors in the differential diagnosis of learning disabilities. The spelling error patterns of learners with dyslexia have been found to be quite similar to those of younger learners who are matched for intelligence and level of reading achievement (Moats, 1983; Bruck & Waters, 1988).

TEXT-LEVEL READING MODULE

Definitions and Scientific Support

Text-level reading is a complex process that requires the rapid integration of multiple skills and sources of knowledge. The learner must be able to (1) connect segments of information in the text to differentiate peripheral from central points, (2) monitor his or her ability to comprehend the text, (3) recall and integrate new information with previously read information, and (4) engage in metalinguistic reasoning such as drawing inferences. All this must be accomplished while reading fluently by paying little attention to words' pronunciations. Hence, comprehension is determined, in large part, by the learner's lexical knowledge (i.e., understanding of words' meanings) and the speed with which the learner can retrieve the phonological representation of words (i.e., words' pronunciations) (Perfetti, 1985; Perfetti &

Hart, 2001). The two major components of text reading that are routinely evaluated in struggling readers are reading fluency and reading comprehension.

Text-Level Reading Fluency

Nearly three decades ago, Allington (1983) identified fluency as the neglected goal of reading. Today, however, reading fluency is viewed as a complex, multidimensional skill that is enhanced or constrained by semantic knowledge, decoding and word identification ability, processing speed ability, level of text complexity, and the learner's practice with reading text.

Reading fluency refers to the speed and accuracy of the learner's ability to translate text into speech (Fuchs, Fuchs, Hosp, & Jenkins, 2001). Meyer and Felton (1999) defined fluency as "the ability to read connected text rapidly, smoothly, effortlessly, and automatically with little attention to the mechanics of reading, such as decoding" (p. 284). To read fluently, learners must be able to rapidly recognize words learned and to segment and decode words that are unfamiliar (Fuchs et al., 2001). Johns and Berglund (2006) delineated four component skills of fluency: (1) speed (number of words read correctly per minute), (2) accuracy (correct pronunciation of words), (3) expression (accurate phrasing, tone, and pitch when reading aloud), and (4) comprehension (understanding the meaning of text).

Fluency functions as a bridge between word recognition and reading comprehension (National Reading Panel, 2000). The speed with which the learner can retrieve the *phonological and semantic representa-tions* of words (i.e., words' pronunciation) (Perfetti, 1985; Perfetti & Hart, 2001) im-pacts both reading fluency and reading com-prehension. Reading fluency is correlated highly with reading comprehension (Carver, 1997, 2000; Fuchs et al., 2001; Kame'enui & Simmons, 2001; Wolf & Katzir-Cohen, 2001). This high correlation is presumed to be strongly related to the way in which cog-nitive resources are allocated during oral text reading. The less attention needed to access word pronunciations, the greater the avail-able resources for attending to the meaning of the text (Stanovich, 1980, 2000).

Reading fluency is typically measured by assessing the learner's rate and accuracy of words read per minute in grade-level oral reading passages; however, some measure-ments of fluency take into account number and length of pauses in between words and prosodic qualities such as phasing and ex-pression (Fuchs, Fuchs, & Kazdan, 1999; Meyer & Felton, 1999; Rasinski & Hoffman, 2003). Over the last decade, educators and researchers have begun to define the con-struct of fluency as a process that is integral to all components of reading (Adams, 1990; National Reading Panel, 2000). Pikulski and Chard (2005) contrast historical or "sur-face" definitions of fluency as a construct that refers to only the accuracy, speed, and prosody of oral reading with more recent, complex, and "deep" definitions in which fluency is viewed "far more broadly as part of a developmental process of building de-coding skills that will form a bridge to read-ing comprehension and that will have a

reciprocal, causal relationship with reading comprehension" (p. 511).

Recent conceptualizations of fluency have underscored the importance of the *rapid processing of symbols* at both the sub-word (sublexical) and word (lexical) levels to the overall attainment of fluent reading (Breznitz, 2006; LaBerge & Samuels, 1974; Logan, 1988, 1997; Wolf & Katz-Cohen, 2001; Kame'enui & Simmons, 2001; Katzir et al., 2006). Learners' abilities to name printed letters rapidly or to associate sounds with printed letters rapidly are measures of their orthographic fluency at the sublexical level, and their ability to read words rap-idly or to decode nonsense words rapidly are measures of their orthographic fluency at the lexical level. As discussed earlier, in-terconnections between words' pronuncia-tions, spellings, and meanings contribute to automatic word recognition, which in turn contributes to fluent reading. Furthermore, research supports a strong relationship be-tween oral reading fluency and reading com-prehension (Carver, 1997; Carver & David, 2001; Fuchs, Fuchs, Hosp, & Jenkins, 2001; Fuchs, Fuchs, & Maxwell, 1988; Kame'enui & Simmons, 2001; Spear-Swerling, 2006). In a longitudinal study of third- and fourth-grade students, Spear-Swerling (2006) found that oral reading fluency predicted reading comprehension even on "easy texts." Single-word reading speed contributed unique variance to oral reading fluency and oral language comprehension contributed unique variance to reading comprehension.

There is evidence of a reciprocal re-lationship between oral reading fluency and reading comprehension from the elementary through the junior high grades (Fuchs et al., 2001). This relationship appears to decline between second and sixth grade (ranging between 0.83 and 0.86 in grades 2–4 and declining to 0.67 in grade 6) as reading comprehension becomes more closely associated with language comprehension than word recognition (Jenkins & Jewell, 1993).

Reflecting this expanded view of reading fluency, Hudson, Pullen, Lane, and Torgesen (2009) presented a multidimensional model of reading fluency that details the subprocesses of reading fluency along with implications for instructional practices. Using this comprehensive model along with Carver's rauding diagnostic model (2000), Figure 2-7 was designed to illustrate a developmental scheme for organizing the levels of automaticity across the components of reading.

Text-Level Reading Comprehension

Reading comprehension refers to the learner's knowledge of words' meanings in the context of text. Reading comprehension occurs as the culmination of word recognition, vocabulary, listening comprehension, and cognition such as reasoning and memory, along with world knowledge. Relationships between spoken language and reading grow stronger beyond the initial stages of word reading (de Jong & van der Leij, 2002), and knowledge across all spoken language domains (e. g., vocabulary, syntax, discourse) contributes to learners' comprehension of texts (Cain & Oakhill,

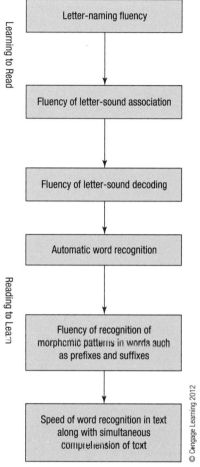

FIGURE 2-7 Developmental scheme for sublexical, lexical, and text fluency

2006; Oakhill & Cain, 2007a; Kintsch & Rawson, 2005; Perfetti, Landi, & Oakhill, 2005). Spoken language proficiency makes a critical contribution to reading ability because listening comprehension, the ability to understand spoken language, sets the ceiling for how well learners will comprehend written text (Biemiller, 2003).

Once learners progress through the stages of learning to read (refer to Figure 2-7), the goal of reading shifts to the acquisition of information though reading comprehension. Wilson and Rupley (1997) state that

> . . . comprehension is a multivariate construct that varies by individual for different kinds of text. For the early elementary years, narrative text (story-oriented text) is almost the only type of text children are presented. By grade 4 however, students are commonly introduced to different kinds of text, most commonly expository text; expository text presents information-dense materials on which students are expected to perform various fairly high-level and complex cognitive processes to extract, summarize, and synthesize information. (p. 48)

Wilson and Rupley (1997) showed a shift in comprehension strategies across grades 2 through 6 using a structural model to depict relationships between background knowledge, phonemic knowledge, and strategy knowledge in children's reading comprehension of academic texts. Narrative tests were used for grades 2 and 3 and both narrative and expository texts were used for grades 4 though 6. They found that in grades 2 and 3, narrative-based text comprehension is driven primarily by phonemic knowledge followed by background knowledge; in grades 3 and 4 background knowledge is the primary factor with strategy knowledge gaining importance; and in grades 5 and 6 strategy knowledge emerges as the dominant factor in determining reading comprehension ability. These findings suggest that as children

develop more experience with reading, it is the strategies that they use in approaching the task, rather than specific knowledge about the content area, that has the largest impact on their reading comprehension.

By the late elementary and middle grades, more advanced discourse-level reasoning skills such as the ability to draw inferences and to understand story structures are associated with text-level comprehension (Oakhill & Cain, 2007b). At the discourse level, learners must develop a network of skills to recall how events are interconnected to yield a coherent and cohesive picture of the content conveyed through listening or through reading text. These skills include using prior knowledge of facts or events to interpret new information, making accurate causal inferences, identifying appropriate referents, understanding how ideas conveyed through speech and print are related to each other through story structures, and forming mental pictures that enable the reader to form visual representations between different segments of text (Kendeou, van den Broek, White, & Lynch, 2007; Kendeou et al., 2006; Oakhill & Cain, 2007b; Cain & Oakhill, 2007a; van den Broek & Kremer, 1999). Lastly, reading comprehension appears to be constrained by working memory in many individuals who have reading difficulties (Berninger, 2008; Swanson, Zheng, & Jerman, 2009). Although the nature of the relationship between reading difficulties and working memory has been debated on various theoretical grounds (Just & Carpenter, 1992; Stanovich, 1990), it appears that students who have linguistic deficits are often limited by the simultaneous demands of processing and storing information. To illustrate this trade-off between processing and storage demands, McCutchen (1996) explains that "in complex tasks such as reading, processing, and storage functions compete for resources as partial linguistic information is stored during the processing of each new segment of text. When demands exceed resources, storage can be affected and information lost from working memory (for example, when a poor reader cannot maintain a sense of sentence context because word identification is extremely effortful)" (p. 302).

TEXT-LEVEL WRITING MODULE

Definitions and Scientific Support

Text-level writing represents a complex integration of linguistic knowledge, working and long-term memory resources, spelling knowledge, and knowledge of writing conventions. Models of the writing process (Berninger et al., 1992; Berninger & Swanson, 1994 [reported in McCutchen, 1996]; Hayes & Flower, 1980, 1987; Hayes, 1996) have provided a framework for categorizing writing skills into three basic types of skills: (1) transcriptional skills that include spelling, punctuation, and handwriting; (2) text generation skills that represent the translation of spoken words into their corresponding orthographic representations (e.g., writing to dictation, written retelling of a story, composing as writing); and (3) advanced compositional skills that require planning, execution, and revising of text.

Linking Reading and Writing

Although they are separate skills, reading and writing share many cognitive processes that connect these two domains of written language. For example, Fitzgerald and Shanahan (2000) identify several links between reading and writing such as the sound-letter correspondence knowledge needed for both skills. Additionally, reading and writing are linked by their relationships to cognitive processes such as working memory. For example, just as working memory has been shown to constrain reading skills (de Jong, 1998; Cain, Oakhill, & Bryant, 2004; Just & Carpenter, 1992; Swanson, 1999; Swanson & O'Connor, 2009), working memory also constrains writing skills (Bereiter & Scardamalia, 1987; Berninger, 1999; McCutchen, 1994 [as reported in McCutchen, 1996]; Swanson et al., 2009).

Although writing occurs much later in development, the developmental sequence of writing is parallel to the sequence for speaking in that children who are learning to write first produce letters, followed in a later stage by words, clauses, sentences, and larger discourse units (Berninger, Fuller, & Whitaker, 1996) Children's development of writing has been studied and described in the context of two approaches: the *product approach*, in which samples of writing collected across different contexts are evaluated on measures of quantity (e.g., length of composition, number of words per sentences), and quality (e.g., organization of the text, use of appropriate semantic and syntactic forms) and the *process approach*, in which learners' knowledge about the act of composing (such as planning, translating ideas into text, and revising text) is studied to determine their understanding and use of these processes. Scardamalia and Bereiter (1986) suggest that this distinction may be an artificial dichotomy because it is through writing (producing a product) that the writer learns how to use cognitive strategies (planning, editing) that shape and refine the written product.

Fitzgerald and Shanahan (2000) described four types of shared knowledge between reading and writing: metaknowledge (pragmatic knowledge); world and domain knowledge (semantic knowledge); universal text attribute knowledge; and procedural knowledge. Furthermore, reading and writing share many of the same neurobiological cognitive underpinnings and constraints described earlier, including reasoning aptitude, language processing, verbal working memory, and processing speed (McCutchen, 1996; Berninger,1999). While several papers have addressed the theoretically and instructionally provocative topic of reading and writing connections (Shanahan & Lomax, 1986), the focus of this module is on the skills and processes that diagnosticians are most likely to evaluate in order to determine strengths and weaknesses that impact their students' writing achievement.

The most commonly cited model of writing processes comes from the work of Hayes and Flower (1980, 1987), who created a schematic for describing factors that influence the written compositions of skilled adults. Their model contained three major elements: the *task environment* (topic, audience-motivating cues, text produced so far); the *writer's long-term memory* (knowledge of the topic, knowledge of the audience, and stored writing plans); and the *writing process*. This original model can be found in numerous papers on the cognitive processes of writing. The three writing process components that drive this model are (1) the *planning* component, which represents the writer's generation of ideas, setting of goals, and organization of text; (2) the *translation* component, which represents the encoding of ideas from an oral to a printed form; and (3) the *reviewing* component, which represents the writer's ability to monitor, reconsider, and revise what she has written. Although this model has been substantially modified (Hayes, 1996), the original components of the model have been retained (Hayes, 1996) and have been used in research studies of the writing development of typically developing students and students who have learning disabilities (Berninger et al., 1992; Graham, Berninger, Abbott, Abbott, & Whitaker, 1997).

Based on their study of children's writings, Berninger et al. (1992) and Berninger, Fuller, and Whitaker (1996) noted that the Hayes and Flower model did not capture developmental aspects of writing that are central to the evaluation of young children's developing writing skills. They proposed several detailed modifications of the Hayes and Flower model for beginning and developing writing, including (1) clarifying the distinction between idea generation (ideas) and text generation (expressing ideas through language); (2) dividing the translational process into two components, a low-level *transcription* component that reflects the translation of language into its written counterpart and a high-level *text generation* component that reflects the translation of ideas into language representations; and (3) underscoring the key roles of language and working memory skills in accounting for individual differences in the development of writing. An adapted version of their revised model for school-age children is shown in Figure 2-8.

Berninger (1999) emphasizes the importance and limitations of working memory in coordinating transcription and text generation skills. Working memory has only a limited capacity for orchestrating these skills simultaneously. Hence, the greater the working memory space needed for transcribing, the less working memory space available for text generation. In fact, transcription processes such as retrieval of letters for spelling and handwriting fluency have been shown to constrain text generation (Berninger et al., 1992; Graham, Harris, & Fink, 2000), and all aspects of planning,

organizing, and revising can be constrained by a learner's language learning disabilities (Singer & Bashir, 2004).

In discussing the development of these processes, Berninger, Fuller, and Whitaker (1996) note that "Planning, translating, and revising are not fully operative in beginning writing, but emerge systematically during the course of writing development" and that "In beginning and developing writers, each of these processes is still developing and each process is on its own trajectory, developing at its own rate" (p. 198). Berninger and Swanson (1994, as cited in Berninger, Fuller, & Whitaker, 1996) proposed a developmental scheme that shows the relative order of the emergence of these skills.

In the primary grades:

- Translation is the first process to emerge
- Transcription emerges before text generation
- Text generation follows a parallel sequence to expressive language acquisition. First words alone are written, then words are combined into sentences, and then sentences are combined into narrative text.

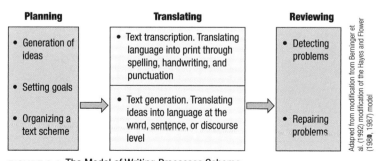

FIGURE 2-8 The Model of Writing Processes Scheme

Ideas evolve while writing (on-line planning) before preplanning a text scheme.

- On-line revising emerges after on-line planning

In the intermediate grades:

- Advanced preplanning of text emerges
- Transcription is an automatic skill
- Text generation expands in form (length of text) and genre to include more advanced types of discourse such as expository writing
- Revising can be accomplished after reviewing written text

Learners with reading deficits can manifest problems in any one or more of the components of the writing process (i.e., planning, translating, reviewing) or in any one or more of the subprocesses within these components (i.e., generating ideas, transcribing, revising). By analyzing the learner's writing skills from this multidimensional perspective, the practitioner will be able to determine the nature and severity of the learner's writing difficulties for (1) making a differential diagnosis, (2) considering how a deficit in one writing process such as transcription can constrain development in higher level writing processes, and (3) developing optimal strategies for intervention. Some learners who have reading disabilities have great difficulty with transcriptional skills alone, some have difficulty with both text transcription and text generation, and others have more difficulty with planning and reviewing than with generating text. Graham and Harris (1997) point out some reasons that may contribute to these difficulties. Students may (1) lack knowledge of the topic that they are required to discuss in writing, (2) lack motivation to write on a topic that they find uninteresting, or (3) fail to generate the ideas that represent their knowledge because their cognitive resources are being used to focus on the mechanical aspects of writing (spelling, punctuation, and handwriting). Issues of this nature underscore the importance of assessing each of the processes that contribute to fluent writing to determine the potential impact of a deficit in one process of writing on skill development in other processes of writing.

READING ACHIEVEMENT

Definitions and Scientific Support

Both reading and writing are developmental skills that evolve in a systematic way and require the complex coordination of basic neurocognitive processes such as language progressing, long-term and working memory, rapid processing of information (e.g., translating letters into sounds or sound into letters); sensory and motor processes (e.g., visual and fine-motor movements); knowledge of the forms and functions of linguistic processes (e.g., phonologic, semantic, syntactic); awareness of linguistic conventions associated with each type of activity; and the social context in which the activity occurs. Reading and writing evolve shortly before or during the primary grades and continue to develop throughout high school, provided that students are given adequate instructional content and intensity of instruction and that they possess the motivation to use print as a vehicle for acquiring information, accomplishing goals, generating ideas, and establishing and maintaining social connections.

Components of Reading Achievement

Grade-level performance in each of the modules above should result in adequate reading achievement. The learner's level of reading achievement is determined by the grade level at which that learner is reading fluently and comprehending accurately. Reading achievement is strongly influenced by three basic factors: (1) the nature of the learner's academic instruction, (2) the cognitive processing abilities of the learner, and (3) the degree to which the learner engages in reading as a source of pleasure and as a means for learning new information. Reading achievement is typically determined by the student's performance on standardized tests. Writing achievement is typically determined by performance on a range of tasks that may include essay composition for quality and fluency, sentence-level construction, editing, spelling, punctuation, and handwriting. Figures 2-9 and 2-10 provide graphic representations of the basic processes that contribute to reading and writing achievement, respectively.

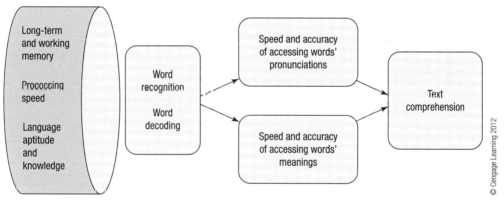

FIGURE 2-9 Basic Factors and Skills that Contribute to Grade-Level Reading Achievement

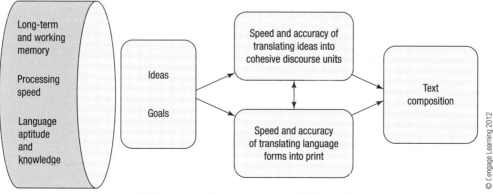

FIGURE 2-10 Basic Factors and Skills that Contribute to Grade-Level Writing Achievement

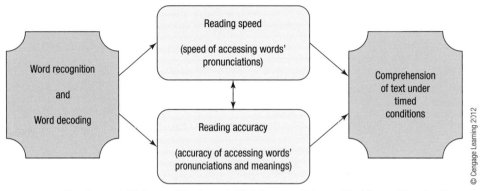

FIGURE 2-11 Developmental Scheme of Fundamental Relationships Between Word Recognition, Reading Fluency, and Reading Comprehension

Using Carver's Rauding Model (2000) of reading achievement along with the Fuchs et al.'s (2001) synthesis of theories and empirical data on issues that apply to reading fluency, Figure 2-11 shows a simple developmental scheme of the hierarchical relationships between word recognition, reading fluency, and reading comprehension that contribute to overall reading achievement.

SUMMARY OF CONSTRUCTS NEEDED FOR READING

Learning to read is a gradual process that begins when learners first come to understand that spoken words and syllables can be broken down into individual sounds or phonemes and that these sounds correspond to the letters or graphemes in printed words. Once learners identify words in print through decoding and rapid sight-word recognition, their reading vocabularies expand rapidly, paving the way for improved reading comprehension. In large part, this vocabulary expansion and enhanced reading com-

prehension results from greater knowledge of the morphological structure of words, which allows learners to "discover" new word meanings.

Adequate listening comprehension skills are critical for the achievement of basic levels of reading comprehension, especially at the sentence level. For more advanced levels of reading comprehension, learners must be able to integrate events into cohesive "mental maps" for all types of texts (e.g., narrative and expository). To become truly skilled readers, they must also achieve reading fluency—the accurate, effortless, and automatic processing at all levels of print—letters, words, and text (Kame'enui, Simmons, Good, & Harn, 2001). Kirby, Desrochers, Roth, and Lai (2008) provide an excellent synthesis of the skills that influence and, in some cases, predict future reading achievement.

Learning to write is also a gradual process and begins when learners are able to translate ideas into text. Learning to write is a complex skill that requires the coordination of not only cognitive and linguistic processes but also the graphomotor skills needed for writing. Children's grasp of the structure of narratives during the preschool years prepares them to apply their knowledge of spoken language, such as the structure used to tell a story, to their early composition of text. As they progress from the elementary to the intermediate grades, students in the early grades develop the ability to reflect or preplan the ideas they wish to convey and adopt an organizational scheme for generating their ideas. They also become capable of moving beyond writing simple narrative formats, such as narrative compositions, to producing expository compositions they are capable of preplanning, transcribing fluently, reflecting on, and revising.

CHAPTER THREE

Application of the Multidimensional Assessment of Reading and Writing Disorders to the Diagnostic Process

THIS CHAPTER AIMS TO:

- Provide practitioners with a selection of standardized tests and other procedures for gathering test data on the skills represented in the Multidimensional Model for Assessing Reading and Writing (MAR^{w}R) modules described in Chapter 2.

- Assist practitioners in (1) identifying the learner's core areas of weakness that impact his or her ability to advance as expected in the acquisition of skilled reading, (2) addressing important issues surrounding the selection of formal and informal reading and writing test procedures, and (3) informing their selection of intervention goals.

GENERAL PRINCIPLES FOR ASSESSING READING AND RELATED PROCESSES

This chapter addresses standardized tests and informal evaluation procedures that can be used to assess the neurocognitive, environmental, and achievement skill factors that are often associated with reading impairments and that are addressed in the Multidimensional Model for Assessing Reading and Writing Disorders (MAR^wR). MAR^wR was designed to serve as a blueprint for conducting a differential assessment of the learner's strengths and weaknesses in reading and other cognitive skills. Table 3-1 shows skills targeted in this model. A MAR^wR checklist, found at the end of this chapter in Appendix 3-1, can be used as a template for developing individualized assessment batteries or as a summary sheet for highlighting learners' strengths and weaknesses.

The tests discussed in this chapter can be used to achieve any number of goals that a practitioner might have for conducting a reading evaluation, including: (1) determining if deficient reading is causally related to a learner's overall poor academic performance; (2) determining the precise areas of weakness in a learner who is struggling to read at grade level based on benchmark or high-stakes test results; (3) determining the precise areas of weakness in a learner who is struggling with reading in spite of showing adequate performance on benchmark or high-stakes tests; (4) determining if a learner who is only struggling with spelling or other mechanics of handwriting has a weakness in one or more components of reading (e.g., decoding); (5) determining if a learner with a history of oral language impairment is also showing deficits in written language; (6) determining if a learner's attentional or behavioral problems in the classroom are related to language learning difficulties; (7) determining if a learner who is struggling with reading or writing qualifies for speech-language therapy services or special education services in public schools; and (8) diagnosing a learner with an ICD-9-CM code (i.e, the *International Classification of Diseases, Ninth Revision, Clinical Modification* [U.S. Department of Health and Human Services, Centers for Disease Control and Prevention, and the Centers for Medicare and Medicaid Services (2009–2010)], discussed in Chapter 4).

Oftentimes, the practitioner's goal in performing a reading assessment is strongly influenced by his or her professional role. For example, in public school systems throughout the United States, learners who are struggling with reading may be tested by different school personnel, such as the school psychologist or reading resource specialist, to determine if the learner qualifies for special education services. However, in many private practices and in clinical settings associated with rehabilitation services, hospitals, or university training clinics, clinical psychologists and speech-language pathologists conduct diagnostic testing to determine the reason for a learner's reading

TABLE 3-1 Skills Targeted in MAR^WR

Language Knowledge	
Vocabulary	Understanding of words and word meanings in both spoken and written language
Word retrieval	Accessing pronunciations of words or sound patterns stored in memory
Morphological awareness	Understanding that morphemic units exist in words and contribute to the meanings of words
Syntactic knowledge	Understanding how to use grammatical rules and to adhere to word order, morphological markers, and other syntactic constraints of one's language
Discourse skills	Understanding causal connections and inferences in spoken and written language
Print Knowledge	
Print awareness	Knowledge of book conventions, concept of word in print, and print mechanics
Letter knowledge	Knowledge of letter names and ability to write letters that represent letter names
Word awareness	Knowledge that words can be segmented into separate units that represent individual spoken words
Phonological Knowledge	
Phonological awareness	Awareness that the stream of speech can be broken down into smaller units
Grapho-phonemic Integration	
Phonics knowledge	Ability to map phonemes (sounds) onto graphemes (letters) and to use graphemes to represent phonemes
Invented spelling	Knowledge that sounds are represented by letters in some consistent way and use of this knowledge to create spellings prior to conventional instruction
Word-Level Reading and Spelling	
Decoding	Ability to segment letters in words into corresponding sounds, then blending sounds to create real words or nonsense words
Word recognition	Ability to recognize familiar words in print (sight-word recognition) such that sight of spelling patterns results in immediate word recognition
Spelling	Ability to use accurate spelling patterns for sound units (e.g., -ight sounds like /ai/) and knowledge of rules that determine word pronunciations (e.g., silent e dictates the pronunciation of *site*)
Text-Level Reading	
Reading comprehension	Ability to understand the meaning of information conveyed in text discourse
Reading fluency	Ability to read words and text accurately and effortlessly
Text-Level Writing	
Mechanics and conventions	Use of legible handwriting and accurate punctuation
Composition	Ability to plan, translate, and review written text

difficulties, followed by specific recommendations for reading intervention.

The product of an assessment may be a comprehensive diagnostic report, a two- to four-page description of test findings, conclusions, and recommendations, or a very brief report of test results with conclusions and recommendations. This will depend on the goal of the assessment and the setting in which it is conducted.

THE EVALUATION PROCESS

Evaluation procedures for each of the areas within the MAR^{w}R are provided for learners who are at the emergent literacy stages of development (learners ranging 4–7 years of age) (see Table 3-2) and for older learners who have been given instruction in reading but are failing to keep pace with their peers (learners in the second semester of first grade and beyond first grade) (see Table 3-3).

TABLE 3-2 Constructs, Domains within Constructs, and Tests for Assessing Emergent Readers from Preschool through Early First Grade (Ages 4–7 Years)

	Tests for Emergent Readers (Ages 4-7 years)
Skill Domains	Measurement Procedures
Neurocognitive Module	
Reasoning	WJ III COG: concept formation, analysis-synthesis *
	WISC-IV: matrix reasoning, block design, picture concepts, picture completion
Verbal Processing	WJ III COG: verbal comprehension*
	WISC-IV: comprehension, similarities, vocabulary
Working Memory	WJ III COG: numbers reversed, auditory working memory*
	WJ III COG: visual-auditory learning (long-term storage and retrieval test of associative memory for words and symbols)*
	WISC-IV: digit span backward, letter-number sequencing
	WMTB-C: phonological loop composite (digit recall, word list matching, word list recall, nonword recall)
Processing Speed	WJ III COG: visual matching, decision speed*
	WISC-IV: symbol search, coding, cancellation
Spoken Language Module	
Vocabulary	ALL: receptive vocabulary; basic concepts*
	ERDA-2: receptive vocabulary, expressive vocabulary
	TOLD-P:3: picture vocabulary; relational vocabulary; oral vocabulary*
	CELF Preschool-2: language content*
	DELV: semantics*
	WIAT-3:expressive vocabulary, oral word fluency*
	WIAT-3: receptive vocabulary*

Morphological Structures and other Sentence Structures	ALL: parallel sentence structures* CELF Preschool-2: language structure* SPELT-P2* TOLD-P:4: morphological completion, syntactic understanding*
Oral Discourse • **Listening Comprehension** • **Story Re-telling** • **Narrative Productions**	ALL: listening comprehension* ELLA: story re-telling* PAL-RW: story retell TNL: test of narrative language
Word Finding **Rapid Serial Naming**	TWF-2: picture naming nouns, sentence completion naming, picture naming verbs, picture naming categories ALL: rapid naming (criterion-referenced)
Phonological Knowledge	
Phonological Awareness	ALL: rhyme knowledge, sound categorization, elision* ERDA-2: syllables ELLA: rhyming, initial sound identification, blending, segmenting, deletion, and substitution* TOPEL: phonological awareness* DAR-2: rhyming, segmenting words, identifying initial consonant sounds, identifying final consonant sounds PAL-RW: rhyming, syllables, phonemes, rimes CTOPP: phonological awareness composite
Print Knowledge	
Print Awareness and Conventions	ALL: matching symbols, book handling, concept of word (criterion-referenced)* ELLA: environmental symbols* TOPEL: print knowledge* TERA-3: print conventions* DAR-2: matching letters
Grapho-phonemic Integration	
Alphabet Knowledge	ALL: letter knowledge (identification and writing)* PAL-RW: alphabet writing, receptive coding, expressive coding ELLA: letter-symbol identification* TOPEL: print knowledge* TERA-3: alphabet* DAR-2: naming lowercase letters
Phonics Knowledge	ALL: phonics knowledge* ELLA: letter-sound identification* TOPEL: print knowledge * TERA-3: alphabet* ALL: invented spelling*

(*Continues*)

TABLE 3-2 Continued

Word-Level Reading	
Word Decoding	ALL: decoding nonsense words (under phonics knowledge)*
	PALS-RW: pseudoword decoding
	ELLA: blending sounds, segmenting sounds*
	ERDA-2: pseudoword decoding
	WJ III ACH: word attack
	WAIT-III: pseudoword decoding
Word Reading	ALL: sight word recognition*
	EDRA-2: word reading
	WJ III ACH: letter-word identification
	WIAT-III: word reading
Meaning-Print Associations	TERA-3: meanings of printed words*
	DAR-2: word meaning
Word-Level Spelling	
Spelling	PALS-RW: word choice (spelling recognition)
	WJ III ACH: spelling
	WIAT-III: spelling
	DAR-2: writing words, spelling
Text-Level reading	
Sentence Comprehension Completion Format	WJ III ACH: passage comprehension
Comprehension of Passage	DAR-2: silent reading comprehension
	ERDA-2: reading comprehension
	GORT-4: reading comprehension
	WIAT-III: reading comprehension
Reading Fluency	GORT-4: passage fluency
	ERDA-2: passage fluency

*appropriate for children at 4 years of age
Test Measures:
ALL: Assessment of Literacy and Language (Lombardino, Lieberman, & Brown, 2005).
CELF Preschool-2: Clinical Evaluation of Language Fundamentals for Preschool (Semel, Wiig, & Secord, 2004).
CTOPP: Comprehensive Test of Phonological Processing (Wagner, Torgesen, & Rashotte, 1999).
DAR-Second Edition, Diagnostic Assessment of Reading (Roswell, Chall, Curtis, & Kearns, 2005).
DELV: Diagnostic Evaluation of Language Variation (Seymour, Roeper, de Villiers, & de Villiers, 2005).
ELLA: Emerging Literacy & Language Assessment (Wiig & Secord, 2006).
ERDA-2, Early Reading Diagnostic Assessment (The Psychological Corporation, 2009).
KBIT-2: Kaufman Brief Intelligence Test (Kaufman & Kaufman, 2004).
PALS-RW: The Process Assessment of the Learner-Test Battery for Reading and Writing (Berninger, 2001).
SPELT-P2: Structured Photographic Expressive Language Test-Preschool (Dawson, Stout, Eyer, Tattersall, Fonkalsrud, & Croley, 2005).
TERA-3: Test of Early Reading Ability (Reid, Hresko, & Hammill, 2001).
TOLD-P:3: Test of Language Development-Primary (Newcomer & Hammill, 1988).
TOPEL: Test of Preschool Early Literacy (Lonigan, Wagner, Torgesen, & Rashotte, 2007).
TWF-2: Test of Word Finding (German, 2000).
WIAT-III: Wechsler Individual Achievement Test (Pearson, 2009).
WISC-IV: Wechsler Individual Scale for Children (Wechsler, 2004).
WJ-COG-III: Woodcock Johnson Test of Cognitive Abilities (Woodcock, McGrew, & Mather, 2001).
WMTB-C: Working Memory Test Battery for Children (Gathercole & Pickering, 2001).

TABLE 3-3 Constructs, Domains within Constructs, and Tests for Assessing Language and Literacy in School-Age Children from Late First Grade and Beyond

Assessment Procedures for School-Age Children from Late First Grade and Beyond

Skill Domains	Measurement Procedures
Neurocognitive Module	
Reasoning	WJ III COG: concept formation, analysis-synthesis
	WISC-IV: matrix reasoning, block design
Verbal Aptitude	WJ III COG: verbal comprehension
	WISC-IV: comprehension, similarities, vocabulary
Verbal Working Memory	WJ III COG: numbers reversed, auditory working memory, visual-auditory learning (long-term storage and retrieval test of associative memory for words and symbols)
	WISC-IV: digit span backward, letter-number sequencing
	CTOPP: nonword repetition, digit span
	CELF-4: number repetition forward
Processing Speed	WJ III COG: visual matching, decision speed, pair cancellation
	WISC-IV: symbol search, coding, cancellation
Language Knowledge Module	
Word Meanings	CELF-4: expressive vocabulary, word definitions, word classes receptive, word classes expressive
	CASL: antonyms, synonyms
	ITPA-3: spoken vocabulary, spoken analogies
	WJ III ACH: picture vocabulary
	WJ III DRB: oral vocabulary
	WIAT-III: oral expression
Morphological Structures and Sentence Structures	CELF 4: word structure
	CASL: grammatical morphemes
	ITPA-3: morphological closure
	SPELT-3: morphology and syntax
	CELF-4: formulated sentences
	CASL: grammaticality judgment, syntax construction
Listening Comprehension (may also measure verbal working memory)	CELF-4: understanding spoken paragraphs
	CASL: sentence comprehension, paragraph comprehension
	WJ III ACH: oral comprehension
	WJ III ACH: story recall
	WJ III DRB: oral comprehension
	WIAT-III: listening comprehension

(Continues)

TABLE 3-3 Continued

Word Finding	TWF-2: picture-naming nouns, sentence-completion naming, picture-naming verbs, picture-naming categories
	TAWF: picture-naming nouns, sentence-completion naming, picture-naming verbs, picture-naming categories
	CTOPP: rapid naming of letters and digits
Serial Naming Speed	CELF-4: rapid automatic naming
	RAN/RAS: rapid automatized naming and alternate naming
Grapho-phonemic Integration Module	
Phonemic Awareness	CTOPP: elision
	ITPA-3: sound deletion
	CELF-4: phonological awareness
Word-Level Reading Module	
Word Decoding	WJ III ACH: word attack
	WIAT-III: pseudoword decoding
	WRMT-R: word attack
	WJ III DRB: word attack
Word Recognition	WJ III ACH: letter-word identification
	WIAT-III: word reading
	WRMT-R: word identification
	WJ DRB III: letter-word identification
	WRAT-4: word reading
Word-Knowledge	WJ III ACH: reading vocabulary
	WJ III DRB: reading vocabulary
	ITPA-3: written vocabulary
Word-Level Spelling Module	
Spelling	WJ III ACH: spelling
	WRMT-R spelling
	WJ III DRB: spelling
	WIAT-III: spelling
	WRAT-4: spelling
	ITPA-3: sound spelling, sight spelling
	SPELL-2: software evaluation of spelling error patterns

Text-Level Reading Module	
Text-Level Reading Comprehension	WJ III ACH: passage comprehension
	WJ III DRB: passage comprehension
	WRMT-R: passage comprehension
	WIAT-III: reading comprehension
	GORT-4: reading comprehension
Text-Level Reading Speed	WJ III ACH: reading fluency
	WJ III DRB: reading fluency
	GORT-4: fluency
	WIAT-III: oral reading fluency
	Oral reading fluency norms (Hasbrouck & Tindal, 2006)
Text-Level Writing Module	
Writing	WIAT-III: essay composition, sentence combining, sentence building
	WJ III ACH: writing fluency, writing samples, editing, punctuation, capitalization
	TEWL-2: writing mechanics, story construction (age 4–11 years)
	TOAL-4: sentence combining, orthographic usage (age 12–24 years)

WJ III COG: Woodcock Johnson III Tests of Cognitive Ability (Woodcock, McGrew, & Mather, 2001b).
WIAT-III: Wechsler Individual Achievement Test–III (Wechsler, 2009).
WJ III ACH: Woodcock Johnson III Tests of Achievement (Woodcock, McGrew, & Mather, 2001a).
WJ III DRB: Woodcock Johnson III Diagnostic Reading Battery (Woodcock, Mather, & Schrank, 2004).
CELF-4: Clinical Evaluation of Language Fundamentals–Fourth Edition (Semel, Wiig, & Secord, 2003).
CASL: Comprehensive Assessment of Spoken Language (Carrow-Woolfolk, 1999).
WRAT-4: Wide Range Achievement Test–Fourth Edition (Wilkinson & Robertson, 2006).
CTOPP: Comprehensive Test of Phonological Processing (Wagner, Torgesen, & Rashotte, 1999a).
WRMT-R: Woodcock Reading Mastery Tests–Revised (Woodcock & Pines, 1998).
GORT-4: Gray Oral Reading Test–Fourth Edition (Wiederholt & Bryant, 2001).
TOWRE: Test of Word Reading Efficiency (Wagner, Torgesen, & Rashotte, 1999b).
ITPA-3: Illinois Test of Psycholinguistic Abilities (Dawson, Stout, & Eyer, 2003).
SPELT-3: Structured Photographic Expressive Language Test–3 (Dawson, Stout, & Eyer, 2003).
TWF-2: Test of Word Finding–Second Edition (German, 2000).
TAWF: Test of Adolescent/Adult Word Finding (German, 1990).
SPELL-2: Spelling Performance Evaluation For Language And Literacy (Masterson, Apel, & Wasowicz, 2006).
TEWL-2: Test of Early Written Language (Hresko, Herron, & Peak, 1996).
TOAL-4: Test of Adolescent and Adult Language Fourth Edition (Hammill, Brown, Larsen, & Wiederholt, 2007).
WISC-IV: Wechsler Intelligence Scale for Children–IV (Wechsler,, 2003).
RAN/RAS: Rapid Automatized Naming and Rapid Alternating Stimulus Tests (Wolf & Denkla, 2005).

No one test or battery of tests has been shown to be superior in identifying all types reading disabilities. A test battery should be individualized as needed and selected based on its psychometric properties, standardization sample, and its probability of identifying the learner's areas of strength and weakness. Interviewing primary caregivers and teachers along with reviewing previous test findings should lead to a judicious selection of tests. Caregiver/teacher questionnaires can provide extremely valuable information to guide the practitioner in choosing a test battery that is most appropriate for the learner and will help the practitioner develop hypotheses about the cause(s) and nature of the learner's difficulties. The caregiver/teacher questionnaire in Appendix 3-2 of this chapter is designed for learners from approximately 4 to 7 years of age and the questionnaire in Appendix 3-3 is designed for learners in the second semester of first grade and beyond. These questionnaires should be used as interview protocols when caregivers are known or suspected to have limited literacy skills in English.

Learners who are observed to show consistent signs of inattention, impulsivity, or hyperactivity should be referred to a professional who can evaluate attention deficit disorder (ADD). Reading disabilities (RDs) and attention deficit disorder frequently co-occur; both are highly heritable (Gilger, Pennington, & Defries, 1992; Semrud-Clikeman et al., 1992). Willcutt and Pennington (2000) report that twin pairs with comorbid RD and ADHD are at higher risk for disruptive behavior problems such as oppositional defiant behavior and conduct disorder than non-RD twins, and that RD is more likely to co-occur with inattention symptoms of ADHD than with hyperactivity/impulsivity symptoms.

Screening may be warranted for learners who are not showing any signs of difficulty in learning spoken language or in accomplishing age-appropriate academic tasks *but* who may be at risk for later learning difficulties due to risk factors associated with sociocultural experiences, developmental difficulties, or family history. In such cases, it should be sufficient to use a truncated battery of tests to determine if further testing is needed. The tests chosen in each of these general areas will depend on the age and/or grade level of the learner.

The tests listed in Tables 3-2 and 3-3 are *not exhaustive lists*; they represent many of the most commonly used tests that compose diagnostic batteries for testing reading, and they correspond to processes and skills integral to the reading processes identified in the MAR^{w}R. Reading screening tests such as the commonly used *Dynamic Indicators of Basic Early Literacy Skills* (DIBELS) and the *Florida Assessments for Instruction in Reading* (FAIR) are not listed, but should be used extensively to identify learners who may be at risk for reading difficulties. Other diagnostic tests are available that can be used to accomplish these same objectives.

The assessment procedures listed in this chapter are primarily standardized tests; however, some criterion-referenced tests are included along with informal approaches for testing areas in which few formal tests are available, such as oral and written discourse. For diagnostic purposes, it is best to compare the learner's skills across subtests that share the same standardization data; however, this is not always possible given the wide range of skills that fall within a comprehensive model and the variability in types of tests and population samples used for collecting normative data.

In Tables 3-2 and 3-3 an attempt was made to compartmentalize tests that represent similar constructs (e.g., listening comprehension, reading comprehension); however, it is essential that practitioners be aware of the fact that tests that appear to be assessing the same construct may be testing different processes as a result of the nature of the stimuli used or the format of the test construction. For example, a learner who has a verbal working memory deficit may do poorly on listening comprehension tests that require holding several temporal details of a story in memory and then answering open-ended questions, but may perform within normal limits on a test that requires filling in a missing word or phrase in a cloze listening comprehension procedure. When comparing performances on different types of reading comprehension tasks, Keenan, Betjemann, & Olson (2008) found that (1) learners' performance on difference tests of reading comprehension are not necessarily highly correlated; (2) learners' *decoding* skills have a greater influence than oral comprehension skills on learners' reading comprehension when it is tested in cloze (i.e., fill-in words) procedures, whereas *oral comprehension* skills have a greater influence on reading comprehension when tested using multiple-choice and or retell procedures; and (3) tests designed to measure reading comprehension can measure different skills when used to test learners at different reading levels.

Many tests used to assess language and literacy skills are tapping into processes that are unidentified by test developers, such as attention, memory, and processing speed. These factors may be causally related to a learner's deficient reading; therefore, it is essential that practitioners analyze the learner's test performance very carefully, much like one would put together the pieces of a puzzle, in an attempt to determine the underpinnings of the learner's reading deficit.

In the following section, tests that can be used to evaluate skills in each of the MAR^{w}R modules are shown for two developmental groups of learners, preschoolers through first graders who range between 4 and 7 years of age and learners in late first grade and beyond who are already struggling with reading.

Formal Assessment Procedures for Preschoolers through Grade 1

Only a few of the tests shown in this section were developed to assess literacy skills in learners under 5 years of age. The tests listed in Table 3-2 yield either a standard score or a criterion-referenced score. Some of the tests are designed to evaluate learners younger than 4 years of age or older than 7 years of age. These tests are marked with an asterisk. For example, both the *Woodcock Johnson III Tests of Achievement* (WJ III ACH; Woodcock, McGrew, & Mather, 2001a) and the *Wechsler Individual Achievement Test-III* (WIAT-III; Wechsler, 2009) are standardized on populations that range from preschool through adulthood. Similarly, the *Woodcock Johnson III Tests of Cognition* (WJ III COG; Woodcock, McGrew, & Mather, 2001b) and the *Wechsler Intelligence Scale for Children* (WISC-IV; Wechsler, 2003) are used widely to assess cognitive abilities in learners from ages 6 to 16 and from preschool to adulthood, respectively. It is not always necessary to evaluate the emergent literacy learner in each one of these areas to determine whether the learner is lacking in specific skills that could impact later reading success. However, the more constructs that are assessed, the more data the practitioner has available to determine the learner's cognitive and linguistic strengths and weaknesses and to develop a profile of the learner's skills across the core component areas of reading.

In Tables 3-2 and 3-3, subtests from test batteries and individual assessment instruments are shown that represent the constructs listed. In many cases, an *index* or *composite* score can be obtained in a specific domain on batteries for tests of cognition (e.g., WJ III COG, Woodcock, McGrew, & Mather, 2001b; WISC-IV, Wechsler, 2003), tests of achievement (WJ III ACH, Woodcock, McGrew, & Mather, 2001a; WIAT-III, Wecshler, 2009), and tests of spoken language (e.g., CELF 4, Semel, Wiig, & Secord, 2003). While learners' test profiles from subtest scores alone have not been shown to accurately differentiate among diagnostic groups (Watkins, 2005), performance on subtests (e.g., processing speed) along with performance on all core

components of reading and writing language discourse contribute many of the pieces of the puzzle needed to create an accurate and comprehensive profile of the learner's strengths and weaknesses and to make a differential diagnosis.

Formal Assessment Procedures for Late Grade 1 and Beyond

Table 3-3 provides a sample of standardized test measures that can be used to identify reading deficits and to diagnose reading disabilities in struggling learners from first grade on. As in Table 3-2, this table is organized to represent the processes or skills highlighted in each of the MAR^wR modules. Again, because age ranges for tests vary, practitioners must examine the normative data for each test and each subtest within a battery of tests to determine its appropriateness for the individual learner.

When conducting a comprehensive evaluation on learners who have been taught to read but are reading below grade level, the practitioner should consider evaluating the learner's abilities in each of the MAR^wR modules, with the exception of those listed under the phonological knowledge and print knowledge modules. Although there may be rare instances when skills in these two areas are not developed and should be assessed, the phonological and orthographic skills that should be evaluated by the end of first grade are found within the grapho-phonemic integration module.

As noted above, although it is not necessary to test the learner in each of these areas to identify a reading deficit, it is critical that the practioner possess a clear understanding of a learner's strengths and weaknesses. For example, a learner who has average or above expressive and receptive language skills and relatively good reading comprehension, in spite of depressed word reading, spelling, and reading fluency, will require different intervention goals than a learner who has adequate expressive and receptive language and good word reading, in spite of difficulties with reading comprehension (refer to classifications in Chapter 4). Oftentimes, parents and teachers can identify marked discrepancies in a learner's ability and this information can serve to focus the practioner on targeting a specific dimension of reading for assessment.

GOALS OF CRITERION-REFERENCED ASSESSMENT AND DIAGNOSTIC PROCEDURES

Criterion-referenced assessment procedures are most useful when diagnosing reading disabilities in domains of language and literacy for which there are few formal assessment procedures, or when the content or task formats on standardized tests fail to provide an adequate profile of the learner's strengths because of a (1) limited number of items for testing a particular construct, (2) limited contexts for testing a construct is tested, (3) limitations of the scoring system (e.g., some writing assessments are scored without taking spelling and punctuation errors into account), (4) need to adapt the tasks to the learner's attentional, sensory, or motor limitations, or (5) lack of standardized tests to assess a specific domain. For example, skills in oral discourse and written composition are strongly associated with reading skills, particularly in the advanced grades, yet very few standardized test procedures are available in these areas.

Informal reading inventories (IRIs) are used frequently by educators to evaluate learners' word-reading fluency and reading comprehension. IRIs are criterion-referenced assessments that are individually administered and are designed to evaluate the learner's skills on a range of reading components so that grade-level achievement can be determined. For example, the *Qualitative Reading Inventory,* 5th edition (QRI-5; Leslie & Caldwell, 2001), is a commonly used IRI that is designed to evaluate literacy skills from preprimer through high school levels using graded word lists and text passages. The QRI-5 and similar informal reading inventories can be used to identify the learner's reading level using narrative and expository passages, to determine the learner's strengths and weakness for component reading skills (e.g., word-level reading, decoding, comprehension), and to determine growth in reading skills over time. IRIs are particularly useful in determining the learner's grade-level skills across component reading skills.

Informal Tests for Diagnosing Specific Reading Problems (Pavlak, 1985) and *Alternative Assessment Techniques for Reading and Writing* (Miller, 1995) are two informative books on informal assessment procedures (with reproducible materials).

Informal Assessment Measures for Spoken and Written Discourse

There are very few standardized methods for assessing learners' production and comprehension of narrative discourse. In her recent book on *Language and Literacy Disorders*, Nelson (2010) notes that "narrative comprehension and production draw on discourse-level skills and can be assessed in tandem by asking a learner to listen to a story and then retell it" (p. 392). Further information on the learner's spoken and written language can be obtained by collecting a sample of the learner's ability to retell a story both orally and in writing. For example, on the listening comprehension subtest from the Assessment of Literacy and Language (ALL) battery, young learners are asked to retell a story read to them before they are asked to answer questions about the story. This procedure could be extended to include (a) features for analyzing components of spoken language story retell and (b) features for analyzing components of written language story. As an example of this informal procedure, a listening comprehension story from the ALL, called *Oscar's Morning*, is shown in Box 3-1 and a list of the key 13 ideas in the story is shown in Box 3-2. Box 3-3 shows an example of a typical first grader's retell of the *Oscar's Morning* story and Box 3-4 shows an example of another first grader who was suspected of having a language disorder. In both cases, the learners were told the story by a speech-language pathologist one time and then asked to retell the story.

BOX 3-1   **The *Oscar's Morning* Story from the ALL Listening Comprehension Subtest**

Oscar is having a terrible morning. First, he wakes up late because he watched a long movie the night before. Then, he finds the dog has chewed a hole in his left shoe. Finally, he reaches school and remembers that his class is going on a field trip today. "Oh boy," says Oscar, "today isn't so terrible after all." Then his teacher asks, "Oscar, did you remember your permission slip?" Oscar's smile changes to a frown.

Although there is no standardized procedure for scoring the two learners' story retell performance on this task using metrics such as the number of ideas, the number of syntactic errors, and the diversity of vocabulary used in the retell can provide a framework for approximating the overall adequacy and age appropriateness of the learners' spoken and written discourse.

Spoken and Written Discourse Language Samples from Learners with a Reading Disability

Additional examples of using an informal story retell procedure to sample the spoken and written language of two boys diagnosed with dyslexia are shown below. The stories used were taken from the *Analytical Reading Inventory* (Woods & Moe, 1989). The story of a mouse, told to the 7-year-old boy, is shown in Box 3-5. The boy's oral retell of the story is shown in Box 3-6, and his written retell is shown in Figure 3-1. A more advanced story

BOX 3-2   **Checklist of the Ideas in the *Oscar's Morning* Story**

1. ___ Child calls Oscar by name one or more times when retelling the story.

2. ___ Child calls the teacher by name one or more times when retelling the story.

3. ___ Child retells that Oscar had a terrible morning.

4. ___ Child retells that Oscar woke up up late.

5. ___ Child retells that Oscar watched a long movie the night before.

6. ___ Child retells that Oscar finds his dog chewed a hole in his shoe.

7. ___ Child retells that the hole is in Oscar's left shoe.

8. ___ Child retells that Oscar arrives at school.

9. ___ Child retells that Oscar remembers that his class is going on a field trip.

10. ___ Child retells that, at first, Oscar feels good about the trip.

11. ___ Child retells that Oscar's teacher asks if he remembered his permission slip.

12. ___ Child retells that Oscar's smile changes to a frown.

13. ___ Child retells the story in an overall correct sequence.

Total Points for Ideas — 13

BOX 3-3   **Example of a Typically Developing First Grader's Story Retell of *Oscar's Morning***

Oscar's Morning

Oscar had a bad morning. His dog bit a hole in his left shoe. Finally, he reached school and he remembers that his class is going on a field trip and he says, "Oh, this isn't a bad day after all." Oscar's teacher asked if he remembered his permission slip. Oscar's smile turned to a frown.

BOX 3-4   **Example of a Story Retell of *Oscar's Morning* by a First Grader who Was Suspected of Having a Language Impairment**

The dog bited the shoe and he forgot the slip.

BOX 3-5   **Original Passage from the *Analytic Reading Inventory***

Swish! My pet mouse ran straight under our neighbor's chair! Out neighbor didn't hear him, because he is quiet, as a mouse should be. If she had seen him, she would have yelled her head off.

Zoom! Now my clever gray mouse is bouncing off the jam jar on the breakfast table. He is sliding on the milk left around my glass! He is dancing on my cupcake.

He loves drinking lemonade. He eats lots of honey and blueberries. He is silly, different, and really quite funny. I'll always love my dear little mouse.

Say, have you seen my sweet gray friend? You better look now because he's right under your chair!

Woods and Moe, 1998

BOX 3-6   **Spoken Language Retell For 7-Year-Old Boy with Dyslexia**

A boy has a mouse, that's like, really funny. And likes to hide under chairs, and likes lemonade. And he likes to dance on top of cupcakes.

BOX 3-7   **Original Passage taken from the *Analytic Reading Inventory***

About 300 years ago, the English started 13 colonies in North America. These colonies later became our first states.

The people in those colonies had difficult lives. For transportation they often walked. Sometimes they used boats if they lived near water. Since there were no cars, it was hard for the early colonists to travel very far.

The colonial houses were much different from our houses. The houses had one large room with a fireplace. This room was used as a kitchen, a dining room, and a living room. Also it was often used as a bedroom because of the fireplace. There were no electric lights. Water had to be carried into the house.

Life for the colonists was very difficult, yet colonists thought they had a good life.

Woods and Moe, 1998

about historical times, shown in Box 3-7, was told to the 15-year-old boy. His oral retell is shown in Box 3-8 and his written retell is shown in Figure 3-2. In both cases, the learners were instructed by a speech-language pathologist to:

Listen to this story (narrative or expository)

Listen to the story one more time

Retell the story to me

Listen to the same story one more time

Retell the story to me in writing

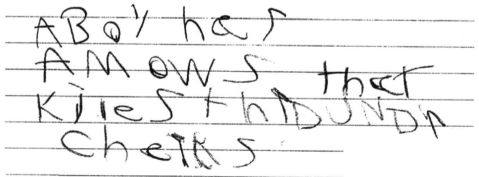

© Cengage Learning 2012

FIGURE 3-1 Written language story retell for the same 7-year-old boy with dyslexia

BOX 3-8 **Spoken language Story Retell for 15-Year-Old Boy with Dyslexia**

(um) About 300 years ago, the English founded colonies which later became our thirteen states or 13 original states or colonies or something like that. (um) Transportation was hard for most of the colonists. They had to walk or used boats if they lived by the ocean. (um) Houses were different then. (Um) They had one large (um) room by the fireplace which was used for dining or for sleeping because of the fireplace.

Because the therapist was interested in evaluating spoken and written language production while placing minimal constraints on memory, the learners were given three opportunities to listen to the story.

An informal inspection of the oral and written samples of the 7-year-old suggests that this learner could convey more information about the story orally than he could in writing. His writing was slow and labored, and appeared to be constrained in his ability to transmit at least as much information about the story as conveyed in his spoken retell.

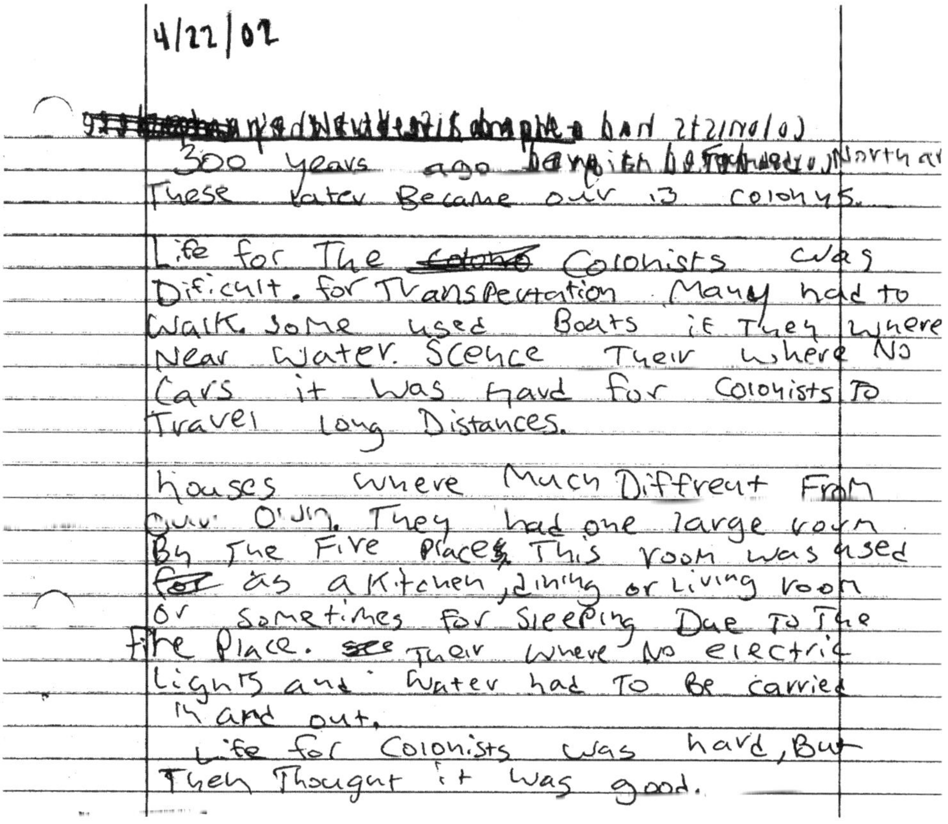

FIGURE 3-2 Written language story retell for the same 15-year-old boy with dyslexia

© Cengage Learning 2012

Inspection of the 15-year-old learner's oral and written retelling of this expository text indicates that he recalled more information about the story in writing after hearing it three times. However, his writing was slow and labored. His translational skills of spelling, punctuation, and handwriting were poor. It was very apparent during testing that his ability to transmit his recall of the story was much more difficult for him in writing than in speaking. The contrast of this learner's well-developed recall in both his spoken and written samples with his poor writing abilities pinpoints his weaknesses in the mechanics of writing, spelling, punctuation, and handwriting. Procedures of this nature are particularly useful when the performance of a learner who is struggling is compared to the performance of peers who are not showing difficulties with written language.

Inspection of a 13-year-old's written expository text (Figure 3-3) shows many spelling errors, lack of punctuation, poor syntax,

missing morphological inflections, poor organization, and many fewer details than provided in the original story (Box 3-9).

Evaluating Text Genres in Speaking

Narrative analyses include an evaluation of both the microstructure and the macrostructure elements of a story. Microstructure components include the number of words and clauses in a story (Strong, 1998); macrostructures include story grammar elements and complexity of story episodes (Hedberg & Westby, 1993). Nelson (2010) provides informative discussions of informal procedures that can be used to evaluate learners' narrative abilities and presents an observational tool for assessing narratives from different developmental schemes. Strong (1998) developed a story-retell procedure that involves listening to an audiotaped story and answering inferential and factual questions. Also, Hedberg and Westby (1993) created a developmental framework for analyzing components of story structures.

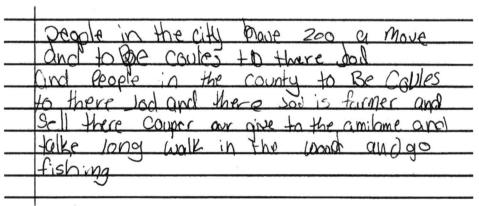

© Cengage Learning 2012

FIGURE 3-3 Written language story retell from a 13-year-old boy with a language learning disability and an early diagnosis of specific language impairment

| BOX 3-9 | Original Passage from the Qualitative Reading Inventory–3 |

People live in different places. Some people live in a city while others live in the country. Still other people live in the areas between the city and the country, which are called suburbs.

People live in the city to be near their jobs. Cities have lots of factories, schools, and offices. If people don't want to drive a long way to their jobs, they live in the city. There are many things to do in the city such as visit museums and zoos. They also have many movie theaters.

People live in the country to be close to their jobs, too. Many people who live in the country are farmers. They plant crops on their land. They may sell their crops or may use them to feed the animals that live on the farm. Farmers raise cows, pigs, and chickens. Although life in the country is quiet, there are other things to do. You can find a river to fish in or take walks in the woods.

Many people live in the suburbs. Some people think that people who live in the suburbs have the best of both worlds. It doesn't take as long to get to either the city or the country. The suburbs are more crowded than the country but less crowded than the city. Where people live depends upon what they like most.

Leslie and Caldwell, 2006

Most recently, Petersen, Gillam, and Gillam (2008) developed a narrative complexity scoring system for quantifying each of the components of a story separately (e.g., characters, setting) using a scale from 0 to 3.

Learners with histories of language impairment are at risk for deficits in higher-level discourse skills (Boudreau, 2008), and procedures of this nature are more informative than standardized tests for establishing evidence-based treatment goals.

Evaluating Text Genres in Writing

Westby (2005) and Scott (2005) have presented detailed and comprehensive systems for assessing writing in narrative, expository, and persuasive genres. For diagnostic purposes, a process model of writing is most useful in differentiating the writing abilities of learners who have different types of reading disability profiles. Learners who have dyslexia typically show greater strengths in the planning process of writing (i.e., generating ideas, setting goals, organizing content) as compared to the translational processes of writing (i.e., transferring thoughts into print, spelling), whereas other learners who have writing difficulties may show greater strengths in the translational than in the planning processes.

Different types of writing genres require different types of evaluations. For example, when evaluating a learner's narrative writings, elements such as (1) characters, (2) setting, (3) plots, (4) problems, and (5) resolutions or conclusions are central to this genre of writing. In contrast, in expository writings (1) text organization, (2) content, (3) style of writing (vocabulary, syntax, and cohesion), (4) writing conventions, and (5) awareness of audience needs and perspectives are central features in this type of genre (Westby & Clauser, 2006).

There are numerous frameworks for evaluating the elements of learners' text composition and these systems vary greatly. Some are holistic in nature and others are designed to assign scores to specific traits (Westby, 2005). Westby (2005) describes developmental rubrics that can be used to score the traits or elements of the learner's writing; procedures of this nature should be helpful in determining the nature of the learner's major hurdles in the writing process across different genres (narrative, expository, and persuasive texts). The "6 = 1 Trait® Writing Model of Instruction & Assessment, developed by the Northwest Regional Educational Laboratory (NWREL; http://educationnorthwest.org/traits), is used quite widely in school districts across the country. This system evaluates six writing traits (conventions, ideas, organization, word choice, sentence fluency, and voice) using a six-point rating scale. Although it is research-based and provides a systematic way to rate multiple dimensions of writing, Spence (2010) cautions that this and other analytic rubrics often fail to adequately address the sociocultural aspects of writing in English language learners. A discussion of assessing reading in English language learners is beyond the scope of this book; however, the reader can refer to a report by Slavin and Cheung (2005) on a best-evidence synthesis of reading programs for English language learners.

Using the modifications by Berninger et al. (1992) to the original Hayes and Flower model of writing (1980, 1987) as a foundation, a simple informal system, such as the one shown in Table 3-4, can be used to conduct a qualitative assessment of written language skill strengths and weaknesses at different points in the learner's written discourse development.

FACTORS TO CONSIDER WHEN DIAGNOSING READING AND WRITING DISORDERS

Because of the variability in reading and writing skills among learners with broad or specific (e.g., dyslexia) language learning disabilities, the following factors should be considered before making a diagnosis:

1. Investigate sociocultural issues that could impact the learner's experience with reading skills or motivation to acquire such skills.

2. Investigate familial history for spoken language, reading, spelling, or writing difficulties.

3. Look for incongruences between the learner's sociocultural experiences, desire to read, overall reasoning and language abilities, and the learner's ability to read, spell, and compose written text.

4. Look for incongruences between the learner's ability to process language through different modalities (i.e., listening, speaking, reading, writing).

5. Examine cognitive processes (e.g., processing speed, verbal working memory) that have been shown to be depressed in some individuals with learning disabilities.

TABLE 3-4 Sample Format for Indicating Strengths and Weaknesses in Three Stages of the Writing Process

Type of Genre	Narrative	Expository	Persuasive
Planning (Middle School, High School)			
Idea Generation			
Goal Setting			
Organization			
Translating (Early Elementary, Middle School, Junior High School)			
Text Generation			
Spelling			
Handwriting			
Reviewing (Junior High, High School)			
Editing			
Reviewing			

6. Look for incongruences between the learner's reasoning abilities and verbal knowledge.

7. Look for incongruences between the learner's reasoning and language abilities and the learner's processing speed or working memory.

8. Examine the components of spoken language (e.g., vocabulary, syntax, listening comprehension) and written language (e.g., spelling, punctuation, handwriting, composition) that have been shown in the scientific literature to be associated with reading difficulties and reading disabilities.

9. Look for differences in a learner's performance on timed tasks as compared to untimed tasks

10. Look for answers when parents' and or teachers' concerns are not validated

by the learner's test performance; this happens frequently when:

- Learners have improved their reading and writing skills significantly through intervention but have test scores that fall within the average range.

- Learners are bright and develop strategies that camouflage their deficits (e.g., memorizing spelling words for tests).

- Learners are not tested in neurocognitive areas.

- Inadequate attention is given to the learner's written language skills for transcription, generation of ideas, and compositional abilities.

Appendix 3-1   MAR^WR Checklist

Skills within MAR^WR Modules	S	W	Comments
Neurocognitive Processes Related to Reading			
Reasoning			
Verbal working memory			
Processing speed			
Spoken Language Knowledge			
Vocabulary skills			
Morphological awareness skills			
Syntactic skills			
Discourse			
Word retrieval skills			
Phonological Knowledge			
Word awareness			
Syllable awareness			
Onset-rime awareness			
Sound categorization			
Grapho-phonemic Integration Knowledge			
Alphabetic principle			
Word-Level Reading			
Full alphabetic reading (decoding) skills			
Word recognition skills			
Word-Level Spelling			
Within word patterns spelling skills			
Syllables and affixes skills			
Derivational relations skills			
Text-Level Reading			
Reading comprehension skills			
Reading fluency skills			
Text-Level Writing			
Text planning skills			
Text translating skills			
Text reviewing skills			

Notes: S= strength; W=weakness
Quantitative or qualitative assessment data can be used to complete this profile summary form.

Parent/Guardian/Teacher Questionnaire for Emergent Readers (Ages 4–7)

Background Information			
Learner's name			
Learner's age and grade			
Learner's date of birth			
Reason for concern			
Please add any other details you think are important for us to know.			

Previous Services	Yes	No	Don't know
Has this learner been labeled or diagnosed with any type of learning difficulty?			
Has this learner received services for any learning problems in the past?			
Is this learner receiving services for any learning problems now?			
Has this learner had any specific health problems that might interfere with his/her development of speech, language, or early literacy skills?			
Has this learner had any emotional struggles that might interfere with his/her development of speech, language, or early literacy skills?			
Please add any other details you think are important for us to know.			

APPENDIX 3-2, CONT.

Parent/Guardian/Teacher Questionnaire for Emergent Readers (Ages 4–7)

Family History	Yes	No	Don't know
Did this learner's mother or guardian graduate from high school?			
Did this learner's mother or guardian attend college?			
Did this learner's mother or guardian graduate from college?			
Does this learner have any brothers or sisters who have learning difficulties in speaking, reading, or writing?			
Does this learner have a *biological* mother or a father who has had similar learning difficulties in speaking, reading, or writing?			
Does this learner's *biological* mother or father have relatives who have similar learning difficulties in speaking, reading, or writing?			
Is the learner's first language English?			
Is more than one language spoken in the home?			
Please list all the languages spoken in the home other than English.			
Do you feel that this learner is having difficulty learning to speak English?			
Please add any other details you think are important for us to know.			

Exposure to Books in the Home Environment	Yes	No	Don't know
Is there a dictionary in the learner's home?			
Are there more than 5 books in the learner's home?			
Are newspapers read by anyone in the learner's home?			
Are there magazines in the learner's home?			
Does the learner have books of his or her own?			
If yes, about how many books does the learner have of his or her own?			
Does this learner ask you to read to him or her?			
If yes, about how often?			
Does anyone in this learner's home read to him or her on a weekly basis?			
If yes, about how often?			
Please add any other details you think are important for us to know.			

APPENDIX 3-2, CONT.

Parent/Guardian/Teacher Questionnaire for Emergent Readers (Ages 4–7)

Hearing, Speaking, Listening, & Attending	Yes	No	Don't know
Has this learner ever had his/her hearing tested?			
If yes, when was this testing done?			
If yes, did this learner pass this test?			
Has this learner had any delays in his/her use of speech sounds?			
Has this learner had any difficulties with using speech to put words together into sentences?			
Does this learner have any difficulty understanding or following directions?			
Does this learner have any difficulty telling stories or remembering stories?			
Does this learner have difficulty attending to activities the way other learners do?			
Does this learner have any difficulty with his/her level of activity?			
Please add any other details you think are important for us to know.			

Knowledge of Sounds in Speech	Yes	No	Don't know
Can this learner tell you how many words are in the sentence "I like animals"?			
Can this learner tell you the beginning letter or sound of his name?			
Can this learner tell you if the word *baseball* has one or two parts?			
Can this learner tell you if two words such as *pie* and *eye* sound alike or rime?			
Can this learner tell you how many sounds are in simple words like *up* and *see*?			
Please add any other details you think are important for us to know.			

APPENDIX 3-2, CONT.

Parent/Guardian/Teacher Questionnaire for Emergent Readers (Ages 4–7)

Knowledge of Print	Yes	No	Don't know
Can this learner name at least 5 letters of the alphabet?			
Can this learner name all or nearly all of the letters in the alphabet?			
Does this learner know the sounds of any letters in the alphabet?			
Does this learner know the sounds of more than 10 letters?			
Can this learner write down the first letter in his/her name?			
Can this learner write down more than one letter in his/her name?			
Can this learner find his/her name when it is printed on paper along with other names?			
Can this learner recognize any common words like *the* or *milk?*			
Can this learner use phonics skills to sound out a pretend word like "bik"?			
Can this learner attempt to spell some words by using at least some of the correct letters?			
Please add any other details you think are important for us to know.			

Performance of Learner Compared to Other Learners	Yes	No	Don't know
Do you feel that this learner's speech sounds are as clear as other learners his/her age?			
Do you feel that this learner's ability to use words in sentences is as good as other learners his/her age?			
Do you feel that this learner can tell you a story as well as other learners his/her age?			
Do you feel that this learner's knowledge of letters and words in print is as good as other learners his/her age?			
Do you feel that this learner's interest in books is similar to other learners his/her age?			
Please add any other details you think are important for us to know.			

Appendix 3-3

Questionnaire for Grade 1 and Above

Caregiver/Teacher Questionaire for School-Age Learners (second semester of 1st Grade and beyond)

Background Information
Learner's name
Learner's age and grade
Learner's date of birth
Parent's, guardian's, or teacher's name
Parent's, guardian's, or teacher's phone number
Reason for concern
Please add any other details you think are important for us to know.

Developmental History	Yes	No	Don't know
Were there concerns about this learner's academic progress in the past?			
Has this learner been diagnosed with a speech disorder?			
Has this learner been diagnosed with a spoken language disorder?			
Has this learner been diagnosed with a reading disorder?			
Has this learner been diagnosed with a hearing loss?			
Has this learner been diagnosed with a central auditory processing disorder?			
Has this learner been diagnosed with an attention deficit disorder?			
Has this learner experienced any problems associated with a serious head injury?			
Has this learner been diagnosed with any other type of learning problem that is not mentioned above?			
Has this learner participated in any special classes or tutoring for school work or in supplemental reading instruction?			
Has this learner had his/her hearing tested within the past year?			
If yes, did he or she pass this test?			

APPENDIX 3-3, CONT.

Does this learner complain that things far away are blurry, despite proper glasses (if needed)?			
Does this learner complain of blurry vision when reading, despite proper glasses (if needed)?			
Does this learner complain of headaches when reading?			
Does this learner complain that the words seem to move around on the page when reading?			
Does this learner complain that it is hard to stay on a line when reading?			
Please add any other details that you think are important for us to know.			

Family History	Yes	No	Don't know
Did this learner's mother or guardian graduate from high school?			
Did this learner's mother or guardian attend college?			
Did this learner's mother or guardian graduate from college?			
Does this learner have any brothers or sisters who have learning difficulties in areas such as speaking, reading, and spelling?			
Does this learner have a *biological* mother or a father who has similar learning difficulties in areas such as speaking, reading, and spelling?			
Does this learner's mother or father have *biological* relatives who have similar learning difficulties?			
Is this learner's home environment structured so that his/her guardians oversee the learner's homework and help him/her with homework on a regular basis?			
Is the learner's first language English?			
Is more than one language spoken in the home?			
Please list all the languages spoken in the home other than English.			
Do you feel that this learner is having difficulty learning English?			
Please add any other details you think are important for us to know.			

APPENDIX 3-3, CONT.

Current Academic Issues	Yes	No	Don't know
Is this learner receiving special service for learning difficulties at school, such as special classes, tutoring, or extra time for tests?			
Does this learner show an interest in reading?			
Does this learner have a spoken language vocabulary that is similar to the vocabulary of his peers?			
Does this learner have difficulty expressing his or her thoughts?			
Does this learner have any difficulty with understanding/following directions?			
Does this learner have difficulty telling stories in a clear and well-ordered way?			
Does this learner have difficulty remembering information that he/she has heard in the classroom?			
Does this learner know that he/she is having difficulty with reading?			
Does this learner ever ask for help with reading or writing?			
Does this learner have difficulty sounding out words that he/she does not recognize?			
Does this learner have difficulty recognizing words that he/she should know?			
Does this learner have difficulty comprehending what he/she reads?			
Does this learner have difficulty understanding information that is read to him/her?			
Does this learner often fail to give close attention to details or make careless mistakes in schoolwork or other activities?			
Does this learner have difficulty organizing tasks and activities?			
Does this learner often fail to listen to what is being said to him or her?			
Does this learner struggle with getting his or her thoughts down on paper?			
Do you feel that this learner knows much more information than he or she conveys or produces when asked to complete a writing assignment?			
Is this learner's writing reasonably legible?			
Does this learner have difficulty forming letters while writing and writing within the expected space on a page?			
Does this learner often fail to follow through on instructions and fail to finish schoolwork, chores, or duties in the workplace (not due to oppositional behavior or failure to understand instructions)?			
Is this learner often easily distracted by extraneous stimuli?			

APPENDIX 3-3, CONT.

Is this learner often forgetful when attempting to complete daily activities?			
Does this learner often fidget with hands or feet or squirm in his/her seat?			

Please add any other details you think are important for us to know.

Please check below to indicate which areas you feel represent a strength or weakness for this learner	Yes- strength	No- weakness	Don't Know
Has clear speech			
Uses correct grammar when speaking			
Understands well when listening to directions			
Understands well when listening to a story			
Can tell a story in an organized way			
Has an interest in reading for schoolwork or for pleasure			
Can quickly recognize familiar words when reading			
Can sound out new words when reading			
Can read out loud well			
Can understand what he or she reads			
Can remember how to spell words			
Can express thoughts through writing			
Has good handwriting			
Can remember rote facts such as math multiplication tables			
Can understand concepts in math or in science classes			
Is motivated to succeed in school			
Has good reasoning abilities (such as in figuring out problems)			
Shows creative abilities (such as in drawing or other activities that require a good imagination)			

Please add any other details you think are important for us to know.

Identifying and Classifying Children at Risk for Reading Deficits

CHAPTER FOUR

THIS CHAPTER AIMS TO:

- Provide practitioners with a framework for classifying profiles in young children with normal-range intellectual abilities who are showing difficulties in one or more domains of language during the preschool through first-grade years, placing them at risk for later reading difficulties.
- Provide practitioners with sample assessment protocols and diagnostic reports for three profiles of learners who are at risk for future reading disabilities: mixed spoken language and emergent literacy deficit, emergent literacy deficit, and environmental disadvantage deficit.
- Provide practitioners with guidelines for implementing differentiated intervention or instruction for the different profile types.

USING THE MAR^wR MODEL TO EVALUATE AND DIAGNOSE EMERGENT READERS

Many researchers have addressed the numerous early risk factors associated with later reading impairment and the varied populations of young children most likely to present risk profiles (Bishop, 2008; Snow, Burns, & Griffin, 1998; Vernon-Feagans, Hammer, Miccio, & Manlove, 2001; Scarborough, 2002; Gayán & Olson, 2003; Sénéchal, Ouellette, & Rodney, 2006).

As noted in Chapters 1 and 2, the causes for weaknesses in language and literacy can be genetic, environmental, or a combination of both environmental and genetic factors. Spoken language disorders, especially when associated with speech articulation difficulties (Bishop, 2008) are highly heritable, as are specific reading disabilities (Olson, 2006). Often, distinctions between environmentally based deficits and biologically based deficits can only be determined with certainty after response patterns to intervention are evaluated in controlled environments for sustained periods of time. For example, children whose reading deficits are caused by environmental factors will respond more quickly and easily to concentrated instruction, but children with biologically based deficits are likely to need more repetitive and multisensory intervention. However, even carefully structured intervention over long periods may not always provide the practitioner with a clear perspective on all factors that are causally related to the learner's language and

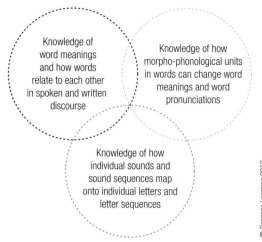

FIGURE 4-1 **Integration of Skills Needed to Develop Skilled Reading**

reading difficulties. Regardless of the root cause(s) underlying emergent literacy challenges, all reading difficulties are associated with weakness in at least one of the three areas shown in Figure 4-1. Integrated and continuously reciprocal interactions among these three areas are needed to develop skilled reading.

As discussed in Chapters 1 and 2, the MAR^wR model consists of select domains of cognitive processing (e.g., working memory) and several specific language-based domains (e.g., spoken language skills, phonological knowledge, word reading) that are fundamental to developing a comprehensive literacy assessment battery and to creating profiles of learners' strengths and weaknesses with precision. Assessment and profiling indices for young learners that are consistent with the MAR^wR are shown in Box 4-1.

| BOX 4-1 | Assessment and Profiling Indices for Preschool Through First-Grade Learners |

- Listening comprehension
- Ability to retell and to generate stories
- Knowledge of word meanings
- Use of sentence structures (e.g., subject-verb agreement)
- Use of morphological structures (e.g., inflectional morphemes such as -ed, -s, -ing)
- Phonological processing skills (i.e., awareness, memory, retrieval)
- Print concepts
- Alphabet knowledge and knowledge of grapheme-phoneme associations for reading and spelling
- Decoding abilities
- Word recognition abilities

LANGUAGE AND EMERGENT LITERACY DEFICIT PROFILES

Different emergent literacy and spoken language profiles can be indicative of potential problems that are likely to emerge in the learner's future reading achievement. General areas of strengths and weaknesses are discussed for the three profiles described in this chapter, *mixed spoken language and emergent literacy deficit, emergent literacy deficit,* and *environmental disadvantage deficit.* Although the profiles do not necessarily represent every learner who possesses adequate aptitude for reading but struggles nonetheless, they should represent the vast majority of learners who are struggling with spoken language or emergent literacy skills between 5 and 7 years of age.

Any learner who is struggling with the spoken language, phonological awareness, or grapho-phonemic constructs that are typically acquired by her chronological age is at risk for a future disability in reading or writing. Regardless of the learner's profile, the primary goal of the practitioner should be to determine if weaknesses exist in one or more of these areas. If weaknesses are identified, early intervention can be instituted as a preventive measure to eliminate, or at least to minimize, the impact of these weaknesses on the learner's future academic achievement.

Profile of Preschool and First-Grade Learners at Risk for Reading Deficits

Diagnostic features and classifications for children between preschool and first grade who are at risk for reading deficits are shown in Tables 4-1 and 4-2, respectively. Sample reports for each diagnostic profile can be found at the end of this chapter along with an interpretation of the assessment findings and general intervention guidelines. When reporting standardized test data for the profiles, two types of scaled scores are used. Typically, composite standardized test scores are based on a mean score of 100 with a standard deviation of ±15 and subtest scores are based on a mean score of 10 with a standard deviation of ±3.

TABLE 4-1 Diagnostic Features Associated with Learners At Risk for Reading Difficulties

	Profile 1 Mixed Spoken Language & Emergent Literacy Deficit	Profile 2 Emergent Literacy Deficit	Profile 3* Environmental Disadvantage Deficit
Spoken Language Knowledge	−	+	−/+
Phonological Knowledge	−/+	−	−/+
Grapheme-Phoneme Knowledge	−/+	−	−/+

(+) = areas of strength, (−) = areas of weakness
*Profile typically associated with learners who have not had adequate sociocultural opportunities.

© Cengage Learning 2012

TABLE 4-2 Classifying Children From 4–7 Years of Age Who Are At Risk for Reading Deficits

Profiles for Children from Preschool–First Grade	
Profile 1a: Mild-Moderate Mixed Language and Emergent Literacy Deficit **Profile 1b:** Severe Mixed Language and Emergent Literacy Deficit	• Mild-to-severe depressed language production or comprehension • Difficulty in one or more phonological processes • Low-normal to above-average nonverbal intelligence • Absence of primary visual, auditory, or motor disabilities
Profile 2: Emergent Literacy Deficit	• Normal language with or without a history of articulation difficulties • Difficulty with emergent literacy skills especially letter knowledge and sound-letter associations • Low-normal to above-average nonverbal intelligence • Absence of primary visual, auditory, or motor disabilities
Profile 3: Environmental Disadvantage Deficit	• Overall depressed preacademic skills with or without previous identification of a language delay or disorder • History of diminished opportunities for exposure to language and to literacy concepts at home or in school • Low-normal to above-average nonverbal intelligence • Absence of primary visual, auditory, or motor disabilities

© Cengage Learning 2012

One type of reading profile not classified in this book as a reading deficit is hyperlexia. Hyperlexia is a behavioral characteristic referred to by Grigorenko, Klin, and Volkmar (2003) as an unexpected and unusual "superability" of some children with developmental disorders to read a large number of words in spite of their depressed intellectual and/or verbal abilities. Children with hyperlexia often present with behavioral characteristics that place them on the continuum of pervasive developmental disorders (PDDs). Hyperlexia represents an extreme pattern of strengths and weaknesses in core reading skills. Learners with hyperlexia are proficient at decoding words but are unable to comprehend the meaning of words at a level that is in any way comparable to their decoding skills. The appearance of hyperlexia in classification models of reading deficits is used to emphasize the degree to which two core reading skills, decoding and comprehension, can be dissociated and represent extreme strengths and weaknesses in the individual learner.

PROFILE 1: MIXED SPOKEN LANGUAGE AND EMERGENT LITERACY DEFICIT

Children who have deficits consistent with this profile are often identified by the age of 4 years with developmental language delays or with specific language impairment (SLI), in spite of having adequate exposure to spoken language and print. SLI is a term used to refer to children who have expressive or receptive language deficits in the absence of primary sensory, motor, or emotional deficits and in spite of exhibiting nonverbal intelligence that is within normal limits (Leonard, 1998). Numerous researchers have identified reading deficits in children who have been diagnosed with SLI and nearly all have reached the same conclusion: these children are at much higher risk for reading difficulties than their typically developing peers (Bishop & Adams, 1990; Bishop, 2001; Catts, Fey, Zhang, & Tomblin, 2001; Stothard, Snowling, Bishop, Chipchase, & Kaplan, 1998; Snowling, Bishop, & Stothard, 2000). Furthermore, children with SLI are at risk for both word-reading and reading comprehension deficits regardless of whether they are diagnosed with expressive SLI or combined receptive and expressive SLI (Simkin & Conti-Ramsden, 2006). Even children initially diagnosed with SLI whose language impairments appear to have been resolved are more likely to demonstrate difficulties with literacy in later years (Scarborough & Dobrich, 1994; Stothard et al., 1998; Snowling et al., 2000; Simkin & Conti-Ramsden, 2006). It appears that the risk and severity of reading disability is related to the severity of the language impairment (Bishop, 2001; Leonard, Lombardino, Giess, & King, 2005). Bishop (2001) reported that SLI children with impairment in one domain of language (e.g., expressive language) were at far less risk than children with impairments in two domains (e.g., expressive and receptive language). Similarly, Simkin and Conti-Ramsden (2006) reported that children with combined receptive and expressive SLI were at greatest risk for reading deficits, followed by children with expressive-only SLI and then children with resolved SLI.

In reference to Bishop and Snowling's (2004) two-dimensional model for classifying developmental language disorders into *phonological deficits* versus *broader language deficits*, Snowling and Hulme (2008) stated that "phonological deficits carry the risk of decoding difficulty, while broader oral language deficits are risk factors for reading comprehension problems" (p. 176). Children with SLI *always* show deficits in nonphonological dimensions of spoken language such as vocabulary or listening comprehension, and *often* show deficits on phonological processing tasks such as sound blending, segmenting, and deleting (Catts, Fey, Zhang & Tomblin, 2001). Sometimes children with SLI exhibit relative strengths in early graphophonemic skills such as phonics; however, even when their phonological awareness and phonics skills are developing at age-appropriate rates, their difficulties with the nonphonological domains of language place them at risk for later deficits in reading comprehension. Profiles 1a and 1b show examples of mixed spoken language and emergent literacy deficits at two levels of severity. Shaded areas in the MAR^wR graphic shown in Figure 4-2 highlight the primary areas of deficit that characterize this profile.

In MAR^wR models shown to represent profile types, *light* shading represents possible deficit areas and *dark* shading represents areas that are not applicable to children within the 5–7 year age range.

PROFILE 2: EMERGENT LITERACY DEFICIT

Children who have deficits consistent with this profile typically are identified later than children with Profile 1a or 1b because often their language appears to be developing normally until they are faced with the challenge of segmenting words into smaller units. These learners may be quite verbal with average or advanced skills in vocabulary. A history of minor mild articulation

problems is not uncommon in these children, but such problems are usually resolved before their literacy difficulties are identified. Typically, their difficulties become apparent during the early stages of literacy acquisition when they are learning names of letters or associations between letter names and their corresponding sounds (Lombardino, Lieberman, & Brown, 2005).

Children with this profile, especially those with a family history of reading difficulties, are often identified as having a learning disability, a "specific reading disability," or dyslexia in the elementary or early middle school grades. Once they are taught to read, their weaknesses are most apparent while reading aloud because of their difficulties with recalling pronunciations of multisyllabic words, and confusing frequently occurring words such as "the" and "this" when spelling because of their difficulties in recalling words' spellings. Although many of these children may have been somewhat late in talking and may have received articulation therapy during the preschool years, few of them have had a previous diagnosis of a specific language impairment. Shaded areas in the MAR^wR graphic in Figure 4-3 highlight the primary areas of deficit that characterize this profile.

PROFILE 3: ENVIRONMENTAL DISADVANTAGE LITERACY DEFICIT

This category is reserved for children who have had inadequate preschool experiences to support the acquisition of a diverse vocabulary, adequate world knowledge, and sufficient exposure to print. Some of them will also have biologically based learning difficulties. It can be difficult to disentangle

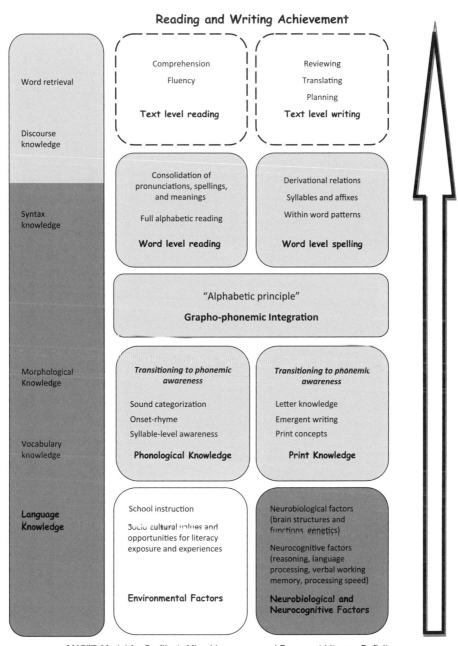

FIGURE 4-2 MAR^WR Model for Profile 1: Mixed Language and Emergent Literacy Deficit
Dark shaded areas in modules: primary deficit skill areas or primary causal factors
Light shaded areas in modules: may or may not be deficit
Dashed line box modules: not assessed in this age range

*Deficits in each of the shaded modules are not necessary for a child's profile to be characterized as representing Profile 1, however, deficits within the domain of spoken language should be apparent.

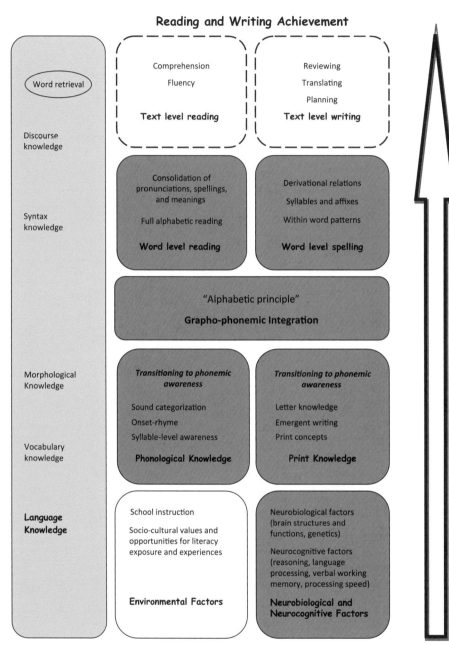

FIGURE 4-3 MAR^WR Model for Profile 2: Emergent Literacy Deficit
Dark shaded areas in modules: primary deficit skill areas or primary causal factors
Light shaded areas in modules: may or may not be deficit
Circled area: key deficit area within a module
Dashed line box modules: not assessed in this age range

*Deficits in each of the shaded modules are not necessary for a child's profile to be characterized as representing Profile 2, however, no primary deficits in spoken language should be apparent.

the causes of their deficits when both environmental disadvantages and biological weaknesses are causal factors underlying their reading difficulties. Only systematic, intensive, and well-designed instruction will help determine if they are experiencing reading deficits with causal roots beyond their environmental disadvantages. Regardless of the degree to which environment and biology may interact in creating roadblocks in literacy learning, these children should show marked improvement in reading achievement with appropriate instruction that targets both the phonological (e.g., phonics) and nonphonological dimensions of language (e.g., vocabulary, comprehension). Shaded areas in the MAR^wR graphic in Figure 4-4 highlight the primary areas of deficit that characterize this profile.

The following sections present sample reports for each of these three profiles. Two samples are given for Profile 1 to show examples of varying levels of severity within a profile type.

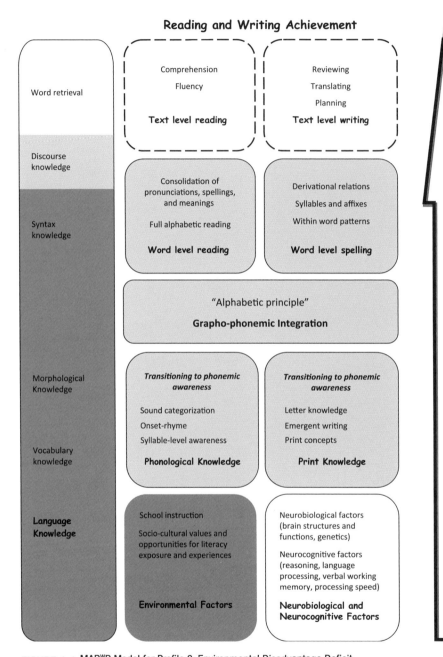

FIGURE 4-4 MAR^{W}R Model for Profile 3: Environmental Disadvantage Deficit
Dark shaded areas in modules: primary deficit skill areas or primary causal factors
Light shaded areas in modules: may or may not be deficit
Dashed line box modules: not assessed in this age range

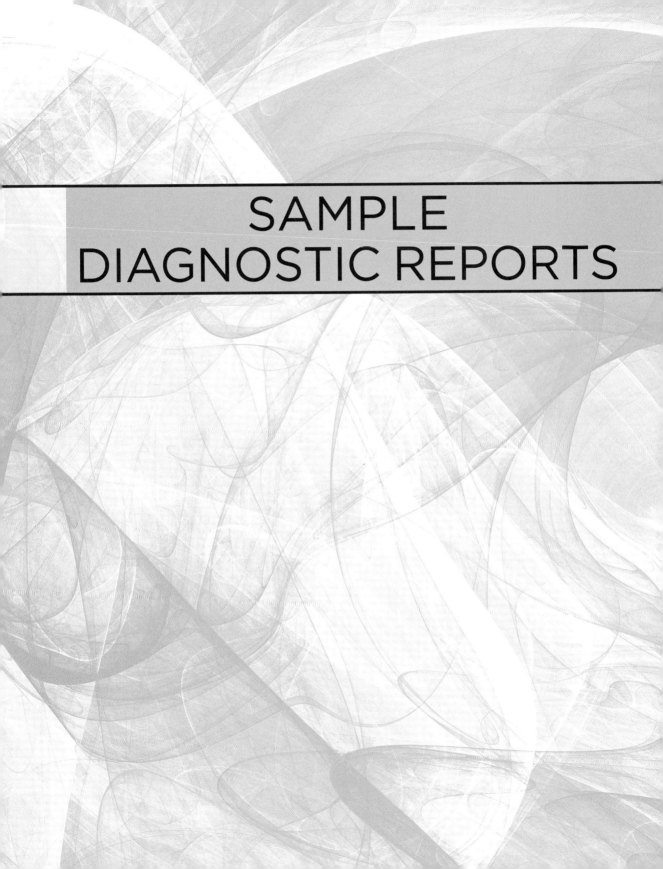

SAMPLE
DIAGNOSTIC REPORTS

Sample Diagnostic Report

SAMPLE DIAGNOSTIC REPORT FOR PROFILE 1A: MILD-TO-MODERATE MIXED SPOKEN LANGUAGE AND EMERGENT LITERACY DEFICIT

Statement of Problem

Amanda Adams, a 6-year, 4-month-old female, was seen at a university language and literacy clinic on April 12, 2009, for an assessment of her spoken language and emergent literacy skills (diagnostic procedure 92506 [evaluation of speech and language]). Amanda is in the last semester of her kindergarten year at the Riker Street Elementary School. Ms. Adams, Amanda's biological mother, indicated that she brought Amanda to this clinic because of Amanda's difficulties with preacademic reading skills being taught in kindergarten. She stated that Amanda often misreads a word after correctly reading it numerous times before and confuses names of letters that sound alike (e.g., says the letter name *b* for *d*). Further, Ms. Adams stated that Amanda's teacher reported that Amanda appears to be struggling with following directions in the classroom. Ms. Adams provided all historical information on Amanda, along with reports from previous testing.

Background Information

Developmental and Medical History

Amanda's birth history is unremarkable. Amanda was a late talker; she began to use single words regularly at about 2 years of age; however, she appeared to "catch up" by the age of 3. Amanda had approximately five middle-ear infections before the age of 3. Her hearing was tested at a university speech and hearing clinic one month ago. Her audiologic report states that she has normal hearing thresholds bilaterally but shows mild difficulty with "binaural integration" and "listening in the presence of background noise." A personal FM system was recommended for classroom use but this accommodation has not yet been implemented.

Environmental and Family History

Amanda attends an elementary school that is rated highly in her school district. Amanda's mother works with Amanda at home on a daily basis. Amanda was tested at her elementary school 6 months ago because she was struggling with her preacademic skills. Her evaluation report from the school's psychologist revealed a composite score of 100 on the *Reynolds Intellectual Assessment Scale*, a composite score of 91 on the *Comprehensive Tests of Nonverbal Intelligence* (CTONI), and composite scores on the *Comprehensive Test of Phonological Processing* (CTOPP) of 109 for phonological awareness, 85 for phonological memory, and 121 for rapid naming.

Amanda's 10-year-old sister was diagnosed with reading comprehension problems when she was 8 years of age and receives special education services at school under a 504 Educational Plan. Amanda's mother and father have college degrees. Neither parent reports having had learning difficulties in school; however, two of Amanda's father's first cousins had difficulty in school and received special services.

Assessment Procedures

Purpose of Testing and Test Measures

The purpose of this assessment was to evaluate Amanda's spoken and written language skills to (a) determine if she is at risk for having difficulties with reading as she progresses through kindergarten and beyond, and (b) provide recommendations for instruction if Amanda is showing signs of being at risk for future reading difficulties. The following tests were used to evaluate Amanda's communication skills:

- *Assessment of Literacy and Language* (ALL; Lombardino, Lieberman, & Brown, 2005)
- *Dynamic Indicators of Basic Early Literacy Skills* (DIBELS; Good & Kaminski, 2002)
- *Test of Narrative Language* (TNL; Gillam & Pearson, 2004)
- *Illinois Test of Psycholinguistic Abilities* (ITPA-3; Hammill, Mather, & Roberts, 2001)

Hearing Screening

Amanda's hearing screening results were within normal limits. Her pure-tone air-conduction thresholds were less than or equal to 20 dB HL (ANSI, 1996) at octave frequencies from 250 through 8000 Hz.

Literacy Screening

The *Dynamic Indicators of Basic Early Literacy Skills* (DIBELS) was used to screen Amanda's reading readiness. Her performance was compared with data for children at the end of the kindergarten school year. Descriptive measures of low risk, emerging, and high risk are used to evaluate performance on the DIBELS. Amanda was given the three DIBELS tests that were appropriate for her grade level: *letter-naming fluency, phoneme segmentation fluency*, and *nonsense-word fluency*. On the letter-naming fluency subtest, Amanda was required to name as many letters as possible in one minute. Her performance on this subtest was in the low-risk range. On the phoneme segmentation fluency subtest, Amanda was required to segment words into individual phonemes. Her performance on this subtest was in the emerging skill range. Finally, on the nonsense-word fluency subtest, Amanda was required to read as many words as possible in one minute. Again, she performed in the low-risk range. Overall, Amanda's performance on the DIBELS suggests that she is meeting the benchmarks for the end of the kindergarten school year.

Spoken Language and Literacy Tests

Assessment of Literacy and Language (ALL)

The *Assessment of Literacy and Language* (ALL) is a screening and diagnostic test for evaluating emergent reading and spoken language skills in preschool through first grade children. Composite scores can be used to create profiles of strengths and weaknesses in both domains. The ALL provides different combinations of tests for different grades. Composite index scores for language and emergent literacy can be calculated for four grade-level periods: preschool, kindergarten fall semester, kindergarten spring semester, and first grade. For children in the spring of their kindergarten year and in first grade, two additional emergent literacy composite scores can be calculated, one for a *phonological composite* (i.e., knowledge and manipulation of sound segments in words) and one for a *phonological-orthographic composite* (i.e., knowledge of phoneme and grapheme associations).

The ALL tests for language include: *basic concepts*: identifying size, color, and place through picture pointing; *receptive vocabulary*: identifying pictures named; *parallel sentence production*: creating parallel syntactic structures through sentence completion; *word relationships*: describing relationships between two words; and *listening comprehension*: answering questions about stories presented orally.

The ALL tests for emergent literacy include: *letter knowledge*: using letter knowledge for letter identification, letter naming, and letter production; *rhyme knowledge*: making rhyme judgements and generating rhymes; *elision*: deleting syllables or sounds to create new words; *phonics knowledge*: associating letters with sounds and reading nonwords; *sound categorization*: identifying words with the same sounds;

and *sight-word recognition*: reading common sight words.

Amanda's standard score on the language composite was 87, which is at the lower end of the average range for her grade. Her subtest scores ranged from depressed to the higher end of average range. Her basic concepts and receptive vocabulary scores are in the below-average range for her grade and her listening comprehension score was depressed.

Amanda's emergent literacy composite was 91, which is within normal limits for her age level. The subtests that comprise these tests yield two separate composite scores, a *phonological composite* score and a *phonological-orthographic composite* score. The phonological composite of 91 was derived from the combined scores for the rhyme knowledge, elision, and sound categorization subtests. The phonological-orthographic composite of 99 was derived from the combined scores for the phonics knowledge and sight-word recognition subtests. Amanda showed greater difficulties with spoken language and phonological skills than with orthographic skills.

The ALL criterion-referenced tests were used to obtain additional information on Amanda's naming and print-related skills. She met grade-level criteria on each of the following five tests: *matching symbols*: matching single letters and numbers as well as sequences of letters, numbers, and four-letter words; *word retrieval*: retrieving associated words rapidly from long-term memory; *rapid automatic naming*: naming serially ordered colors and objects rapidly; *concept of word*: identifying words in print; and *invented spelling*: using phoneme-grapheme knowledge to create word spellings.

Additional Language Tests

The *Illinois Test of Psycholinguistic Abilities* (ITPA-3) for ages 5 to 12 was used to assess Amanda's performance on tasks that assess various linguistic processes. The three subtests from ITPA-3 administered during this evaluation were *spoken analogies*, *spoken vocabulary*, and *morphological closure*.

The spoken analogies subtest measures the ability to complete a phrase by identifying relationships among words. The examiner reads a four-part analogy in which the last part is missing. The child then tells the examiner the missing part. For example, in response to "birds fly, fish _____," the child might say "swim." This subtest assesses verbal reasoning, listening comprehension, oral expression, and semantics. The spoken vocabulary subtest measures the ability to identify spoken words when provided with attributes of words. The examiner says a word that is actually an attribute of some other noun. For example, the examiner may say, "I am thinking of something with a roof," to which the child might respond, "house." This subtest assesses listening or speech comprehension, spoken vocabulary, and semantics. The morphological closure subtest measures the ability to complete a partially formed sentence by applying a final word that is grammatically correct. The

examiner gives an oral prompt with the last part missing. For example, the examiner says "big, bigger, _____," and the child completes the phrase by saying "biggest." This subtest assesses morphology and listening skills.

Amanda's standard scores for the spoken analogies and morphological closure subtests were 10 and 9, respectively, placing her in the average range. In contrast, her score on the spoken vocabulary subtest was 6, placing her greater than one standard deviation below the mean and indicating depressed lexical knowledge.

The *Test of Narrative Language* (TNL) is a norm-referenced test for assessing *narrative comprehension* and *oral narration*. Narrative comprehension measures the ability to understand information in stories produced by others and to make inferences about information not explicitly stated. Oral narration measures the ability to tell a story in a coherent way by tying together characters, actions and events, consequences, and resolutions.

Amanda's performance on the TNL showed a discrepancy between her ability to comprehend a story and her ability to tell a story. Although her narrative comprehension was at the lower end of the average range, her oral narration was depressed, yielding an overall narrative language ability index (NLAI) of 76.

Written Language Sample

Amanda was asked to retell a story in writing. The following story was read to her from a second-grade-level paragraph from the

Analytic Reading Inventory (Woods & Moe, 1989). The passage was read twice to minimize constraints of working memory on her written text performance.

Mouse passage

Swish! My pet mouse ran straight under our neighbor's chair! Our neighbor didn't hear him because he is quiet, as a mouse should be. If she had seen him she would have yelled her head off. Zoom! Now my clever gray mouse is bouncing off the jam jar on the breakfast table. He is sliding on the milk left around my glass! He is dancing on my cupcake. He loves drinking lemonade. He eats lots of honey and blueberries. He is silly, different, and really quite funny. I'll always love my dear little mouse. Say, have you seen my sweet gray friend? You better look now because he's right under your chair!

Amanda's written language sample, reproduced in this section, indicated that she understood the concept of print, she possessed some knowledge of sound-letter associations as demonstrated in her invented spellings (e.g., "mas" for *mouse*), and she recalled a commonly used but irregular word (*the*). However, she produced few ideas from the story.

Evaluation Summary

Amanda Adams, a 6-year, 4-month-old female, was seen at a university language and literacy clinic for a language and literacy evaluation. Previous testing revealed that she functioned in the low average to average range on tests of nonverbal intelligence. In this assessment, Amanda's performance on a battery of language and emergent literacy tests, in conjunction with reports from her mother and teacher, indicates that her profile is characteristic of a mild-to-moderate mixed receptive-expressive language disorder (ICD-9-CM, 315.32). Her deficits in spoken language place her at risk for a developmental reading disorder (ICD-9-CM, 315.00).

Amanda's greatest weaknesses lie in the lexical and the narrative domains of language, particularly when the sequencing of information is required. On the ALL, she exhibited the greatest difficulty with basic concepts, receptive vocabulary, and listening comprehension. Her word-level vocabulary and her knowledge of concepts are weak, her ability to comprehend narratives is depressed, and she has difficulty with discourse cohesion (i.e., connecting words and sentences to create a complete story). A summary of Amanda's test scores are shown in Table 4-3.

Recommendations

It is recommended that:

1. Amanda receive spoken language intervention that targets:

   a. Production and comprehension of age-appropriate language concepts

TABLE 4-3 Summary of Amanda's Scores

Test	Subtest	Standard Score	Percentile Rank	Descriptive Rating
Assessment of Literacy and Language (ALL)				
	Word relationships	5*	5	Depressed
	Listening comprehension	5*	5	Depressed
	Basic concepts	7*	16	Below average
	Receptive vocabulary	7*	16	Below average
	Parallel sentence production	12	75	High average
	Spoken Language Composite	87	19	Low average
	Letter knowledge	9	37	Average
	Rhyme knowledge	9	37	Average
	Elision	8	25	Average
	Phonics knowledge	11	63	Average
	Sound categorization	7*	16	Below average
	Sight-word recognition	10	50	Average
	Emergent Literacy Composite	91	27	Average
	• Phonological composite	87	19	Low average
	• Phonological-orthographic composite	99	47	Average
ALL Supplemental Tests				
	Book handling	CR	—	Met criterion
	Matching symbols	CR	—	Met criterion
	Word retrieval	CR	—	Met criterion
	Rapid automatic naming	CR	—	Met criterion
Dynamic Indicators of Basic Early Literacy Skills (DIBELS)				
	Letter-naming fluency	CR	—	Low risk
	Phoneme segmentation fluency	CR	—	Emerging skill
	Nonsense-word fluency	CR	—	Low risk
The Illinois Test of Psycholinguistic Abilities (ITPA-3)				
	Spoken analogies	10	50	Average
	Spoken vocabulary	6*	9	Depressed
	Morphological closure	9	37	Average
Test of Narrative Language (TNL)				
	Narrative comprehension	8	25	Average
	Oral narration	4*	2	Depressed
	Narrative Language Ability Index	76*	5	Depressed

*Score is at least one standard deviation below mean.

b. Story re-retelling using a framework to facilitate story grammar

c. Story comprehension

2. Use a computerized program daily that can be individually tailored to Amanda's level of phonics knowledge and that extends into broader language concepts such as vocabulary and comprehension. The Language Tune-Up Kit is a research-based phonics software program designed for children 6 years of age or older (http://www.jwor.com), and the Reading Lesson is a phonics-based software program designed to target the letter knowledge and phonics skills of children from 4 to 7 years of age (http://www.readinglesson.com).

3. A return to the clinic for a reevaluation within one year if her mother and teacher feel that she is not progressing at the expected rate to transition to the next grade level.

Suggested Book Resources for Her Parents and Teachers

1. Pinnell, G. S., & Fountas, I. C. (2007). *The continuum of literacy learning (Grades K–2): A guide to teaching.* Portsmouth, NH: Heinemann.

2. Bear, D. R., Invernizzi, M., Templeton, S., & Johnston, F. (2004). *Words their way: Word study for vocabulary, phonics, and spelling instruction* (3rd ed.). Upper Saddle River, NJ: Pearson Prentice Hall.

3. Ganske, K. (2000). *Word journeys: Assessment-guided phonics, spelling, and vocabulary instruction.* New York: Guilford.

SAMPLE DIAGNOSTIC REPORT FOR PROFILE 1B: SEVERE MIXED SPOKEN LANGUAGE AND EMERGENT LITERACY DEFICIT

Statement of Problem

Brittany Brown, a 6-year, 8-month-old female, was seen at a university language and literacy clinic on March 21, 2009, for an assessment of her language and emergent literacy skills (diagnostic procedure 92506 [evaluation of speech and language]). Ms. Brown, Brittany's biological mother, was concerned about Brittany's difficulty with literacy tasks in the classroom, based on reports from Brittany's first-grade teacher. Ms. Brown provided all historical information on Brittany's development.

Background Information

Developmental and Medical History

Brittany's birth history was unremarkable. She appeared to be developing normally until about 12 months of age, when Ms. Brown noted that Brittany was not using any words or wordlike forms to communicate. Brittany produced her first word at 18 months and she began to combine words shortly before her third birthday. Brittany was diagnosed with an overall developmental delay, a spoken language disorder, and attention-deficit/hyperactivity disorder (ADHD) 2 years ago at the First Street Clinic. She received language therapy during individual weekly sessions for one year. Brittany's most recent language evaluation report at the same clinic, 6 months ago, stated that her composite score on the *Comprehensive Tests of Nonverbal Intelligence* (CTONI; Hammill, Pearson, &

Wiederholt, 1997), a nonverbal intelligence test, was 84. However, her receptive language and expressive language scores fell below 1.5 standard deviations of the mean (<78).

Educational and Family History

Brittany lives with her biological parents and her older brother. She attends a regular first-grade class at South Street Elementary School, where she has an Individualized Educational Plan (IEP) and receives pull-out Exceptional Student Education (ESE) services daily for reading and math. She also receives speech and language therapy services at school in small-group 30-minute sessions twice per week. In addition, Brittany receives one 50-minute session of *Lindamood Individualized Phoneme Sequencing* (LiPS) intervention at a local clinic, two times per week.

Brittany's 8-year-old biological brother was diagnosed with "mild-moderate" autism at age 3 and also receives ESE services in school. Ms. Brown has an undergraduate degree in early childhood education and reports a negative history for any learning difficulties. Brittany's father has an associate's degree and works as a building contractor. He experienced learning difficulties throughout school but was not formally identified as having a learning disability and did not receive any special services inside or outside of school.

Assessment Procedures

Purpose of Testing and Test Measures

The purpose of this assessment was to evaluate Brittany's language and emergent literacy abilities. The following tests were used:

- *Assessment of Literacy and Language* (ALL; Lombardino, Lieberman, & Brown, 2005)
- *Comprehensive Test of Phonological Processing* (CTOPP; Wagner, Torgesen, & Rashotte, 1999a)
- *Test of Early Written Language*–2nd Edition (TEWL-2; Hresko, Herron, & Peak, 1996)

Hearing Screening

Brittany's hearing screening results were within normal limits. Her pure-tone air-conduction thresholds were less than or equal to 20 dB HL (ANSI, 1996) at octave frequencies from 250 through 8000 Hz.

Language and Literacy Tests

Assessment of Literacy and Language (ALL)

The *Assessment of Literacy and Language* (ALL) was used to measure Brittany's language and emergent skills (refer to Profile 1a for a description of the ALL). Brittany's *language composite* of 47 and her *emergent literacy composite* of 61 showed that both her spoken language and her emergent literacy skills were very depressed for a child in the spring semester of first grade. Her *phonological composite* score of 66 and her *phonological-orthographic composite* score of 60 indicated that her phonological and orthographic skills were comparably depressed. Also, Brittany did not meet the criterion score for children in the spring semester of first grade on the ALL *invented spelling* subtest.

The *Comprehensive Test of Phonological Processing* (CTOPP for ages 5–6) was used to assess Brittany's phonological awareness, phonological memory, and rapid-naming skills. The seven core subtests used were *elision, blending words, sound matching, memory for digits, nonword repetition, rapid color-naming,* and *rapid object-naming.* Composite scores were calculated for *phonological awareness, phonological memory, and rapid naming.*

The elision subtest measures the ability to say a word and then say what is left of that word after dropping out designated sounds. This test assesses phonemic awareness, a skill that develops in conjunction with early reading acquisition. The blending words subtest measures the ability to combine sounds to form words. The sound matching subtest measures the ability to match a target sound to a picture of an item whose word representation begins or ends with the same target sound. Combined scores from the elision, blending words, and sound matching subtests yield the phonological awareness composite. The memory for digits subtest measures memory by asking the subject to repeat a series of numbers ranging in length from two to eight digits. The nonword repetition subtest measures the ability to repeat nonsense words that range in length from 3 to 15 sounds. Combined scores from the memory for digits and nonword repetition subtests yield the phonological memory composite. The rapid color naming and rapid object naming subtests measure the speed of rapid serial naming for colors and for objects, respectively. Combined scores from the two tests yield the *rapid-naming composite.*

Brittany's scores on the phonological awareness subtests ranged from below average on the sound matching and elision subtests to average on the blending words subtest. These scores yielded a phonological awareness composite of 85. Brittany's scores on the phonological memory subtests ranged from very depressed on the memory for digits subtest to average on the nonword-repetition subtest. These scores yielded a phonological memory composite of 76. On the rapid naming subtests, Brittany's performance ranged from depressed on the rapid color naming subtest to average on the rapid object naming subtest. These scores yielded a rapid naming composite of 76. Her composite scores in all three areas of phonological processing are depressed, although she showed a strength in blending sounds into words.

The Test of Early Written Language–2nd Edition (TEWL-2) assesses early writing ability with two subtests, *basic writing* and *contextual writing.* The basic writing subtest measures the functional or mechanical components of writing that include metalinguistic awareness, directionality, organizational structure, awareness of letter features, punctuation, capitalization, spelling, proofing, sentence combining, and logical sentences. Brittany obtained a basic writing score of 80, which falls in the below average range for her age. She was able to write her name, write numbers, write letters, identify writing instruments, identify written material, and copy words. However, she was unable to write at least 12 letters of the alphabet in correct order, identify cursive and print writing, spell any words correctly, identify a word in a sentence, or identify the beginning and end letter in a word.

The contextual writing subtest measures generative writing skills that include punctuation, capitalization, syntactic maturity, vocabulary, and spelling. For this subtest, Brittany was presented with a picture and asked to write a story about it. She did not achieve a basal level of performance so testing was discontinued. Brittany's writing sample consisted of lines of random letters, starting at the top of the page. The letters she produced were not phonetic representations of the target words and were not grouped together to represent words.

Evaluation Summary

Brittany Brown, a 6-year, 8-month-old female, was seen at a university language and literacy clinic on March 2, 2009, for an assessment of her language and literacy (diagnostic procedure 92506 [evaluation of speech and language]). Brittany was in the second semester of first grade and receiving daily pull-out ESE services for reading and math in small groups every day in addition to language therapy at a private clinic. Brittany's performance on a battery of language and emergent literacy tests in conjunction with reports from her mother and teacher corroborate her previously identified weaknesses in spoken language and indicate that her profile is characteristic of a severe mixed receptive-expressive language disorder (ICD-9-CM, 315.32), placing her at high risk for a developmental reading disorder (ICD-9-CM, 315.00).

Informal observations showed that Brittany's social-communication behaviors were appropriate throughout several hours of testing, and she appeared to enjoy being engaged with the practitioners during testing and break-time activities. However, Brittany's language and emergent literacy skills are very depressed. Her greatest strengths were observed on the CTOPP nonword repetition and blending words subtests. She had the most difficulty with word meanings, as reflected in her very depressed scores on the ALL subtests of basic concepts, receptive vocabulary, listening comprehension, and word relationships. Her emergent literacy skills on the ALL were also very depressed, especially in the areas of rhyme knowledge, and sightword recognition. Her relative strengths in areas of elision and phonics are very likely the result of her LiPS intervention. Finally, Brittany did not meet grade-level criterion for the invented spelling ALL subtest; she often spelled a word with the correct first letter followed by "ay," indicating deficient knowledge of letter-sound correspondences. Many of her attempts to spell words were strings of random letters that were not phonetically similar to the target words. A summary of Brittany's scores are shown in Table 4-4.

Recommendations

It is recommended that:

1. Brittany receive intensive spoken language and emergent literacy intervention in a one-to-one or small-group setting on a daily basis for at least 90 minutes, with an emphasis on word meanings, listening comprehension, word reading and spelling through decoding and analogy

TABLE 4-4 Summary of Brittany's Scores

Test	Subtest	Standard Score	Percentile Rank	Descriptive Rating
Assessment of Literacy and Language (ALL)				
	Word relationships	2*	0.4	Very depressed
	Basic concepts	1*	0.1	Very depressed
	Receptive vocabulary	1*	0.1	Very depressed
	Listening comprehension	1*	0.1	Very depressed
	Parallel sentence production	6*	9	Below average
	Spoken Language Composite	47*	<0.1	Very depressed
	Rhyme knowledge	3*	1	Very depressed
	Elision	6*	9	Below average
	Phonics knowledge	5*	5	Depressed
	Sound categorization	4*	2	Depressed
	Sight-word recognition	1*	0.1	Very depressed
	Emergent Literacy Composite	61*	0.5	Very depressed
	• Phonological composite	66*	1	Very depressed
	• Phonological orthographic composite	60	0.4	Very depressed
	• Invented spelling	CR		Did not meet criterion score
Comprehensive Test of Phonological Processing (CTOPP)				
	Elision	6*	9	Below average
	Blending words	11	63	Average
	Sound matching	6*	9	Below average
	Phonological Awareness Composite	85*	16	Low average
	Memory for digits	3*	1	Very depressed
	Nonword repetition	9	37	Average
	Phonological Memory Composite	85*	16	Low average
	Rapid color-naming	4*	2	Depressed
	Rapid object-naming	8	25	Average
	Rapid-Naming Composite	76*	5	Depressed
Test of Early Written Language–2nd Edition (TEWL-2)				
	Basic writing	80*	10	Below average
	Contextual writing			Unable to obtain basal level

*Score is at least one standard deviation below mean.

strategies, and story recall in oral and written language activities.

2. Mr. and Ms. Brown consider moving Brittany from her current school to the Martha's Montessori charter school for the next school year, where the curriculum is designed specifically for students with language learning disabilities. This school provides a language-rich curriculum and daily LiPS instruction as the foundation for their reading curriculum.

3. Mr. and Ms. Brown consider enrolling Brittany in the Listening and Literacy Summer Camp, where she will be able to receive therapy to facilitate her vocabulary and listening comprehension along with LiPS instruction throughout the summer.

Suggested Book Resources for Brittany's Parents and Teachers

1. Blachman, B. A., Ball, E. W., Black, R., & Tangel, D. M. (2000). *Road to the code: A phonological awareness program for young children*. Baltimore: Paul H. Brookes.

2. Bear, D. R., Invernizzi, M., Templeton, S., & Johnston, F. (2004). *Words their way: Word study for vocabulary, phonics, and spelling instruction* (3rd ed.). Upper Saddle River, NJ: Pearson Prentice Hall.

3. Ganske, K. (2000). *Word journeys: Assessment-guided phonics, spelling, and vocabulary instruction*. New York: Guilford.

4. Lingui Systems (www.linguisystems. com), a publishing company that produces numerous materials (e.g., books, books on CD, software programs) for children who need language intervention.

SAMPLE DIAGNOSTIC REPORT FOR PROFILE 2: EMERGENT LITERACY DEFICIT

Statement of Problem

Carlos Calas, a 5-year, 7-month-old male, was seen at a university language and literacy clinic on March 1, 2009, for an assessment of his language and emergent literacy skills (diagnostic procedure 92506 [evaluation of speech and language]). Ms. Calas, Carlos' biological mother, brought him to this clinic because of the difficulties he is having with learning letter names and letter sounds. She also noted that Carlos struggles with spelling, organization, and following multistep directions. Ms. Calas was concerned about Carlos' potential to succeed in first grade because he is barely passing his kindergarten benchmarks. She came to the clinic to find out if Carlos has dyslexia, another type of learning disability, or if he simply needs more time to learn to read. Ms. Calas provided all historical information on Carlos' development.

Background Information

Developmental and Medical History

Ms. Calas had a long and difficult labor with Carlos. Calos was badly bruised around his eyes, nose, and forehead and exhibited immature eye movements for a short while. Since that time, his development has been uneventful, his communicative and sensorimotor milestones were achieved at appropriate ages, and his overall health has been good.

Ms. Calas reports that Carlos has not shown any difficulties with his speech or language development. He appears to have a good expressive vocabulary and good language comprehension skills. However, his teacher recently stated that Carlos is having difficulty remembering the names of the letters of the alphabet and the sounds that correspond to these letters. Occasionally, he appears to have difficulty remembering a word for an object that he has named many times before.

Environmental and Family History

Carlos lives with his biological parents. He is receiving a good education and his teacher is very attentive to his learning difficulties. Both Mr. and Ms. Calas graduated with associate's degrees from a community college. Ms. Calas has no history of learning difficulties; however, both her biological brothers and her husband, Carlos' biological father, were diagnosed with dyslexia. She noted that her husband reports having had difficulties with reading and spelling as far back as he can remember.

Assessment Procedures

Purpose of Testing and Test Measures

The purpose of this testing was to evaluate Carlos' language and emergent literacy skills and to determine if he shows signs of having a specific reading disability.

Hearing Screening

Carlos' hearing screening results were within normal limits. His pure-tone air-conduction thresholds were less than or equal to 20 dB HL (ANSI, 1996) at octave frequencies from 250 through 8000 Hz.

Language and Literacy Tests

Assessment of Literacy and Language (ALL)

The *Assessment of Literacy and Language* (ALL; Lombardino, Lieberman, & Brown, 2005) was used to evaluate Carlos' skills (refer to Profile 1a for complete description of ALL). The ALL spoken language tests given to Carlos were *basic concepts, receptive vocabulary, parallel sentence production, word relationships,* and *listening comprehension.* His spoken language composite score of 112 fell at the higher end of average for his age and his language subtest scores ranged from average to superior.

The ALL emergent literacy tests given to Carlos were *rhyme knowledge, elision, sound categorization, phonics knowledge,* and *sight word recognition.* His ALL emergent literacy composite score of 76 fell greater than 1.5 standard deviations below the mean. Although his phonological composite score (sound knowledge only) was 91, his phonological-orthographic composite score (sound-letter pattern knowledge) of 68 clearly underscored his difficulties with letter names and letter-sound associations.

Criterion-referenced tests from the ALL were used to assess Carlos' skills for *matching symbols, word retrieval, rapid naming, concept of word,* and *invented spelling.* He did not meet the criterion score for his age on the concept of word and invented spelling tests. Carlos' language composite score is significantly higher than his emergent literacy composite score. This discrepancy is characteristic of young children who are at risk for dyslexia.

Articulation

Carlos did not exhibit any articulation errors in his speech.

Evaluation Summary

Carlos Calas, a 5-year, 7-month-old male, was seen at a university language and literacy clinic for an assessment of his language and emergent literacy skills. His scores from the present evaluation, along with parent and teacher reports of his reading difficulties and his positive family history for dyslexia, indicate that he is at risk for developmental dyslexia (ICD-9-CM, 315.02).

On the ALL, Carlos' scores for the language subtests ranged from average to superior, yielding a language composite score of 112. In contrast, Carlos's emergent literacy composite score of 76 was depressed for his grade. The marked discrepancy between his language and emergent literacy composite scores is clinically significant and is characteristic of a profile that represents a specific reading disability (i.e., dyslexia). This specific reading disability is likely to become very apparent once Carlos is expected to decode words and quickly recall the pronunciation of words learned. A summary of his scores are shown in Table 4-5.

Recommendations

It is recommended that:

1. Carlos be enrolled in a multisensory phonics-based explicit training program for a minimum of four 60-minute sessions weekly, beginning as soon as possible.

2. Carlos' teacher be made aware of his potential difficulties with phonics, decoding, spelling, and word reading and inform Ms. Calas of these difficulties if observed in the classroom.

3. Carlos return to this clinic if he is unable to keep pace with his peers by the middle of his first-grade year.

4. Ms. Calas review recommendations on the International Dyslexia Association (IDA) Web site (http://www.interdys.org) for instructional programs and for tutors located near her home.

Suggested Book Resources for Carlos' Parents and Teachers

1. Hall, S. L., & Moats, L. C. (2002). *Parenting a struggling reader*. New York: Broadway Books.

2. Adams, M. J., Foorman, B. R., Lundberg, I., & Beeler, T. (1998). *Phonemic awareness in young children. A classroom curriculum*. Baltimore: Paul H. Brookes.

3. Blachman, B. A., Ball, E. W., Black, R., & Tangel, D. M. (2000). *Road to the code: A phonological awareness program for young children*. Baltimore: Paul H. Brookes.

TABLE 4-5 Summary of Carlos' Scores

Test	Subtest	Standard Score	Percentile Rank	Descriptive Rating
Assessment of Literacy and Language (ALL)				
	Listening comprehension	10	50	Average
	Word relationships	12	75	High average
	Basic concepts	11	63	Average
	Receptive vocabulary	13	84	Above average
	Parallel sentence production	14	91	Superior
	Spoken Language Composite	112	79	Average
	Letter knowledge	4*	2	Depressed
	Rhyme knowledge	9	37	Average
	Elision	8	25	Average
	Phonics knowledge	4*	2	Depressed
	Sound categorization	9	37	Average
	Sight-word recognition	7*	16	Below average
	Emergent Literacy Composite	76*	5	Depressed
	• Phonological composite	91	27	Average
	• Phonological-orthographic composite	68*	2	Depressed
	Concept of word	CR	—	Did not meet criterion
	Invented spelling	CR	—	Did not meet criterion
	Matching symbols	CR	—	Met criterion
	Word retrieval	CR	—	Met criterion
	Rapid automatic naming	CR	—	Met criterion

CR=criterion-referenced score

*Score is at least one standard deviation below mean.

© Cengage Learning 2012

4. Bear, D. R., Invernizzi, M., Templeton, S., & Johnston, F. (2004). *Words their way: Word study for vocabulary, phonics, and spelling instruction* (3rd ed.). Upper Saddle River, NJ: Pearson Prentice Hall.

5. Language Tune-Up Kit Interactive Reading Software (Orton-Gillingham Curriculum on CD-ROM (www.jwor.com)

SAMPLE DIAGNOSTIC REPORT FOR PROFILE 3: ENVIRONMENTAL DISADVANTAGE DEFICIT

Statement of Problem

Devon Darby, a 5-year, 9-month-old male, was seen at the First Street Elementary School for an evaluation of his language and literacy skills on August 28, 2007, in the fall of his kindergarten year. He was recommended for testing by his teacher because he scored in the lower 20% of his class on tests of preacademic skills related to emerging literacy during the first 6 weeks of his kindergarten year. Devon's teacher was concerned about his depressed emergent literacy skill scores, his lack of interest in books, and his inattention in class during the daily "alphabet time" period. Devon's grandmother provided historical information on his development.

Background Information

Developmental and Medical History

Devon did not experience any difficulties at birth. He talked shortly after his first birthday, and he appeared to be developing well overall. He had occasional ear infections prior to 2 years of age. Devon was screened for speech and language skills while in Head Start. He passed the screening and has not received any special services. Devon's attendance in the Head Start Program was sporadic.

Family History

Currently, Devon lives with his mother, grandmother, and two older siblings. He moved frequently with his mother when he was between 1 and 3 years of age. His mother, who has a high school degree, works as a clerk in a local grocery store. Devon's father is not living in the home and little is known about him other than that he did not complete high school.

Purpose of Testing and Test Measures

The purpose of this assessment was to evaluate Devon's language and emergent literacy skills

prior to his participation in a small-group early literacy intervention program offered by the school's speech-language pathologist. The *Assessment of Literacy and Language* (ALL: Lombardino, Lieberman, & Brown, 2005) was used to evaluate his skills before and after his participation in the program (see Profile 1a for a description of ALL).

Hearing Screening

Devon's hearing screening results were within normal limits. His pure-tone air-conduction thresholds were less than or equal to 20 dB HL (ANSI, 1996) at octave frequencies from 250 through 8000 Hz.

Language and Literacy Intervention Program

Devon received small-group instruction in spoken language, phonics, and spelling skills in 55-minute sessions 4 times per week for 9 months with a speech pathologist. In each session, the clinician spent 15 minutes teaching sound-letter correspondences, 15 minutes writing simple monosyllabic words that contained the sound-letter pairs previously learned, and 20 minutes learning the meaning of words and categorizing words in two ways: (1) by semantic relationships (sad/unhappy) and (2) by phonological segments (rhyme, sound categorization, phoneme segments).

Pre- and Post-program Language and Literacy Testing

Devon's scores on the ALL prior to entering therapy in the fall and after terminating therapy in the spring are shown in Tables 4-6 and 4-7. At the termination of the program (end of the second semester of kindergarten),

TABLE 4-6 Summary of Devon's Pre-intervention Test Scores on the ALL Early in the Fall of His Kindergarten Year

Subtest	Standard Score	Percentile
Basic concepts	3*	1
Receptive vocabulary	4*	2
Parallel sentence production	5*	5
Word relationships	3*	1
Listening comprehension	4*	2
Spoken Language Composite	60*	0.4
Letter knowledge	3*	1
Rhyme knowledge	6*	9
Elision	7*	16
Emergent Literacy Composite	72	3
• Phonological composite	66	1

*Score is at least one standard deviation below the mean.

TABLE 4-7 Summary of Devon's Post-intervention Test Scores on the ALL in the Spring of His Kindergarten Year

Subtest	Standard Score	Percentile
Basic concept	9	37
Receptive vocabulary	10	50
Parallel sentence production	13	84
Word relationships	11	63
Listening comprehension	9	37
Spoken Language Composite	102	55
Letter knowledge	11	63
Rhyme knowledge	10	50
Elision	7*	16
Phonics knowledge	12	75
Sound categorization	10	50
Sight-word recognition	10	50
Emergent Literacy Composite	100	50
• Phonological Composite	94	34
• Phonological-Orthographic Composite	104	61

*Score is at least one standard deviation below the mean.

a *phonological-orthographic composite* score was calculated for Devon in addition to the *phonological composite* score that was also calculated in the fall.

Summary

Devon Darby has shown significant progress during the 9 months that he has attended kindergarten and participated 4 times weekly in small-group literacy intervention sessions. His spoken language and emergent literacy composite scores on the ALL changed from composite scores at or below the 3rd percentile to composite scores at or above the 50th percentile. The only weakness that is apparent in his post-intervention profile is in the area of phoneme manipulation as tested on an elision task.

Devon's progress, as measured by these pre- and post-intervention scores, is consistent with his language and literacy growth in the classroom. Devon's teacher reports that he is functioning in the top 40% of his class and that he is prepared to enter first grade next fall. The rate of Devon's progresss, in conjunction with his teacher's report of his average standing among his peers, supports the conclusion that he does not have an obvious learning disability, but rather needs systematic exposure to foundational skills that he did not possess early in his kindergarten year. The degree to which daily small-group instruction contributed to Devon's growth over and above his classroom instruction cannot be determined, however, his rate of learning was clearly indicative of a learner with adequate potential to function at grade level.

Recommendations

Devon's speech-language pathologist recommended that:

1. He be screened at the beginning, middle, and end of first grade to ensure that he maintains his grade-level performance in reading.

2. His intensive therapy be reinstated if his progress falls below the 30th percentile in reading, to ensure that he does not experience academic failure as he moves through the elementary grades.

3. He participate in the school's summer reading program to help ensure that he has continuous and systematic exposure to grade-level reading instruction.

4. He participate in games in which he is required to create words from scrambled sets of letter tiles by using the tiles to spell words that he knows. Games of this nature should facilitate his phonemic awareness and can be found online and on iPhones.

Identifying and Classifying School-Age Children with Reading Disabilities

CHAPTER FIVE

THIS CHAPTER AIMS TO:

- Provide practioners with an overview of the scientifically-based literature on classifications of reading disorders.
- Provide practitioners with a framework for classifying profiles in school-age children beyond first grade who have normal-range intellectual abilities, who are failing to keep pace with their classroom peers in spite of having had appropriate levels of instruction, who have had adequate sociocultural support and opportunities, and who are motivated to succeed academically.
- Provide practitioners with sample assessment protocols and diagnostic reports for three profiles of reading disabilities: dyslexia, mixed spoken and written language disorder, and reading comprehension disorder.

EVALUATING AND DIAGNOSING SCHOOL-AGE LEARNERS WITH READING DISABILITIES

Attempts have been made to subclassify types of developmental *spoken language impairments* (Bishop & Edmundson, 1987; Conti-Ramsden & Botting, 1999; Conti-Ramsden, Crutchley, & Botting, 1997; Tomblin, 2008) and developmental *reading disabilities* (Aaron, Joshi, & Williams, 1999; King, Giess, & Lombardino, 2007; Carver & Clark, 1998; Catts, Adlof, & Weismer, 2006; Cain & Oakhill, 2006; Fletcher, Morris, & Lyon, 2005; Wolf & Bowers, 1999) when they affect learners who have the intellectual, sociocultural, and academic support to learn language but fail either to develop the spoken language or the written language skills expected for their age, even though their development appears to be normal in all other ways. For many years, these developmental language learning disabilities have been identified by exclusionary criteria and by an IQ-achievement discrepancy standard for performance (Francis, Shaywitz, Stuebing, Shaywitz, & Fletcher, 1996).

While subgrouping learners with specific learning disabilities remains a challenge (Verhoeven & van Balkom, 2004), there is clear evidence that learners with *developmental language impairments*, who are typically identified before they enter school, and learners with *developmental reading disorders*, who are typically identified once they experience reading difficulties, are heterogeneous groups of learners with language disabilities. For both groups, it is likely that their developmental deficits are due to multiple factors, and it is the combination of these factors that determines how their language learning disability is expressed (Bishop & Snowling, 2004; Bishop, 2008; Leonard et al., 2002; Scarborough, 2002; Pennington, 2006; Pennington & Bishop, 2009). Within these two general groups, learners' impairments can range widely in severity, rendering some learners severely impaired and others mildly or moderately impaired. Hence, to meet the instructional needs of children with learning disabilities, the practitioner must have a detailed assessment of the learner's spoken and written language skills in order to choose the optimal scope and sequence of a scientifically validated method for treatment. There is no universal consensus on subtypes of reading disability; however, the three most commonly identified reading disorder profiles in school-age learners are (1) dyslexia, (2) mixed spoken and written language disorder, and (3) reading comprehension disorder. These profiles are discussed in detail and designated as Profiles 4, 5, and 6, respectively, in this chapter.

The International Classification of Diseases, Ninth Revision, Clinical Modification (ICD-9-CM), Sixth Edition diagnostic system codes (U.S. Department of Health and Human Services, Centers for Disease Control and Prevention, and the Centers for Medicare and Medicaid Services, 2009–2010) are commonly used medical designations for classifying types of language and reading disabilities. Diagnostic codes are often required to qualify students for services or to obtain third-party reimbursement for services (see Table 5-1 for these codes). The terminology used to describe or diagnose children with developmental reading disorders often varies across disciplines (e.g., speech-language pathology, educational psychology, clinical psychology), across settings (i.e., educational versus clinical or medical settings), and across goals (instruction, differential diagnosis, research classification). Terminology for describing the same basic profiles of reading disorders can differ, often resulting in confusion for families who are trying to understand the nature of their children's learning difficulties

and to determine the optimal treatment procedures. The ICD-9-CM terminology and corresponding codes used to represent descriptions of reading disabilities are shown in Table 5-1.

Developmental disorders of spoken language that impact reading development and achievement have been studied extensively in the areas of spoken language production, spoken language comprehension, phonological processing, word reading, reading fluency, and reading comprehension in learners from grade 1 through high school (Snowling & Hulme, 2005). In the following sections, three behavioral profiles are presented that

TABLE 5-1 ICD-9-CM Diagnostic Codes for Reading Disorders

Profile	Types of Reading Disability	ICD-9-CM Classification Codes
4	• *Dyslexia** • Reading disability • Specific reading disability • Learning disability	ICD-9-CM: 315.02 (developmental dyslexia)
5	• *Mixed language and literacy disorder** • Learning disability • Language learning disability • Receptive or receptive language disorder • Specific language impairment • Oral and written language learning disability • Auditory processing disorder	ICD-9-CM: 315.32 (mixed receptive-expressive language disorder) *or* ICD-9-CM: 315.00 (reading disorder, unspecified)
6	• *Comprehension disorder** • Poor comprehender • Specific comprehension deficit • Reading disability • Learning disability	ICD-9-CM: 315.00 (reading disorder, unspecified)

*These terms are preferred for use in this book.

represent the patterns of strengths and weaknesses that have been most clearly validated in the scientific literature and that have been observed in the author's diagnostic work in reading disabilities over the past 12 years. In this book, these three profiles are referred to as (1) dyslexia, (2) mixed spoken and written disorder, and (3) reading comprehension disorder. These terms are italicized in each of the three profiles in Table 5-1 and are described in Table 5-2. Learners with characteristics of these profile types have deficits in one or more component skills of reading. Their classifications are determined largely by strengths and weaknesses in the areas of phonemic awareness, rapid automatized naming, nonword decoding, word reading, spelling, reading fluency, listening comprehension, expressive language, and reading comprehension, in addition to their performance on tests of cognitive processes that rely heavily on language knowledge, verbal working memory, and processing speed. In this chapter, detailed descriptions of these three types of reading disorders are presented along with sample diagnostic reports for each profile.

Although some learners with reading disabilities will have profiles that fit neatly into one of the three types of profiles described in Tables 5-1 and 5-2, others may exhibit areas of strength or weakness that are unexpected. For this reason it is critical that the practitioner have knowledge of the learner's overall sociocultural experiences, motivation to learn to read and write, classroom instruction, and the nature of previous interventions in addition to having an assessment of the learner's performance in all

age-appropriate component skills for both spoken and written language. For example, children who have dyslexia, defined by a core deficit in the phonological domain of language, may perform adequately on phonological decoding, and word recognition tasks if they have received intensive tutoring in phonics-based treatment methods, but may continue to experience word-reading difficulties on timed tests of word reading and on tests of reading fluency. A manifestation of their slow lexical access is typically seen in their oral reading rate even when they are able to read accurately and in their rate of written text generation even when their ideas are strong conceptually.

Furthermore, it is critical that the practitioner be flexible when using patterns of strength and weakness to arrive at a diagnosis. Current emphasis on phonological awareness, the alphabetic principle, and word decoding in many kindergarten and first-grade classrooms may obscure signs of a reading disability that will become apparent only once the learner is required to read fluently with comprehension.

READING DISABILITIES AS IDENTIFIED IN MAR^{W}R

Dyslexia Profile

Learners who have deficits consistent with this profile are typically classified as having dyslexia or specific reading disability (SRD). The profiles of these learners are characterized by a primary deficit in the phonological domain of language (Stanovich, 1988a). Their phonological skills are typically lower

TABLE 5-2 Primary Spoken and Written Language Characteristics for Dyslexia, Mixed Spoken and Written Language Disorder, and Comprehension Disorder

Profile Type	Spoken Language Characteristics	Reading and Writing Characteristics
Profile 4a and 4b: Dyslexia	• Deficits in phonological and orthographic coding along with a lack of fluency in reading • Depressed ability to remember the precise oral pronunciations of words learned, particularly when they consist of multisyllabic and complex constructions • Relatively frequent history of short-term articulation therapy • Range of lower end of average to well above average for domain-specific language production and comprehension tasks (e.g., vocabulary, morphology) with overall spoken language scores typically in the average range • Listening comprehension exceeds reading comprehension, although sometimes holding lengthy oral directions in memory is difficult • Listening comprehension exceeds word reading and reading fluency • Language production in terms of vocabulary and complexity of ideas is often an obvious strength in bright and advantaged students who have dyslexia	• Depressed phonological decoding of nonwords, word reading, spelling, and readings fluency • Spelling is always impaired and retention of word spellings can be very difficult • Writing mechanics including punctuation conventions are typically poor • Morphosyntactic deficits such as omitting plural (e.g., *s*) and possessive markers (e.g., *'s*) may be apparent in written language • Handwriting varies from good to very poor • Writing conventions, such as punctuation and capitalization, are often ignored or misused
Profile 5: Mixed Spoken and Written Language Disorder	• Depressed oral language abilities in one or more domains of language (e.g., semantic, syntax, pragmatics); however, deficits in phonological processing (awareness, memory, rapid naming) can be mild • Typically has a history of early language impairment • Often shows deficits in production of oral language narratives and other forms of oral discourse • Often shows deficits in use of morphological and syntactic forms • Language production in terms of vocabulary and complexity of ideas is often an obvious strength in bright and advantaged students who have dyslexia	• Can show relatively good word recognition, reading fluency, and spelling • Depressed reading comprehension • Depressed writing composition in terms of story grammar and other structural elements of discourse • Morphosyntactic and semantic errors are often observed in written composition
Profile 6: Reading Comprehension Disorder	• Typically unidentified with learning difficulties until 4th grade and beyond • Average to strong phonological decoding and word recognition • Relatively weak language comprehension skills at the word and discourse levels • Weaknesses in telling well-structured and integrated stories orally • Variable performance on tasks of working memory	• Word-level reading, decoding, and spelling are all superior to reading comprehension • Depressed reading comprehension skills, particularly beyond the 3rd–4th-grade level • Weaknesses in a well-structured and integrated story in writing

than younger children who are reading at the same general grade level (Stanovich, 1988b), indicating that they are not simply exhibiting a developmental delay but rather a difference in the development of their phonological skills that underpin skilled reading. The phonological processing weaknesses of learners with dyslexia may be evident on oral phonological tasks such as phoneme deletion and on orthographic word-level tasks such as decoding and word recognition. Their spelling skills are always deficient because they must rely solely on their phonological or orthographic memories when generating a word in writing rather than rapidly integrating phonological and orthographic memories—a particularly difficult skill for persons who have dyslexia. They often show deficits on tests of rapid serial word retrieval (e.g., rapid automatized naming [RAN]). While a core deficit in the phonological domain of language is considered to be the "hallmark" of dyslexia, deficits in orthographic knowledge (e.g., the sound segment/shun/ is spelled "tion" or "sion"), verbal working memory (Berninger et al., 2006), and processing speed (Berninger, Abbott, Billingsley, & Nagy, 2001; Catts, Gillispie, Leonard, Kail, & Miller, 2002; Park et al., 2011; Ramus, 2003; Wolf & Bowers, 1999) have also been strongly associated with the cognitive profiles of persons with dyslexia. Lyon, Shaywitz, and Shaywitz (2003) defined dyslexia as

> a specific learning disability that is neurobiological in origin. It is characterized by difficulties with accurate and/or fluent word recognition and by poor

spelling and decoding abilities. These difficulties typically result from a deficit in the phonological component of language that is often unexpected in relation to other cognitive abilities and the provision of effective classroom instruction. Secondary consequences may include problems in reading comprehension and reduced reading experience that can impede growth of vocabulary and background knowledge (p. 2).

In addressing the relatively modular nature of dyslexia, Stanovich (1988b) stated that "phonological awareness is relatively dissociated from other higher-level cognitive skills" (p. 160). Approximately 6%–17% of school-age children with reading difficulties show a primary deficit in nonword reading and present profiles that are consistent with the diagnosis of dyslexia (Fletcher, 2009; Vellutino, Fletcher, Snowling, & Scanlon, 2004). The reading deficits in these learners manifest primarily at the word level, where facility with phonological coding is most critical. The ratio of males to females who have dyslexia is approximately 1.5:1 (Fletcher, 2009; Pennington et al., 2009). Learners with dyslexia are frequently referred to as "poor decoders" (Bishop & Snowling, 2004). Reading deficits in poor decoders are most apparent on untimed and timed tests of word reading; decoding, spelling, and oral fluency and in the transcriptional skills of writing including spelling and punctuation.

There is a continuum of individuals who meet the criteria for having dyslexia (Snowling, 2009). Some learners represent a "classic" case of dyslexia in which phonological deficits are found in the absence of any apparent oral language impairments, whereas others also show some degree of weakness in (1) word-finding difficulties, (2) spontaneous recall of words, and (3) pronunciations of complex words (Lovett, 1987; Vogel, 1977; Lombardino, Riccio, Hynd, & Pinheiro, 1997). Their oral language weaknesses are often not severe enough to warrant a diagnosis of specific language impairment, and are not comparable to the difficulties that these learners with dyslexia are experiencing in reading, spelling, and writing. The shaded areas in Figure 5-1 show the primary areas of deficit that characterize dyslexia in the MAR^{w}R.

Dyslexia and attention-deficit/ hyperactivity disorder (ADHD) co-occur in 25%–40% of learners whose primary diagnosis is either dyslexia or ADHD. Furthermore, dyslexia is often accompanied by dysgraphia, a specific learning disability of written expression that is not nearly as well defined as dyslexia. Dysgraphia is generally characterized by difficulties with letter formation, letter spacing within words and between words on a page, spelling, and overall handwriting quality. The International Dyslexia Association (http://www.interdyc .org; "Fact Sheet on Dysgraphia") states that children with dysgraphia do not have a primary motor deficit but they may have difficulty planning the graphomotor sequences for producing precise letter formations. Although poor spelling is associated with dysgraphia, deficits in spelling alone do not constitute dysgraphia. All individuals with dyslexia have difficulty spelling but not all individuals with dyslexia have

dysgraphia. Dysgraphic writing is characterized by marked difficulties with the formation and consistency of shapes of letters, spatial planning, and overall writing legibility. Dysgraphia can occur in isolation or with a range of other developmental disorders such as mixed spoken language and literacy disability and attention deficit disorder (Berninger, 2008). Figure 5-2 shows a writing sample of an 8-year-old boy who has dyslexia and dysgraphia, and Figure 5-3 shows a writing sample of a 10-year-old boy who has dyslexia without dysgraphia.

Difficulty on tasks of rapid automatized naming (RAN) is frequently associated with dyslexia, and some researchers argue that a rapid-naming speed deficit represents a *second core deficit* that is distinct from the phonological core weakness that is the hallmark of current descriptions of dyslexia (Wolf & Bowers, 1999). Some research literature supports the idea that learners with dyslexia can exhibit isolated deficits in phonological awareness (PA) or in rapid automatized naming (RAN) (Wolf et al., 2002; King, Giess, & Lombardino, 2007). This profile has been referred to as a single-deficit profile (i.e., a deficit in either PA or RAN). Learners with single deficits in naming have less severe impairments than those who exhibit a double-deficit profile (deficits in both PA and RAN). While naming-speed deficits occur frequently in many persons who are diagnosed with dyslexia, Vukovic and Siegel (2006) suggest that there is not enough evidence to support an isolated rapid-naming deficit in persons who have dyslexia. However, in cross-linguistic studies of dyslexia (1) rapid-naming speed differentiates

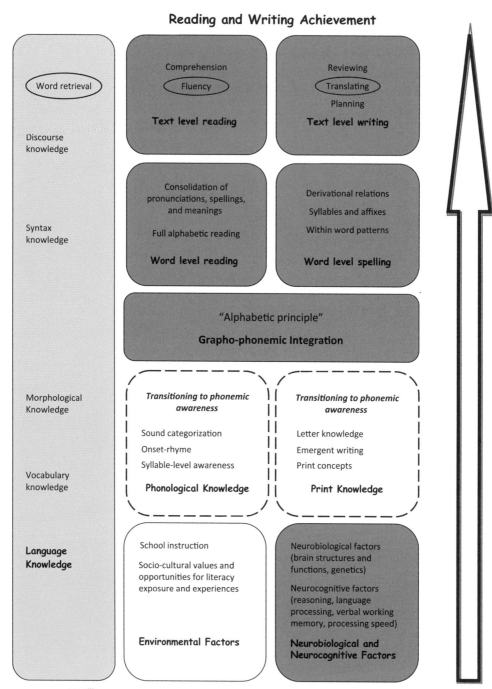

FIGURE 5-1 MAR^WR Model for Profile 4: Dyslexia/Specific Reading Disability
Dark shaded areas in modules: primary deficit skill areas or primary causal factors
Light shaded areas in modules: may or may not be deficit
Circled area: key deficit area within a module
Dashed line box modules: not assessed in this age range

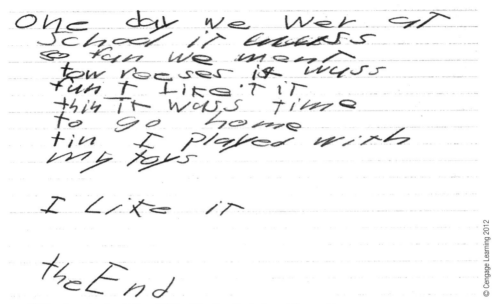

FIGURE 5-2 Writing Sample of an 8-Year-Old Boy Who Has Dyslexia and Dysgraphia

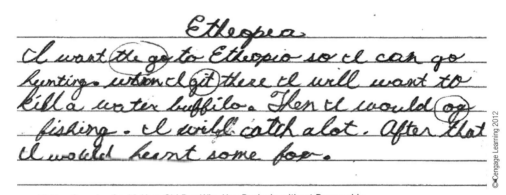

FIGURE 5-3 Writing Sample of a 10-Year-Old Boy Who Has Dyslexia without Dysgraphia

individuals who have dyslexia from typical readers in every language studied (Wolf et al., 2002), and (2) naming speed is a better predictor of reading than phonological decoding beyond the very beginning stages of reading in transparent languages such as Finnish, Dutch, and German, whose phoneme-grapheme relationships are more predictable than they are in English (Caravolas, 2005).

Many high-functioning learners who have dyslexia are not diagnosed. Some are able to compensate for their depressed phonological knowledge by relying on their reasoning abilities and world knowledge to comprehend what they read well enough to go unnoticed until their phonological abilities are taxed by a difficult activity such as learning to read and write in a second language (Difino & Lombardino, 2004; Difino, Johnson, & Lombardino, 2008). Others may not be diagnosed with a reading disability even though they are struggling with reading or writing if their scores on standardized tests of reading are insufficiently discrepant with their IQs, or if their word-reading scores fall within the average range in spite of evidence that their overall cognition is much more advanced than their reading or writing achievement.

Figure 5-4 displays an unedited keyboard writing sample of a bright 13-year-old boy with dyslexia (and dysgraphia) who did not qualify for learning disability services at his school because his composite scores on standardized tests did not show the required discrepancy. This student's expository text was written in response to the assignment "Write a synopsis of a favorite movie along with a personal reaction to the story." This adolescent had well-developed spoken language and reasoning abilities (Wechsler Intelligence Scale for Children [WISC-IV]: general ability index of 117; verbal comprehension index of 121). In contrast, his word-reading and decoding skills were below average and his writing skills, particularly in the translational processes (i.e., spelling and handwriting), were very depressed for his age, sociocultural opportunities, and overall intellectual abilities. A marked discrepancy is very apparent between his strong ability to recall and generate ideas about the movie, *Blood Diamond*, and his difficulties with translating his ideas into writing. The students' grammatical, punctuation, and capitalization errors were not corrected except in one segment in which the idea he was expressing was placed in parenthesis for clarification. The correct spelling of each misspelled word is shown in parentheses to enhance the readability of his story. Figure 5-5 shows an adapted synopsis of this movie (taken from the Internet Movie Database; http://www.imdb.com/title/tt0450259/plot-summary) to underscore the complexity of the multiple plots in *Blood Diamond*.

Most Common Diagnostic Indicators of Dyslexia

Several of the most common indicators of dyslexia are listed below. Some of these indicators are presented as specific areas of deficit and others are described as differences between skill domains. No one of these indicators should be used to make a diagnosis of dyslexia nor should all of these indicators be required to make a diagnosis of dyslexia. Individuals who have dyslexia will exhibit several of these indicators and the ones they manifest will be determined by varying factors including the learner's (a) overall quality of education, (b) language and world knowledge from environmental experiences, (c) instruction in literacy, (d) disorder severity, (e) previous reading intervention, and (f) reasoning and other cognitive abilities.

1. Depressed ability in one or more phonological processing skills, including phonological awareness, verbal short-term or working memory, rapid automatized naming

Blood diamond

Watch (watched) by CS

The year this movie was produced was co-produced and directed by Edward Zwick.

I just wanted to start out saying that this is a vary (very) true, and great movie (this is a true, and very great movie). In fact it might be the beast (best) movie that I have ever seen in my life. The movie starts out explaining thee (the) team (theme) and the time that t (it) takes place in. the (then) it goes to the co charter (character) dijmon hounson witch (which) is a local fisher man (fisherman) who has a vary (very) bright son. The (They) are walking to school when RUF witch (which) stands for revolutionary united front for sierra leaon (leone) attack (attacked) their villager (village) to look for workers, and to cut (missing text: off parts of their bodies to send) a clear message to not vote so that the RUF could gain control of that conflict zone. After he was caputerd (captured) he was forsed (forced) to work.

Then it shows his son getting captured. Then the main charter (character) shows up Danny archer slash smuggler who get (gets) caught and put on (in) jail then it goes to dijimon (djimon) hounson and shows him working in a river and finds a huge dimond (diamond) that will coust(cost) many people lives. Then he goes and try(tries) to hide it then the government troops come in and take him and a lot of ruf people to jail. Theat (That) is when the co (colonel) cahriter (character) meats (meets) with the man (main) chartiter (character). They let Danny go and he bargones (bargains) to get dijmon (djimon) out of jail and for a few days he convises (convinces) him to go get that dimond (diamond) and in reture (return) he will get his son and family back.

So they go out to find his family and hook up with thi (this) reporter and go to a camp were (where) dijimon (djimon) finds out that his son hase (has) been taken by the ruf and that holle (whole) time the movie shows small lips (bits) of the son becoming a solger (soldier) for the ruf.

So then they go with a bunch of repoter (reporters) and get ambushed and then the 3 main chritertier (characters) go find refuge and then the man that helps them gets shot so they go and drive him to the conras (convoy)camp witch (which) is a company hired by the government to kill the ruf. And bijimon (djimon) and danney (danny) sneek (sneak) of (off) so that they can keep the dimond (diamond) all to them self's (themselves) and the (thoy) find the camp were (where) dijimon (djimon) was working at and dijimon (djimon) waits till danney (danny) whent (went) to bed and he took of (off) looking for his son and finds him. But his son was munipulaed (manipulated) in to (into) thinking that his father left him so he was caputed (captured). Danney (Danny) wakes up and the air stricke (strike) comes in and danney (danny) makes his move to find dijimon (djimon) and his son. They do and then are capuserd (captured) by the conors (colonel) who is a sumgular (smuggler) two (too).

They make danney (danny) and dijumande (djimon) find they (the) dimoned (diamond) then they bouth (both) relises (realize) that they will be shot if they find the dimoned (diamond)so the (they) kill all of the grds (guards) and the conarl (colonel). Then danney (danny) and dijumon (djimon) find it and take of (off) and on the way danney (danny) find (finds) that he has been hit and dies. So then dijimon (djimon) and the reporter make a sting operation to prove who is buying illegal stones witch (which) they do and then the operation is exposed and dijumon (djimon) is reniter (reunited) with his family end of the story.

(For me, this true movie, I think very [much] changed the way we see normal diamonds today)

Reation (Reaction)

This is a vary (very) true movie that I think chageed (changed)the way we seen (see) normal dimondes (diamonds) to day (today). **to** *me* I belive (believe) that it does shead (shed) light that Africa is a crule (cruel) and unvergiving (unforgiving) unstable place to be. All so (Also) that it shows how small the atteps (attempts) are to make a differences (difference) that is why they show the unicef people that seem to (too) bissey (busy)to care. The movie all (also) has a secrete (secret) meassege (message) that one person cant (can't) make a differences (difference) it takes a lot of people and time and wester (western) help to infulance (influence) this conflite (conflict)to ctop and start the beqaning (beginning) of ferdom (freedom) and a great place to live for its inhabudens (inhabitants).

FIGURE 5-4 Typed Sample of a Movie Synopsis by a 14-Year-Old Boy with Dyslexia

It is 1999, Sierra Leone, and communities located in the country's coveted diamond-rich region are randomly attacked by rebel forces that use every unimaginable terror tactic to take over these areas controlled by the government militias. The atrocities committed by the rebels are staggering in their scope and the National government is corrupt and abusive in its own right.

The film opens when rebels, the Revolutionary United Front (RUF) attack and ravage another quiet village. Armed with assault rifles and machetes, the rebels are a force of unimaginable brutality. The rebels indiscriminately shoot their way through the village, intimidate potential voters by chopping off their hands, enslave the strong men to mine the diamonds, and the abduct young male children who are drugged and terrorized into being child soldiers readied to kill their parents and neighbors.

Solomon Vandy (Djimon Hounsou), a Mende fisherman is violently separated from his family, and unbeknownst to Solomon, his young son Dia is forcibly taken into the rebel forces and with the use of drugs, manipulation, and terror tactics is turned into a brutal killer who is proud say "I'm a baby killer".

Unlike the other men, Solomon is spared from having his hands chopped-off so he can be used as a laborer mining diamonds under the rebel command of Captain Poison (David Harewood). In the RUF rebel diamond fields, Solomon finds an enormous rare pink diamond and tries to bury the gem in the nearby woods. Government troops launch an attack on the rebel fields. At that very moment Captain Poison sneaks up and puts a gun to Solomon’s head, making him dig up the gem.

Just before Solomon hands over diamond, Captain Poison is shot and injured, giving Solomon time to rebury the stone out of sight of the rebel commander. Moments later, the Government militia rounded up the rebels and enslaved alike laborers, to be taken to prison in Sierra Leone's capital, Freetown.'

Meanwhile, Danny Archer (Leonardo DiCaprio), "Soldier of Fortune", a hired gun who specializes in the sale of so-called "blood diamonds", is arrested and imprisoned for trying to smuggle, the now confiscated, rebel diamonds into bordering Liberia.

Danny had been transporting diamonds to a South African mercenary, Colonel Coetzee (Arnold Vosloo), his former commander in the most decorated unit of the South African Border War. Coetzee is now employed to procure rebel black market diamonds by the infamous South African diamond company executive Van De Kaap (Marius Weyers)

In prison Danny overhears Captain Poison threatening Solomon about the buried pink diamond. Danny realizes getting that rare stone is his only real chance to repay Coetzee for the confiscated diamond cache, and to get out of Africa.

After he secures his own release and pays for Solomon's bail, the two men meet and Solomon cautiously accepts a deal to trade the diamond in exchange for help in finding his family. Danny and Solomon find their way to Maddy Bowen (Jennifer Connelly), an American journalist. In return for Danny giving her proof of Van De Kaap's Diamond Co. collaboration with the rebel black market trade, Maddy agrees to help Solomon find his family, and to use her travel access with the press convoy to go to Kono to find the diamond.

Rebel attacks separate Solomon and Danny from the Press convoy and the two men endure much together before they finally reach the RUF controlled mining camp in a river valley, where Solomon buried the rare diamond.

Danny remains hidden and calls in the Captain Coetzee's mercenary force but the rebels quickly discover Solomon. Captain Poison holds a machete to the neck of Dia, Solomon's expressionless son, to force Solomon into finding the diamond. Feeling silent rage when he sees his destroyed son before him, Solomon takes the shovel Poison gives him for the dig. And in an instant, the sky over the camp is swarming with the South African mercenary force, as it bombards the rebel camp with a massive air strike. RUF rebels are dropping like flies, and the entire camp is in thundering chaos. Caption Poison hits the ground. At that moment, Solomon releases his silent rage and bludgeons Caption Poison to death with shovel. It takes no time for Colonel Coetzee and the surviving rebels to begin their hunt for Danny and Solomon. They will stop at nothing to secure the diamond Danny now has in his possession.

Soon Coetzee is killed by Danny's but Danny is also mortally wounded and will not make it out of the countryside alive. Dia appears from woods and holds a gun on Danny and his father. Dia is ready to kill them both but Solomon calls out to his son. Despite what Dia has become, Solomon affirms that he sees only his son - a son who is still deeply loved by the father before him. Solomon tells Dia

"you are Dia Vandy"

"you are a good boy"

and reminds Dia of his life and his love, and that he can put behind him the horrible things he was made to do.

Dia breaks down and joins his father and Danny. But Danny is dying, and the rebels are on their heels. To set things right, Danny returns the diamond to Solomon, then sends his father and son off to the airstrip to catch a two-seater plane that he had pre-arranged to take them off the continent.

As the plane ascends, Danny makes his last call to the journalist, Maddy Bowen, asking her to take care of Solomon and Dia, secure the sale of their diamond and the reunification of their family. Of course, she does.

FIGURE 5-5 Internet Adapted Synopsis of *Blood Diamond*

Sources used in formulating this synopsis:
Sierra Leone: Case Study
by Janine DiGiovanni February 2001
Crimes of War Project 1999–2003
http://www.crimesofwar.org/archive/archive-sierracase.html

Diamonds and the Devil, Amid the Anguish of Africa
By Manohla Dargis

Published: December 8, 2006
http://movies.nytimes.com/2006/12/08/movies/08diam.html

Blood Diamond: A movie review by James Berardinelli
ReelViews : The Ultimate Guide to the Best 1000 Modern Movie
http://www.reelviews.net/php_review_template.php?identifier=882

2. Impaired rapid word recognition, decoding, and spelling

3. Impaired reading in spite of adequate spoken language, especially listening comprehension

4. Impaired reading accuracy and speed when reading aloud (i.e., reading fluency)

5. Impaired spontaneous spelling, although memorization of spelling words for tests may be adequate

6. Variable reading comprehension is linked to degree of skill in word-level reading

7. Difficulty recalling and often repeating the pronunciations of complex multisyllabic words

8. Impaired written language due largely to spelling errors and omissions, or errors in punctuation

9. Slow writing often characterized by inconsistent spacing between letters, inconsistent letter sizes, and poor legibility

10. Oral language abilities that far exceed reading fluency and transcriptional writing skills (i.e., spelling, punctuation)

11. Reading comprehension abilities that far exceed word-level reading and reading fluency

12. Reasoning or conceptual abilities that far exceed reading and writing skills

13. Reasoning or conceptual abilities that exceed processing speed or working memory

Mixed Spoken and Written Language Disorder Profile

Approximately 50% of learners identified with reading disorders also have oral language impairments (Catts, 1993; McArthur, Hogben, Edwards, Heath, & Mengler, 2000). Berninger, O'Donnell, and Holdnack (2008) refer to these learners has having an oral and written language learning disability (OWL LD) because they show more pervasive oral language difficulties than learners who have dyslexia. Some of these learners have been identified as having specific language impairment (SLI) prior to entering school, some have been identified as having a language learning disability (LLD) in the early grades, and others go unidentified until they begin to exhibit difficulties with reading comprehension. Gough and Tunmer (1986) referred to learners who have comparable levels of difficulty with decoding and comprehension as "garden variety poor readers." The majority of learners who have reading disabilities fall under this classification. Learners with this profile often have reading skill profiles that are very similar to those of younger learners (Stanovich, 1988a).

In contrast to the learners who have dyslexia, many learners with mixed oral and written language disorders exhibit weaknesses across several oral and written language domains. They typically show reasoning and verbal composite scores on the Woodcock Johnson III Tests of Cognitive Ability (WJ III COG; Woodcock, McGrew, & Mather, 2001b) that fall in the low-average range (Park, Kim, & Lombardino, 2009) and always exhibit reading comprehension deficits that are comparable to or greater than their word-level reading deficits. Typically, learners with this profile exhibit overall depressed academic achievement because, unlike learners with dyslexia, their deficits cut across a wider range of domains that affect reading, leaving them with fewer alternative routes for compensating for their processing difficulties.

Although some young children with specific language impairment (SLI) may not show signs of impaired word-level reading in the early grades, Conti-Ramsden & Botting (1999) noted that the majority of children diagnosed with SLI in the early grades, who continue to show characteristics of SLI at 11 to 14 years of age, have depressed reading abilities. Unlike learners with dyslexia, who exhibit a strength in reading comprehension relative to reading accuracy, learners with a history of SLI are more likely to exhibit deficits in reading comprehension than in reading accuracy (Conti-Ramsden & Botting, 1999; Snowling, Bishop, & Stothard, 2000), although they often have deficits in both component areas. In a discussion of differences between children with reading disabilities who have marked language deficits (i.e., mixed spoken and written language deficit) in comparison to those who do not (i.e., dyslexia), Berninger (2008) states:

> Our evidence to date suggests that those whose difficulties surface during the preschool years are more likely to have pervasive metalinguistic problems in phonological, morphological, and syntactic

awareness that interferes with their ability to (1) use decontextualized oral language to understand teachers' instructional language, (2) learn written language, and (3) self-regulate, that is, verbally mediate, the learning process across the academic curriculum. In contrast, children who showed no difficulty in oral language during the preschool years and whose first signs of difficulty in learning written language occurred when letters were introduced, for example, in kindergarten, are most likely to have problems only in phonological awareness (p. 108).

The language deficits of children with SLI are theorized to be caused by or associated with a number of different factors, including deficits in learning the rules of grammar (van der Ley & Ullman, 2001); deficits in temporal auditory processing of rapid speech (Tallal, Miller, & Fitch, 1993) and limitations in phonological working memory (Gathercole & Baddeley, 1990); and in more complex tasks of working memory that requires simultaneously storing and processing spoken language (Montgomery, 1995, 2000). Joanisse (2004) argued that phonological deficits that converge with other domains of language are a likely causal factor of SLI.

Based on the results of brain-imaging studies showing that words appear to be stored in memory in different neural forms, *phonological* word forms, *morphological* word forms, and *orthographic* word forms (Crosson et al., 1999; Richards et al., 2006), Berninger (2008) proposed that mixed spoken and written language deficits, dyslexia, and dysgraphia can be differentiated on the basis of deficits in these areas of word-form storage. She posits that these three types of learning disabilities are associated with different types of memory word-form deficits. Dysgraphia is a case of an isolated deficit in the memory codes that store orthographic word forms. Dyslexia results from deficits in both the phonological and the orthographic memory codes that store word forms, and mixed spoken and written language disabilities are the expression of deficits across all three word-form areas.

Writing difficulties in children with SLI and language learning disabilities (LLDs) have been well documented (Bishop & Clarkson, 2003; Gillam & Johnston, 1992; Scott & Windsor, 2000; Dockrell, Lindsay, & Connelly, 2009; Puranik, Lombardino, & Altmann, 2008). In comparing the written discourse of LLD children with both chronological age (CA) and language age (LA) matched controls, Scott and Windsor (2000) found that the LLD children used fewer total numbers of T-units (i.e., unit similar to a sentence) and fewer total numbers of words in their writing samples, produced a higher degree of grammatical errors, and experienced much more difficulty with expository writing than narrative writing.

In a longitudinal study, Dockrell, Lindsay, and Connelly (2009) examined the longitudinal trajectories of the written language abilities of children with SLI at 8, 11, 12, 14, and 16 years of age and concurrent relationships between their spoken language, reading, and handwriting at 16 years of age. In addressing the question of developmental trajectories, they found that (1) SLI children's writing performance decreased between ages 11 and 16, and (2) handwriting fluency, as measured by the number of alphabet letters written in 1 minute, was the only significant predictor of written language abilities. In addressing the students' performance in writing at age 16, they found that the SLI students (1) performed better on tasks of oral language than on tasks of written language; (2) performed more poorly in written language than in literacy measures of reading comprehension, reading decoding, and spelling; and (3) performed best on measures of grammar and capitalization and most poorly on measures of sentence structure, ideas and development, vocabulary, organization, and coherence.

In a study of two groups of children with learning disabilities, Puranik, Lombardino, and Altmann (2006) showed that learners' written retellings of an expository text differentiated students with a diagnosis of language learning disability (LLD) from students with a diagnosis of developmental dyslexia (DD). The DD group produced a higher number of T-units (sentence-type units), used a higher total number of words and total number of different words, and recalled a larger number of ideas than the LLD participants.

Figure 5-6 shows the primary deficit areas that are characteristic of the mixed spoken and written language disorder profile

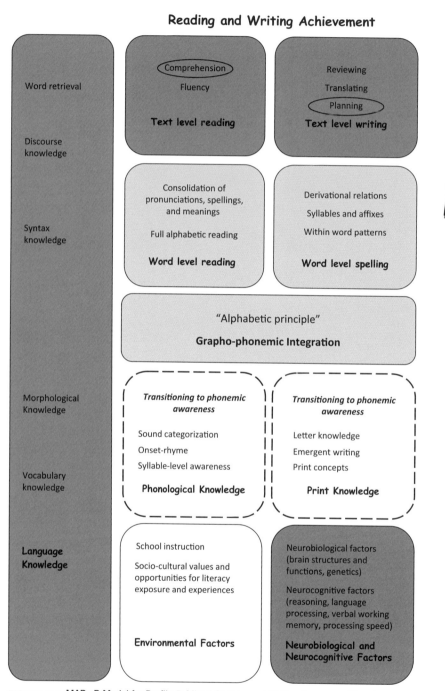

FIGURE 5-6 MARwR Model for Profile 5: Mixed Spoken and Written Language Disorder
Dark shaded areas in modules: primary deficit skill areas or primary causal factors
Light shaded areas in modules: may or may not be deficit
Circled area: key deficit area within a module
Dashed line box modules: not assessed in this age range

in the MAR^wR. Common characteristics of this profile are:

1. History of preschool language difficulties

2. Oral language deficits are observed in more than one domain of spoken language (i.e., word meanings, morphological and syntactic structures, discourse)

3. Receptive language, as measured on tasks of listening comprehension, is typically impaired

4. Narrative abilities are typically impaired

5. Reading comprehension is impaired regardless of whether word decoding is accurate or depressed

6. Overall reading achievement is not widely discrepant with verbal intelligence

7. Verbal reasoning is weak

8. Use of semantic contexts to facilitate understanding and memory is weak

9. Use of semantic contexts from print to facilitate reading comprehension is weak

Reading Comprehension Disorder Profiles

Approximately 20%–40% of learners' reading disorders are not identified until fourth through eighth grade. The majority of these late-emerging learners with reading difficulties have primary deficits in reading comprehension (about 7%), followed by those who have a primary deficit in word reading (about 4.4%) and those who show deficits in both word reading and reading comprehension (about 1.5%) (Compton & Catts, 2009).

Learners with reading comprehension deficits differ from those with a mixed deficit disorder in that they typically exhibit age-appropriate word reading. Their strengths are in the phonologically based word-level components of reading and their weaknesses are evident in the comprehension of connected text (Cain & Oakhill, 2006). Poor reading comprehension is found in about 10% of children in the elementary grades (Nation & Snowling, 1997; Yuill & Oakhill, 1991).

Several studies by Kate Nation and colleagues have shown that learners with impaired reading comprehension have weak oral language abilities (Nation, Adams, Bowyer-Crane, & Snowling, 1999; Nation & Snowling, 1997, 1999). It is now well documented that a subgroup of learners with reading comprehension deficits *do not have deficits* in the domain of phonological processing yet show deficits in the semantic and morphosyntactic domains of oral language. In their study of children with impaired reading comprehension, Nation, Clarke, Marshall, and Durand (2004) found that between 11.5% and 43% of poor comprehenders qualified for a diagnosis of SLI based on varying criteria used to define SLI in previous studies. They stated that "as a group, poor comprehenders have relative weaknesses across a range of language skills that are important to reading comprehension, from understanding the meaning of individual words to understanding figurative expressions" (p. 208).

A few longitudinal studies have provided insight into the developmental profiles of poor comprehenders. Cain and Oakhill (2006) studied good and poor comprehenders from 8 to 11 years of age. They chose poor comprehenders whose word-reading skills were no more than 6 months below their chronological age to help ensure that word-reading skills were not an obvious cause of their comprehension deficits. They reported a substantial degree of heterogeneity in the performance of their poor comprehenders on a range of language and cognitive tasks; however, they identified the following patterns over the 3-year period: (1) most poor comprehenders continued to show depressed comprehension as they progressed in school; (2) most poor comprehenders maintained the ability to understand the meaning of single words to a degree comparable to those of good comprehenders; (3) among the poor comprehenders, general cognitive abilities and receptive language abilities did not appear to affect their reading comprehension scores at 8 years of age, but 3 years later, those with higher cognitive abilities made greater gains in reading comprehension and those with higher receptive vocabulary made greater gains in word reading; (4) poor comprehenders, while functioning at grade-appropriate levels on standardized tests of math and science, generally scored significantly lower than their peers who were skilled in reading comprehension. Overall, Cain and Oakhill's (2006) data suggest that while a heterogeneous profile of strengths and weakness is found in learners who have poor comprehension, weak receptive vocabulary and weak reasoning in early

grades appear to be related to reading comprehension and academic performance in later grades. Figure 5-7 shows the primary areas of deficits that are characteristic of the comprehension deficit profile in the MAR^{w}R.

In a retrospective investigation, Catts et al. (2006) examined the developmental progression of language skills from kindergarten through fourth grade for poor comprehenders in eighth grade. Poor comprehenders were identified as performing below the 25th percentile for reading comprehension and above the 40th percentile for word recognition. Poor comprehenders were best differentiated from poor decoders and typical readers on measures of language comprehension. While considerable heterogeneity existed in this population, it was clear that poor comprehenders, especially beyond the fourth grade, had weaknesses in the nonphonological domains of language.

Furthermore, Wagner and Ridgewell (2009) reported on findings from their large-scale study on specific reading comprehension disability. They examined the percentage of children identified as poor comprehenders who showed adequate decoding only and those who showed both adequate decoding and vocabulary. Over 30,000 first-through third-grade students in Reading First Florida schools were studied. Their data showed that (1) between 1.54% and 23.12% of these children were poor comprehenders, depending on the children's grade levels and the percentile criterion used to determine impaired comprehension (at or below the 5th percentile versus at or below the 20th percentile);

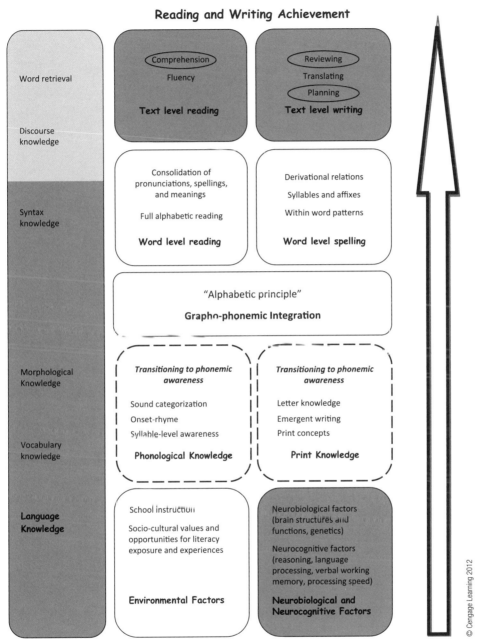

Reading and Writing Achievement

FIGURE 5-7 MAR^WR Model for Profile 6: Reading Comprehension Disorder
Dark shaded areas in modules: primary deficit skill areas or primary causal factors
Light shaded areas in modules: may or may not be deficit
Circled area: key deficit area within a module
Dashed line box modules: not assessed in this age range

(2) less than 1% to over 5% of the poor comprehenders had adequate decoding; and (3) only 0.07%–0.66% of the poor comprehenders showed both adequate decoding and vocabulary. Their data are consistent with other findings that poor comprehension is associated with weaknesses in oral language. The authors argued that a specific deficit in reading comprehension isolated from weaknesses in oral language knowledge is very infrequent. Given the unexpected appearance of reading difficulties that are identified in grade 4 and beyond, it is quite possible that poor comprehenders who are identified later have weaknesses in language that are most apparent when the complexity of content in the academic curriculum becomes more dependent on interactions between higher-order language knowledge (e.g., vocabulary, written discourse) with other cognitive skills (e.g., inferencing, monitoring comprehension), identified by Cain and Oakhill (2007).

Finally, in a treatment study of poorer comprehenders with age-appropriate phonological skills, Nation, Snowling, and Clarke (2007) found that the poor comprehenders learned to make phonological matches with novel word forms much like their control group, but they exhibited much more difficulty when required to make associations between semantic information and novel objects. These findings support previous data suggesting that the primary deficit in poor comprehenders with good decoding skills lies in the realm of consolidating new meaning, a semantic deficit that is largely dissociated from phonological skills.

SUMMARY OF READING PROFILES: ISSUES AND PRINCIPLES

The overlap in areas of deficit among learners with dyslexia, mixed spoken and written language disorder, and reading comprehension disorder can obscure the strengths in skills that differentiate the learner's assessment profiles unless a comprehensive evaluation is conducted to examine the wide range of abilities across their spoken and written language. Table 5-3 provides a summary of these characteristics across groups for each of the areas addressed in the MAR^{w}R.

SUMMARY OF IMPLICATIONS FOR IDENTIFYING PROFILES OF STRENGTHS AND WEAKNESSES

Reading relies on the integration of multiple domains of oral and written language knowledge (Hoover & Gough, 1990; Foorman, Francis, Shaywitz, Shaywitz, & Fletcher, 1997). Along with essential experiences and knowledge from their environmental supports, learners bring their own particular neurobiological makeup to the task of bridging and melding their knowledge of spoken and written language. The combination of these two powerful influences, biology and environment, determines the extent to which learners become proficient in their oral and written language skills. Fletcher and Lyon (2008) hold that "dyslexia results from an interaction of neurobiological factors that make the brain at risk and environmental factors that moderate this risk" (p. 30). This same

TABLE 5-3 Characteristics Across Groups for Areas Addressed in MAR^WR

Relative Areas of Strength and Weakness for Three Profiles of Reading Disability (Dyslexia, Mixed Spoken and Written Language Disorder, and Reading Comprehension Disorder) Across MAR^WR Domains

	Dyslexia	Mixed Spoken and Written Language Disorder	Comprehension Disorder
Cognitive Processes			
Reasoning	Varies from the average to superior range Always superior to word-reading and reading-fluency skills Often superior to verbal aptitude score	Within the average range but often at the lower end of this range Can be superior to or commensurate with verbal abilities	Within the average range
Verbal Working Memory	Often depressed, especially on more complex tasks of working memory	Often depressed, especially on more complex tasks of working memory	Insufficient data available
Processing Speed	Frequently slow on simple tasks of symbol matching or symbol associations	Frequently slow on simple tasks of symbol matching or symbol associations	Insufficient data available
Spoken Language Skills			
Vocabulary Knowledge	Superior to reading abilities, assuming adequate environmental enrichment	Often commensurate with reading ability Even when broad word meanings are adequate, difficulties may be seen in "depth" of word meanings, such as in words with multiple meanings or in using words figuratively	Variable. May not qualify for speech-language pathology services in early grades but later testing is likely to reveal weaknesses in word meanings.
Word Retrieval	Word-retrieval problems are often reported as occurring in spontaneous language. When tested in the context of RAN, slower than expected naming speeds are often observed	Word-retrieval problems are often reported as occurring in spontaneous language. When tested in the context of RAN, slower than expected naming speeds are often observed	Insufficient data available
Morphosyntactic Knowledge	Typically not well tested but has been reported to be somewhat depressed in some individuals with dyslexia although difficulties are not apparent in spoken language	Depressed spoken language production is a hallmark of specific language impairment	May not qualify for language intervention services in early grades but later testing reveals weaknesses in oral language production

(*continues*)

TABLE 5-3 (*continued*)

Listening Comprehension	A clear strength unless working memory is taxed	Depressed spoken language comprehension is a hallmark of specific language impairment	May not qualify for language intervention services in early grades but later testing reveals weaknesses in oral language comprehension
Discourse	Usually well developed in spite of some difficulty organizing thoughts quickly and in retrieving words quickly	Variable and dependent on the nature of the discourse skills tested but frequently weak in story telling and in using cohesive devices to bind elements of a story	Likely to be somewhat weak in the vocabulary and cohesion aspects of oral discourse
Phonological Knowledge			
Phonological Awareness	Core deficit area most apparent on tasks of phoneme manipulation	Deficits are frequently but not always observed	Variable. Many poor comprehenders show adequate phonological awareness abilities but others show deficits
Word Reading			
Decoding (Timed and Untimed)	Automaticity of decoding is a hallmark, especially in the less-transparent alphabetic languages such as English High-functioning students may score within the average range on untimed decoding measures but often show depressed scores on timed tests	Typically depressed	Typically, decoding skills are adequate. Decoding is superior to reading comprehension
Word Recognition (Timed and Untimed)	Automaticity of word recognition is a hallmark, especially in the less transparent alphabetic languages such as English High-functioning students may score within the average range on untimed word recognition measures but rarely on timed measures	Typically depressed	Typically, word recognition is adequate Word recognition is superior to reading comprehension
Word Spelling			
Spelling	Hallmark deficit area even after considerable practice; errors are often phonetically plausible	Typically depressed and are similar to those of younger children with comparable reading skills	Variable Can fall within the normal range

Text-Level Reading			
Reading Comprehension	May appear weak until decoding skills improve, but is typically a strength beyond the earliest stages of reading Ability to take advantage of contextual cues and world knowledge often provides adequate comprehension under untimed conditions	Weakness due to difficulties with reading at the word and text levels Weakness may be due to difficulties with verbal memory and difficulties in taking advantage of context to infer meaning	Most apparent reading component deficit beyond 3rd grade and continues throughout school Comprehension of individual words exceeds comprehension of text
Reading Fluency	Typically laborious with many errors or miscues Fluency increases with improvements in decoding and automatic word recognition	Typically slow and depends on word recognition skills and complexity of text. Fluency can be superior to reading comprehension	Typically good because of adequate decoding and word recognition
Text-Level Writing			
Punctuation	Depressed, especially relative to text content and organization	Superior to text content and organization	Insufficient data
Handwriting	Often characterized by errors in letter formation, letter spacing, and inconsistent spatial orientation	Varied	Insufficient data
Composition	Very problematic with greatest difficulties in the mechanics of writing Good at generating ideas/content (e.g., number of different words, number of ideas). Transcriptional skills are most impaired and often restrict vocabulary usage and length of composition. Some syntactic errors are noted and most appear to be due to difficulties in word retrieval, which can impact text organization and fluency	Very problematic with greatest problems in the vocabulary and cohesive dimensions of writing and often emerges as greatest area of weakness Weaknesses are typically noted in content (e.g., number of different words, number of ideas), form (e.g., sentence structure), generation and organization of ideas, knowledge of what the reader needs to know, and transcriptional skills (e.g., spelling)	Weakness in content-based aspects of written discourse, such as level of vocabulary used and knowledge of writing, that takes into account what the reader needs to know

position aptly characterizes all learning disabilities.

The links between oral and written language are irrefutable and have been addressed in many resources on reading development and reading disabilities (Catts & Kamhi, 2003; Neuman & Dickinson, 2002; Dickinson & Neuman; 2006; Snowling & Hulme, 2005). Although the profiles of persons with reading deficits are varied in nature, clinical and experimental data provide descriptions of commonly occurring patterns of strengths and weaknesses that allow practitioners to *better identify* the strengths and weaknesses of learners who are already manifesting reading deficits and *more precisely target* core reading-deficit areas in treatment.

SAMPLE DIAGNOSTIC REPORTS

Sample Diagnostic Reports

SAMPLE DIAGNOSTIC REPORT FOR PROFILE 4A: DYSLEXIA

Statement of Problem

Evan Edsen, a 10-year-old male, was seen at a university language and literacy clinic on June 1, 2004, for an assessment of his reading, spelling, and oral language skills (diagnostic procedure: 92506 [evaluation of speech and language]). Evan's mother, Mrs. Edsen, brought him to the clinic because she was very concerned about the difficulty he was experiencing with reading, writing, and spelling, and she wanted to know what could be done to help him learn these skills more efficiently. Furthermore, she was concerned about his inability to attend in school for long periods of time and his overall high level of activity.

Background Information

Developmental and Medical History

Evan is the youngest of three children. He lives at home with his mother, father, and two siblings, ages 17 and 14 years. Mrs. Edsen reported that she had an unremarkable pregnancy and delivery with Evan. She stated that Evan's general health is excellent and that he has had no serious injuries. Mrs. Edsen also reported that Evan has good coordination and is very active. All of Evan's developmental and communication milestones were reported to be achieved at the appropriate ages or earlier than expected.

Environmental and Educational History

Evan has been homeschooled since first grade. According to his mother, Evan is currently working at the third-grade level in all subjects except reading, writing, and spelling. She feels that he is functioning below the third-grade level in these areas. Based on Evan's age and years of homeschooling, he should be performing on the fourth-grade level in all academic work. Evan's siblings have not experienced any difficulty with reading and spelling; however, Mrs. Edsen reported that Evan's father has always had great difficulty with spelling; and reported that he has always been a slower reader in spite of his completion of a graduate degree in anthropology.

Speech-Language History

Mrs. Edsen stated that Evan's production and comprehension of spoken language appears to be very good. She has noticed recently that Evan appears to have difficulty recalling specific words at times, but he shows no other signs of having difficulty with his spoken language. Mrs. Edsen stated that she first became concerned about Evan's reading ability 2 years ago. She stated that his letter-sound recognition is weak and inconsistent and that he gets frustrated with reading and spelling. She noted that Evan does not enjoy reading but does enjoy being read to. She also noted that Evan has no difficulty understanding math concepts, but has difficulty with math problems that require remembering a sequence of operations. She stated that he continues to have difficulty memorizing his multiplication tables.

Assessment Procedures

Purpose of Testing and Test Measures

The purpose of this assessment was to evaluate Evan's written language abilities in conjunction with his overall cognitive abilities to determine if he exhibits a reading disability and to make recommendations for intervention, if needed. The following tests were used to evaluate Evan's reading and reading-related skills:

- Woodcock Johnson Tests of Achievement–Third Edition (WJ III ACH; Woodcock, McGrew, & Mather, 2001a)

- Woodcock Johnson Tests of Cognitive Abilities–Third Edition (WJ III COG; Woodcock, McGrew, & Mather, 2001b)

- Gray Oral Reading Mastery Test–Fourth Edition (GORT-4; Wiederholt & Bryant, 2001)

- Comprehensive Test of Phonological Processing (CTOPP; Wagner, Torgesen, & Rashotte, 1999a)

- Test of Word Reading Efficiency (TOWRE; Wagner, Torgesen, & Rashotte, 1999b)

Hearing Screening

Evan's hearing was screened and found to be within normal limits bilaterally. His pure-tone air-conduction thresholds were less than or equal to 20 dB HL (ANSI, 1996) at octave frequencies from 250 through 8000 Hz.

Phonological Processing Testing

The CTOPP for ages 7 through 24 was used to assess Evan's phonological awareness, phonological memory, and rapid-naming skills. The following six core subtests from the CTOPP were used to assess Evan's phonological processing abilities: *elision*, *blending words*, *memory for digits*, *rapid digit-naming*, *nonword repetition*, and *rapid letter-naming*.

Evan's scores on the phonological awareness subtests ranged from depressed on the elision subtest (5; 5th percentile) to high average on the blending-words subtest (12; 75th percentile), yielding a *phonological awareness composite* score of 91 (27th percentile). This score was at the lower end of the average range for his age and indicated a weakness in his ability to perform phonological manipulations. He performed in the average range on the memory-for-digits subtest (standard score of 9; 37th percentile) and on the nonword-repetition subtest (standard score of 11; 63rd percentile). These subtests yielded a *phonological memory composite* score of 100 (50th percentile). His scores were very depressed on both the rapid digit-naming (5; 5th percentile) and rapid letter-naming (5; 5th percentile) subtests, corresponding to a *rapid-naming composite* score of 70 (2nd percentile). This score fell in the very depressed range for his age. His performance on this test indicates that both his phonological awareness manipulation skills (i.e., elision) and his ability to quickly retrieve lexical information stored in long-term memory (i.e., RAN) are weak. Both of these domains of phonological processing contribute to reading fluency.

Psychoeducational Cognitive Testing

Seven subtests from the WJ III COG were used to assess Evan's cognitive processing abilities: *verbal comprehension* (measures the recall of vocabulary, synonyms, and antonyms, as well as the completion of analogies); *visual-auditory learning* (measures the ability to associate words with novel symbols in order to read sentences formed by the symbols); *spatial relations* (measures the ability to discern which shapes construct a particular whole); *sound blending* (measures the ability to provide a whole word when given the individual sounds of that word); *concept formation* (measures the ability to form rules and concepts based on visually presented stimuli); *visual matching* (measures the speed of identifying two numbers in a line of numbers that are similar); and *numbers reversed* (measures the ability to attend to spoken numbers, hold them in memory, and then repeat them in reverse order). Combinations of WJ III COG subtest standard scores were used to derive composite scores for *verbal ability, thinking ability, cognitive efficiency,* and *general intellectual ability* (GIA).

For six of the seven WJ III COG subtests, Evan's standard scores fell in the average range for his age. He obtained a standard score of 90 (25th percentile) on the visual-auditory learning subtest, 92 (30th percentile) on the spatial relations subtest, 96 (39th percentile) on the verbal comprehension subtest, 97 (43rd percentile) on the numbers reversed subtest, 107 (68th percentile) on the concept formation subtest, and 112 (80th percentile) on the sound blending subtest. On the visual matching subtest, Evan obtained a standard score of 60 (0.4 percentile), indicating that his visual processing speed is very depressed.

Both Evan's thinking ability composite score (a measure of the ability to employ alternate thinking strategies when information in short-term memory cannot be processed automatically) of 95 (41st percentile) and verbal ability composite score (a measure of spoken language that includes comprehension of individual words and the comprehension of relationships between words) of 96 (39th percentile) are in the average range for his age. However, his cognitive efficiency composite score (a measure of the speed or automaticity with which one engages in certain cognitive or academic maneuvers) of 77 (6th percentile) is in the depressed range for his age. Evan's general intellectual ability composite score of 91 (28th percentile) is at the lower end of the average range for his age.

Psychoeducational Achievement Testing

Nine subtests from the WJ III ACH were used to measure Evan's academic achievement in the domains of reading, spelling and mathematics. The *letter-word identification* subtest measured his sight vocabulary. *Reading fluency* measured his ability to read and answer yes/no questions both quickly and accurately. *Math fluency* measured his speed and automaticity in the retrieval of basic arithmetic facts; both of these subtests are timed. The *math calculation* subtest measured his computational skills under untimed contexts. The *spelling* subtest measured his ability to apply orthographic principles in the spelling of real words. The *writing fluency* subtest measured his ability to write a sentence using three specific words. The *writing samples* subtest measured his ability to write a sentence about a picture shown. The *word attack* subtest measured his skill to sound-out phonetically regular nonsense words. The *oral comprehension* subtest measured his ability to use syntactic and semantic cues to complete a short passage.

Evan's subtest scores ranged from very depressed to average for his age. He had the most difficulty on tasks involving reading, writing, and spelling, especially on tasks performed under timed conditions. Evan demonstrated significantly depressed abilities on the letter-word identification (64; 1st percentile) and spelling (61; 0.5 percentile) subtests, on timed tasks of reading fluency (61; 0.5), math fluency (62; 1st percentile), and writing fluency (62; 1st percentile). On the reading-fluency subtest, he completed only 3 questions in 3 minutes. On the math fluency subtest, he completed only 17 simple math problems (e.g., 1 − 1 = __, 0 + 3 = __) in 3 minutes. On the writing fluency subtest, he produced only 3 complete sentences in 7 minutes. In contrast, on the writing samples subtest, Evan obtained a standard score of 89 (22nd percentile). This score falls in the low-average range for his age. It should be noted that this subtest was

not timed and only the content of Evan's sentences were scored. His sentences were characterized by capitalization, punctuation, and spelling errors. Evan performed in the low-average range on the calculation (85; 16th percentile) and word attack (84; 14th percentile) subtests. He performed in the average range for his age on the oral comprehension (98; 45th percentile) subtest, demonstrating a strength in this area.

Evan's overall levels of achievement are significantly lower than predicted from his verbal ability composite and his thinking-ability composite scores. Table 5-4 shows his subtest and composite standard scores for the WJ III ACH.

Word-Level and Text-Level Reading Testing

The TOWRE was used to measure Evan's ability to pronounce printed words in isolation accurately and fluently under timed conditions. The *sight word efficiency* subtest was used to measure his ability to recognize familiar words as whole units (aka sight words). The *phonemic decoding efficiency* subtest was used to measure his ability to decode nonwords. Each test measures the number of word units read in 45 seconds. The average standard score is 100 with a standard deviation of ±15. Evan read 15 words correctly in 45 seconds, resulting in a very depressed sight word efficiency score of <55 (<1st percentile). He read 8 nonwords correctly in 45 seconds, resulting in a phonemic decoding efficiency score of 72 (3rd percentile). This score indicates that his decoding skills exceed his word recognition skills yet decoding is also depressed for his age.

TABLE 5-4 Evan's Test Scores

Test	Subtest	Standard Score	Percentile Rank	Descriptive Rating
Test of Word Reading Efficiency (TOWRE)				
	Sight word efficiency	<55	<1	very depressed
	Phonemic decoding efficiency	72	3	depressed
	Total Word Reading Efficiency	56	<1	very depressed
Comprehensive Test of Phonological Processings (CTOPP)				
	Elision	5*	5	depressed
	Blending words	12	75	high average
	Phonological Awareness Composite	91	27	average
	Memory for digits	9	37	average
	Nonword repetition	11	63	average
	Phonological Memory Composite	100	50	average
	Rapid letter-naming	5*	5	depressed
	Rapid digit-naming	5*	5	depressed
	Rapid-Naming Composite	70*	2	very depressed
Gray Oral Reading Test–4th Edition (GORT-4)				
	Rate	2*	<1	very depressed
	Accuracy	1*	<1	very depressed
	Fluency (Rate + Accuracy)	1*	<1	very depressed
	Passage comprehension	8	25	low average
	Oral Reading Quotient	67*	1	very depressed
Woodcock Johnson Tests of Achievement–3rd Edition (WJ ACH III)				
	Letter-word identification	64*	1	very depressed
	Reading fluency	61*	0.5	very depressed
	Calculation	85	16	below average
	Math fluency	62*	1	very depressed
	Spelling	61*	0.5	very depressed
	Writing fluency	62*	1	very depressed
	Writing samples	89	22	low average
	Word attack	84*	14	below averaged
	Oral comprehension	98	45	average
Woodcock Johnson Tests of Cognitive Abilities–3rd Edition (WJ III COG)				
	Verbal comprehension	96	39	average
	Visual-auditory learning	90	25	lower end of average
	Spatial relations	92	30	average
	Sound bending	112	80	higher end of average
	Concept formation	107	68	average
	Visual matching	60*	0.4	very depressed
	Numbers reversed	97	43	average
	Verbal Ability Composite	96	39	average
	Thinking Ability Composite	95	41	average
	Cognitive Efficiency Composite	77*	6	depressed
	General Intellectual Ability	91	28	lower end of average

*Score is at or below one standard deviation below the mean.

These two subtest scores were combined to yield a *total word reading efficiency* score of 56 (<1st percentile).

The GORT-4 was used to assess Evan's reading fluency and comprehension. The GORT-4 consists of a series of stories beginning with the first grade level and progressing to advanced levels. Evan was asked to read a story aloud as quickly and accurately as possible and then answer five multiple-choice questions related to the story. A *fluency* score was computed for each story by combining his scores obtained for *rate* (time taken to read the passage) and *accuracy* (number of errors made). The mean score for these subtests is 10 with a standard deviation of ±3. These scores were combined to derive an *oral reading quotient*, which has a mean of 100 and a standard deviation of ±15. Evan's scores on the GORT-4 varied from very depressed to low average for his age. He obtained a reading rate score of 2 (<1st percentile) and an accuracy score of 1 (<1st percentile). These scores were combined to yield a very depressed range for his age and were combined to yield a very depressed fluency score of 1 (<1st percentile). In contrast, his *reading comprehension* score was 8 (25th percentile), which falls at the lower end of the average range for his age. These scores corresponded to an oral reading quotient of 67 (1st percentile), indicating that his oral reading skills were significantly depressed for his age. While reading aloud, Evan attempted to sound out most of the words in the passage. However, his attempts were frequently inaccurate showing limited word recognition ability. Despite his slow and inaccurate reading, he was able to comprehend the text, suggesting that he was able to use his world knowledge to comprehend the story even though he was not able to quickly identify the majority of the words.

Articulation

Evan did not exhibit any articulation errors in his speech.

Evaluation Summary

Evan Edsen is a 10-year-old male whose reading and reading-related abilities were assessed in the domains of phonological awareness, word recognition, decoding, spelling, reading comprehension, writing, reading fluency, and various math skills along with a number of other neurocognitive processing skills. Evan's scores from the present evaluation, along with parent observations, educational difficulties, and family history are consistent with a diagnosis of developmental dyslexia (ICD-9-CD, 315.02), along with a with a number of other neurocognitive processing skills. Evan's behavioral symptoms include depressed skills in the areas of phonological awareness; word reading; and nonword decoding in timed and untimed conditions; spelling; reading rate and accuracy in reading text; and in writing fluency. Evan demonstrated better reading comprehension than reading rate and accuracy, a classic sign of developmental dyslexia. Furthermore, he demonstrated a processing speed deficit on several tasks including the visual matching test on the WJ III COG, the RAN, and on all of the fluency tasks (reading, writing, math) on the WJ III ACH, in spite of his average composite scores on the WJ III COG for both thinking and verbal ability. Evan's scores are shown in Table 5-4 and a summary of his primary areas of strength and weakness is shown in Table 5-5.

TABLE 5-5 Summary of Evan's Primary Areas of Strength and Weakness

	Processing Speed	Working Memory	Verbal Abilities	Word Recognition	Fluency in Reading, Writing, Math	Rapid Naming	Reading Comprehension
Weakness	✓			✓	✓	✓	
Strength		✓	✓				✓

© Cengage Learning 2012

Recommendations

Since Evan presents with developmental dyslexia, academic accommodations and intensive, multisensory, or explicit intervention are essential for him to achieve his full potential. He will be able to advance his reading, writing, and spelling skills if appropriate instructional strategies and academic accommodations are instituted.

There is a high incidence of secondary emotional difficulties, such as frustration and depression, in students with learning disabilities who do not receive adequate instructional accommodations. Evan needs to be provided with alternative and appropriate instructional plan for reading and writing, as well as appropriate support in the areas in which he does well and enjoys.

It is recommended that:

1. Evan be enrolled in a multisensory phonics- and fluency-based instructional program, which provides intense one-on-one intervention. The International Dyslexia Association recommends that individuals with dyslexia be instructed in reading and spelling in a way that is direct, explicit, and simultaneously multisensory. The instruction should begin with phonemic awareness instruction, followed by a systematic approach to phonics, both analytic and synthetic. It should also teach reading and spelling as related subjects, with intense practice and constant weaving of the concepts taught. There are several multisensory structured language programs to choose from; some have been developed for individual tutoring and others have been developed for classroom use. Some examples are:

- Orton-Gillingham Method (Gillingham & Stillman, 1997)
- Barton Reading and Spelling Program (Barton, 2000)
- Lindamood Individualized Phoneme Sequencing Program (LiPS; Lindamood & Lindamood, 1998) (Note: This program focuses on phonological instruction.)
- Wilson Reading System (Wilson & Rupley, 1997)
- Specialized Program Individualizing Reading Excellence (S.P.I.R.E; Clark-Edmands, http://www.esp .schoolspecialty.com)
- Slingerland Multisensory Approach (Slingerland, 1971)
- Herman Approach
- Alphabetic Phonics (http://www.eps .schoolspecialty.com)

2. Lexercise (http://www.lexercise.com/), an advanced Web-based treatment program for children who have dyslexia or other language-based learning disabilities that result in reading difficulties at the word level, can be used. Under the direction of a practitioner, Lexercise can be used in schools, clinics, or home environments to practice the sequence of constructs that are taught in all Orton-Gillingham-based approaches to reading. These constructs are taught through carefully developed games that can be played at varying levels of complexity and speech. The games target a range of core reading components: (1) sounds and letters, (2) reading and spelling, (3) word parts, and (4) vocabulary. The various domains' targets and the specific skills and processes that are facilitated for each game within each domain are shown in Table 5-6.

3. Evan's parents consider a computer-based program such as the *Touchmath* program (http://**www.epsbooks.com**) to assist in facilitating his math fluency skills. This program uses a multisensory approach to teaching basic math skills.

4. Evan's parents read grade-level books to him or have him listen to grade-level books on tape in order to support his vocabulary growth. Some ideas for grade-level books can be found on http://www.bookadventure.org. On this Web site Evan can find a list of books at his reading level that interest him and also earn points for each book he reads that can be redeemed for awards and prizes.

5. Mrs. Edsen should have Evan tested for attention-deficit/hyperactivity disorder (ADHD) in light of her concern over his high activity level and the fact that he has difficulty sitting still. There is a high incidence of ADHD in children who have dyslexia.

It is also recommended that Mrs. Edsen visit the following Web sites: International Dyslexia Association (http://www.interdys.org) and Family Solutions for Dyslexia (http://www.dyslexiaanswers.com)

School-Based Accommodations

The nature of Evan's reading disability creates an impairment that substantially limits several major life activities, including reading and writing, and the potential for academic success. Because Evan is currently being homeschooled, Mrs. Edsen has the opportunity to tailor Evan's learning environment to best meet his needs. The following accommodations may be beneficial in helping Evan learn at home. In addition, if Evan attends public school in the future, he will need such accommodations in the classroom to meet his educational needs as adequately as a child without a disability. These accommodations can be provided through an Individualized Educational Plan (IEP) or a 504 plan.

1. Evan should have all textbooks available to him on audiotape to ensure that he is able to quickly access the content for each class that requires reading. Textbooks and other reading material can be accessed through Recording for the Blind & Dyslexic

TABLE 5-6 Sample of Lexercise Activities

1. Sounds & Letters	Isolator	Phonemic awareness: speech sound isolation and sequencing in two to five sound words
		Working memory for single spoken words and single speech sounds
		Rapid processing of speech sounds
	MatchStar: Sounds	Matching identical speech sounds
		Working memory for speech sounds
		Rapid processing of speech sounds
	MatchStar: Letters	Matching identical letters (graphemes)
		Working memory for letter (graphemes)
		Rapid processing of letters
	MatchStar: Sounds to Letters	Matching speech sounds (phonemes) with their letter symbols (graphemes)
		Working memory for speech sounds and their letter symbols
		Rapid processing of speech sounds and letter symbols
2. Reading & Spelling	MatchStar: Words Printed	Matching Identical printed words
		Working memory for printed words
		Rapid processing of printed words
	MatchStar: Words Spoken	Matching identical spoken words
		Working memory for spoken words
		Rapid processing of spoken words
	MatchStar: Words Spoken to Words Printed	Matching spoken words to printed words
		Working memory for spoken and printed words
		Rapid processing of spoken and printed words
3. Word Parts	MatchStar: Suffixes	Matching two forms of the same word: the base word and the word with a suffix
		Rapid processing of printed words
4. Vocabulary	DefineStar	Matching a spoken definition to a printed word
		Working memory for a spoken definition
		Reading single words accurately and quickly

(RFB&D) (http://www.learningally .org), which provides digitally recorded materials.

2. Evan should be given more time on tests and other class work and be given tests orally that require grade-level reading.

3. Evan should be allowed to use a calculator for his math assignments and tests. Students with dyslexia have a particularly difficult time memorizing rote facts such as addition and subtraction facts and the multiplication tables.

4. Evan's math instruction should focus on understanding math concepts and not on math calculation. Students with dyslexia can excel in understanding math concepts, especially those involving spatial relationships.

5. Evan should be allowed to dictate or type written assignments and be provided with Ginger software (http:// www.gingersoftware.com) for all written assignments. This software is designed to correct spelling and grammar errors and can be purchased with text-to-speech capabilities.

6. Evan should not be required to copy from the board or from a book. A peer note-taker should be provided, or the teacher should provide a copy of his own notes.

7. Evan should be given reduced homework assignments in all of his subjects.

8. These accommodations should be provided for all standardized tests.

Suggested Resources for Parents and Teachers

1. The Florida Center for Reading Research (http://www.fcrr.org) is an excellent resource for research information.

2. Moats, L. C., & Dakin, K. E. (2008). *Basic facts about dyslexia.* International Dyslexia Association Bookstore, Baltimore: International Dyslexia Association.

3. Hall, S. M., & Moats, L. C. (2002). *Parenting a struggling reader.* New York: Broadway Books.

4. Shaywitz, S. (2003). *Overcoming dyslexia: A new and complete science-based program for reading problems at any level.* New York: Knopf.

5. Ginger software for home and school use (http://www.gingersoftware.com).

SAMPLE DIAGNOSTIC REPORT FOR PROFILE 4B: DYSLEXIA (FOLLOW-UP EVALUATION)

Statement of Problem

Frank Fadino, an 11-year, 4-month-old male, was seen at a university language and literacy clinic on October 1, 2005 for a reevaluation of his reading and spelling skills (diagnostic procedure: 92506 [evaluation of speech and language]). Mr. Fadino, Frank's father, brought him to the clinic to determine his current level of functioning and to get updated recommendations.

Background Information

Frank was first seen at this university clinic 2 years ago for a reading evaluation. Results of the evaluation were consistent with a diagnosis of developmental dyslexia. Soon after, Frank began receiving intensive intervention using the Lindamood Phoneme Sequencing Program (LiPS) for 3 months, 6 hours a day. Mrs. Fadino reported that Frank's classroom performance significantly improved as a result of this intervention.

Frank is currently in fourth grade at First Street School in Key County, Florida. Mrs. Fadino reports that he is doing well in school but continues to demonstrate difficulty with spelling. Frank reported that he is receiving good grades and is on the Honor Roll. He stated that his favorite subjects are history, math, and physical education, and his least favorite subjects are writing and band. As for classroom accommodations in school, Frank receives extra time on tests as needed and he is not penalized for spelling errors on writing assignments. In addition, he is not required to take a foreign language. Since terminating the LiPS program, Frank has received weekly tutoring with one of his LiPS tutors. Frank stated that during their sessions they read together and practice writing. Frank reports that he spends 1 to 2 hours per night on homework and about 2 hours if he is studying for a test. Mr. Fadino reported that he reads with Frank every night.

Assessment Procedures

- Woodcock-Johnson Tests of Achievement–3rd Edition (WJ III ACH; Woodcock, McGrew, & Mather, 2001a)

- Gray Oral Reading Mastery Test–4 (GORT-4; Wiederholt & Bryant, 2001)

- Comprehensive Test of Phonological Processing (CTOPP; Wagner, Torgesen, & Rashotte, 1999a)

- Test of Word Reading Efficiency (TOWRE; Wagner, Torgesen, & Rashotte, 1999b)

- Written Language Sample (nonstandardized task)

Phonological Awareness Testing

The *Comprehensive Test of Phonological Processing* for ages 7 through 24 was used to assess phonological awareness, phonological memory, and rapid naming skills. The six core CTOPP subtests were given (refer to Profile 4a).

Frank's scores on the phonological awareness subtests ranged from below average on the *elision* (7; 16th percentile) subtest to average on the *sound blending* (9; 37th percentile) subtest, yielding *phonological awareness composite* of 88 (21st percentile). His scores on the phonological memory subtests ranged from below average on the *memory for digits* (7; 16th percentile) subtest to low average on the *nonword repetition* (8; 25th percentile) subtest, yielding *a phonological memory composite* of 85 (16th percentile).

The *rapid naming* subtest scores ranged from below average on the *rapid digit naming* (7; 16th percentile) subtest to low-average on the *rapid letter naming* (8; 25th percentile) subtest, yielding a *rapid naming composite* of 85 (16th percentile). Frank's performance on this test indicates that his ability to rapidly retrieve familiar words remains weak; however his composite scores for phonological awareness and rapid naming have improved since he was tested in 2008.

Reading Testing

The *Test of Word Reading Efficiency* (TOWRE) was used to measure Frank's ability to pronounce printed words in isolation accurately and fluently under timed conditions (refer to Profile 4a). Frank read 47 words correctly in 45 seconds, corresponding to a depressed *sight word efficiency* score of 79 (8th percentile). Similarly, he read 13 nonwords correctly in 45 seconds, corresponding to a depressed *phonemic decoding efficiency* score of 76 (6th percentile). These combined subtest scores yielded a *total word reading efficiency* score of 73 (4th percentile), which falls in the depressed range for his age. Frank's performance on this test indicates that his word-level reading fluency continues to be depressed.

The *Gray Oral Reading Test–4* is a test used to assess reading rate, accuracy, fluency, and comprehension (refer to Profile 4a). Frank's reading rate (4; 2nd percentile) and reading accuracy (3; 1st percentile) fell in the depressed range for his age. These scores combined yielded a very depressed reading fluency (2; <1st percentile) score. His

very depressed reading fluency underscores the difficulty of developing this skill even in learners who have had intensive word level intervention. In contrast, Frank's *reading comprehension* (11; 63rd percentile) fell within the average score. When his scores for fluency and comprehension were combined to yield an *oral reading quotient*, his overall score fell well below average (79; 8th percentile). Frank read the paragraphs very slowly and inaccurately. He did not recognize most words automatically. As Frank read aloud, he skipped words and often substituted words that were consistent with the content of the narratives showing that he was taking advantage of contextual cues and reading for meaning. Even though he did not accurately and automatically recognize many of the words in the passages, he was able to derive meaning from the passages by making good predictions and by using his background knowledge to compensate for his depressed word recognition.

Psychoeducational Tests of Academic Achievement

Eight subtests of the *Woodcock Johnson III Test of Achievement* (WJ III ACH) were administered to measure Frank's basic academic achievement in the domains of reading, spelling, and writing (refer to Profile 4a). The subtest standard scores were combined to obtain composite scores for *broad reading; broad written language; basic reading skills; basic writing skills,* and *written expression*.

On the WJ III ACH, Frank performed in the average range on the *writing samples* subtest (94; 34th percentile). He performed in the low average range on the *letter-word identification* (87; 19th percentile), *writing fluency* (83; 13th percentile), *passage comprehension* (82; 12th percentile), *word attack* (86; 18th percentile), and *editing* (86; 18th percentile) subtests. Frank's scores on the *reading fluency* (78; 8th percentile) and *spelling* (76; 6th percentile) subtests were depressed. He demonstrated the most difficulty with the spelling subtest. Examples of Frank's spelling errors are: "tadle" for *table*, "coked" for *cooked*, "flore" for *floor*, "secned" for *second*, "lear" for *early*, "reworde" for *rewards*, and "addvencher" for *adventure*. His errors experienced that he was using a phonics strategy in his attempts to spell. Also, Frank demonstrated spelling difficulties on the writing fluency and writing samples subtests, although these errors, along with capitalization and punctuation errors, were not counted off as these subtests are scored on content only. Frank did not use any proper capitalization with the exception of *I* on both writing subtests. Spelling errors on these writing subtests included "hacking" for *hatching*, "animle" for *animal*, "use" for *us*, "onpeing" for *opening*, and "con" for *come*. Frank's performance on the subtests yielded low average scores for the following composites: broad reading (80; 9th percentile), broad written language (80; 10th percentile), basic reading skills (86; 18th percentile), basic writing skills (82; 11th percentile), and written expression (86; 18th percentile).

Spontaneous Writing Sample

The WJ III ACH Writing Evaluation Scale was used to analyze Frank's writing sample.

The scoring system for this scale is a 4-point Likert scale in which 0 represents very poor performance and 4 represents very good performance for nine individual writing skills: handwriting, spelling, punctuation and capitalization, vocabulary, syntax/usage, narrative text structure, expository or event text structure, sense of audience, and affect.

Frank was asked to write about a topic of his choosing. He chose to write about the history of football and the first Super Bowl. His writing sample consisted of seven sentences. His paragraph was well organized with a clear beginning and ending. In addition, he used correct punctuation and age-appropriate vocabulary. In contrast, his sample contained many spelling errors. For example, he wrote "tack" for *took*, "rornid" for *forming*, and "fist" for *first*. Writing weaknesses were found with his handwriting and use of proper capitalization. His writing sample is shown in Figure 5-8.

Using the Handwriting Legibility Scale, Frank's handwriting on the writing samples subtest and his spontaneous writing sample was assessed. This analysis was based on the six elements that affect handwriting quality: slant, spacing, size, horizontal alignment, letter formation, and line quality. The scale ranges from 100 (artistic) to 0 (illegible) in 10-point increments. Frank received a rating of 20, which is considered fair. His handwriting was characterized by inconsistent letter slant, too-wide letter spacing within words and between words, uneven horizontal alignment, and poor general letter formation. His letter size and line quality were satisfactory.

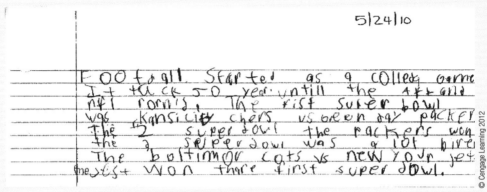

FIGURE 5-8 Frank's Writing Sample

Evaluation Summary

Frank Fadino, an 11-year, 4-month-old male, was evaluated for his reading and reading-related abilities in the areas of phonemic awareness, phonological memory, rapid naming, word recognition, word decoding, spelling, reading comprehension, writing, and reading fluency. His scores from this evaluation are consistent with a diagnosis of developmental dyslexia (ICD-9-CD, 315.02) that was given in 2008. This is expected because dyslexia is a lifelong condition. Individuals with dyslexia, even after intervention, typically continue to show weaknesses in reading and spelling, although they may make marked progress in their literacy skills.

Frank continues to demonstrate weaknesses in phonological processing, sight word recognition, decoding (phonics), encoding (spelling), reading fluency, and writing. In contrast, he has demonstrates well-developed reading comprehension skills. This discrepancy between reading fluency and reading comprehension is a classic sign of developmental dyslexia. Frank showed the greatest gains in reading comprehension since the last evaluation. His strong reading comprehension is consistent with his strong oral language skills. These strengths allow him to compensate for his weaknesses in word level reading and to perform well in the classroom. Frank's test scores from this evaluation and from his previous evaluation are shown in Table 5-7, and a summary of his primary areas of strength and weakness is shown in Table 5-8.

Recommendations

Frank continues to present with reading and spelling difficulties that are consistent with his previous diagnosis of dyslexia. Intensive, multisensory, explicit intervention and academic accommodations are essential for him to continue to succeed in both academic and personal environments.

It is recommended that:

1. Frank be enrolled in an Orton-Gillingham-based instructional reading program because of its

TABLE 5-7 Frank's Test Scores from Current and Previous Evaluations

	Current Test Scores (2010)			Previous Test Scores (2008)		
CTOPP	Standard Score	Percentile	Descriptive Rating	Standard Score	Percentile	Descriptive Rating
Elision	7*	16	below average	6*	9	depressed
Sound blending	9	37	average	8	25	low average
Phonological Awareness	88	21	lower end of average	82*	12	below average
Memory for digits	7*	16	below average	7*	16	below average
Nonword repetition	8	25	low average	8	25	low average
Phonological Memory	85*	16	below average	85*	16	below average
Rapid digit naming	7*	16	below average	6*	9	depressed
Rapid letter naming	8	25	low average	7*	16	below average
Rapid Naming	85*	16	below average	79*	8	depressed
TOWRE	Standard Score	Percentile	Descriptive Rating	Standard Score	Percentile	Descriptive Rating
Sight word efficiency	79*	8	depressed	67**	1	very depressed
Phonemic decoding efficiency	76*	6	depressed	82*	12	below average
Total Word Reading Efficiency	73*	4	depressed	69**	2	very depressed
GORT-4	Standard Score	Percentile	Descriptive Rating	Standard Score	Percentile	Descriptive Rating
Rate	4**	2	very depressed	2**	<1	very depressed
Accuracy	3**	1	very depressed	1**	<1	very depressed
Fluency (rate + accuracy)	2**	<1	very depressed	1**	<1	very depressed
Comprehension	11	63	average	6	9	depressed
Oral Reading Quotient	79*	8	depressed	61*	<1	very depressed
WJ III ACH	Standard Score	Percentile	Descriptive Rating	Standard Score	Percentile	Descriptive Rating
Letter-word identification	87	19	lower end of average	77*	2	depressed
Passage comprehension	82*	12	below average	78*	7	depressed
Spelling	76*	6	depressed	70**	2	very depressed
Writing fluency	83*	13	below average	63**	1	very depressed
Writing samples	94	34	average	80*	9	below average

(*continues*)

TABLE 5-7 (*continued*)

WJ III ACH	Standard Score	Percentile	Descriptive Rating	Standard Score	Percentile	Descriptive Rating
Word attack	86	18	low average	81*	10	low average
Reading fluency	78*	8	below average	70**	2	very depressed
Editing	86	18	low average	NA	NA	
Broad Reading Skills	80*	9	below average	68**	2	very depressed
Broad Written Language	80*	10	average	64**	1	far below average
Basic Reading Skills	86	18	low average	74*	4	below average
Basic Writing Skills	82*	11	below average	N/A	N/A	
Written Expression	86	18	low average	65**	1	far below average
CELF-4	Standard Score	Percentile	Descriptive Rating	Standard Score	Percentile	Descriptive Rating
Core Language Score	NA	NA	NA	12	75	higher end of average

* Score is more than one standard deviation below the mean or average score
** Score is more than two standard deviations below the mean or average score

© Cengage Learning 2012

TABLE 5-8 Frank's Primary Areas of Strength and Weakness

	Short-term Memory	Word Recognition	Decoding	Spelling	Fluency in Reading and Writing	Reading Comprehension	Spoken Language
Weakness	✓	✓		✓	✓		
Strength			✓			✓	✓

© Cengage Learning 2012

simultaneous emphasis on reading and spelling real words in isolation and in sentences, and its focus on orthographic patterns. Orton-Gillingham-based systems begin with instruction of phonemic awareness, followed by a systematic approach to phonics, both analytic and synthetic. These systems also teach reading and spelling skills simultaneously. Orton-Gillingham-based systems provide multisensory phonics and fluency-based instruction. Programs that meet these requirements include the

Barton Reading and Spelling System, Alphabetic Phonics, Spalding Reading Method, and the Wilson Reading Program. Therapy should be for 1 hour 2–3 times per week after school or on the weekends if during school is not possible (see Recommendation 3 below). The Lexercise supplemental instructional program (http://www.lexercise.com/) should be considered to augment weekly intervention sessions.

2. Programs such as the *Read Naturally One Minute Reader* (http://www.readnaturally.com) or *Quick Reads: A Research-Based Fluency Program* (http://www.pearsonlearning.com) can be used to facilitate improved reading fluency.

3. Mr. and Mrs. Fadino share the results of this evaluation with pertinent school personnel. Ideally, Frank should receive intervention in school, through reading and writing lab pull-outs on a daily basis using an Orton-Gillingham-based reading program. As academic demands continue to increase throughout the elementary and middle school years, Frank may need additional assistance (e.g., tutoring) for academic coursework, especially as the complexity of words in his reading curricula increase.

4. Frank be allowed to access school accommodations that can provide him with additional assistance to promote his academic success. Academic demands will continue to increase as Frank gets older, so more assistance may be needed in order to ensure his academic success. Below is a list of classroom accommodations that Frank may find beneficial. Some of these accommodations may be appropriate now, or may become necessary as Frank advances in school:

- Frank should be given more time on tests and other class work. This includes more time on all standardized tests.

- Because of his reading difficulty, oral administration of tests may be necessary.

- Frank should use a computer for all written assignments so that he can use a spell-check program (see Ginger writing software). He should not be penalized for errors in spelling, grammar, punctuation, and capitalization.

- Frank should not be required to read aloud in class, participate in spelling bees, or exchange papers for grading.

- Frank should be provided with books on audiotape for all reading assignments when needed.

- Frank should not be required to copy from the board or from a book. A peer note-taker should be provided, or the teacher should provide a copy of his own notes.

- Math instruction should focus on memorization. For math problems that require a sequence of steps to solve, he should be given a list of these steps. Students with dyslexia can excel in understanding math concepts, especially those involving spatial relationships.

- If Frank does not recognize words from grade-level texts, a list of these words should be created and practiced.

- Frank is encouraged to find books at his reading level (not grade level) and read for at least 20 minutes per day. One way to encourage Frank to continue reading and to find appropriate grade-level books is to use the http://www.bookadventure.org Web site. On this Web site, Frank can find a list of books at his reading level that interest him and also earn points for each book he reads.

5. Mr. and Mrs. Fadino continue to read grade-level books to Frank or have him listen to books on tape in order to support vocabulary growth.

6. Mr. and Mrs. Fadino look into the *Language Tune-Up Kit* at *Home Reading Software* (jwor@jwor.com). This Orton-Gillingham-based software assists individuals from 6 years through adulthood to hone their reading skills at home.

7. Mr. and Mrs. Fadino and Frank might want to explore the *Confident Reader Program.* (http://www.confidentreader.com). This program, which consists of assistive reading software, converts electronic text to speech using a natural-sounding, computer-generated voice. The Confident Reader reads electronic text (such as e-books, Web pages, pdf files, Microsoft Word documents). The typing-echo feature recites text automatically by letter, word, or sentences so mistakes in typing are heard and can be corrected.

8. A list of qualified tutors in their residential area can be found on the International Dyslexia Association's (http://www.interdys.org) along with numerous resources on reading disorders. Additionally, numerous scientifically based resources for treating reading disabilities can be found at the Florida Center for Reading Research (http://www.fcrr.org).

SAMPLE DIAGNOSTIC REPORT FOR PROFILE 5: MIXED SPOKEN LANGUAGE AND READING

Statement of Problem

Gail Gomez, an 8-year, 8-month-old female, was seen at a university language and literacy clinic on June 1, 2010 (diagnostic procedure: 92506 [evaluation of speech and language]). Mrs. Gomez, Gail's biological mother, brought her daughter to the clinic for a reading evaluation because she has been struggling with class work, taking substantially longer than other students in the class to complete assignments, and showing a lack of focus and organization during tasks. Gail's pediatrician recommended that she have her reading skills evaluated to rule out a language learning disability before further testing for attention deficit disorder.

Background Information

Developmental and Medical History

Mrs. Gomez reported that her pregnancy was free of complications, except that Gail was born 1 month premature. She was healthy at the time of her birth. Gail reached all communication and developmental milestones at the appropriate ages. Mrs. Gomez rated her daughter's general health as good, although she has been diagnosed with asthma. Gail's hearing has been found to be normal. Mrs. Gomez reported a negative family history for learning difficulties. Gail has been raised in a bilingual environment and she has been speaking English fluently since 2 years of age. Although her grandparents often speak to her in Spanish, both her parents speak to her in English only.

Educational History

Gail just completed second grade at Fifth Street School in Keys County, Florida, and is going into third grade in the fall. Mrs. Gomez reported that Gail did well academically in prekindergarten, kindergarten, first, and second grade. She stated that Gail has maintained good grades throughout but has shown difficulty focusing on tasks and getting assignments completed in a timely manner. Mrs. Gomez stated that Gail was in the middle reading group in her second grade class. Mrs. Gomez was told by Gail's teacher that Gail often "zones out" in class, often acts very tired during the school day, and sometimes falls asleep in class, even after sleeping over 8 hours the night before. Mrs. Gomez also reported that homework has been an especially difficult area, as Gail tends to lose focus and needs hours to complete assignments.

Assessment Procedures

The purpose of this assessment was to evaluate Gail's spoken and written language abilities in conjunction with her general cognitive abilities to determine if she has a reading disability. The following tests were used:

- Woodcock-Johnson Tests of Achievement 3rd Edition Form A (WJ III ACH; Woodcock, McGrew, & Mather, 2001a)
- Woodcock-Johnson Tests of Cognitive Abilities–3rd Edition (WJ III COG; Woodcock, McGrew, & Mather, 2001b)
- Gray Oral Reading Mastery Test–4 (GORT-4; Wiederholt & Bryant, 2001)

- Comprehensive Test of Phonological Processing (CTOPP; Wagner, Torgesen, & Rashotte, 1999a)

- Test of Word Reading Efficiency (TOWRE; Wagner, Torgesen, & Rashotte, 1999b)

- Clinical Evaluation of Language Fundamentals–4 (CELF-4; Semel, Wiig, & Secord, 2003)

- Written Language Sample (nonstandardized task)

Psychoeducational Cognitive Testing

Three subtests from the Woodcock-Johnson Tests of Cognitive Abilities-3rd Edition (WJ III COG) were used to obtain a composite score for *brief intellectual ability* (BIA). These subtests measured *verbal comprehension*, *concept formation*, and *visual matching* (refer to Profile 4a). Gail performed in the low range on the verbal comprehension (77; 7th percentile) and visual matching (79; 8th percentile) subtests, and at the lower end of the average range on the concept formation (87; 20th percentile) subtest. Her subtest scores were combined to yield a below average BIA composite (78; 7th percentile). Gail's performance on this test indicates that she has weak oral vocabulary and processing speed, with a relative strength in reasoning.

Phonological Awareness Testing

The *Comprehensive Test of Phonological Processing* for ages 7 through 24 was used to assess *phonological awareness*, *phonological memory*, and *rapid naming* skills (refer to

Profile 4a). Gail's scores on the phonological awareness subtests ranged from average (*elision*, 10; 50th percentile) to above average (*blending words*, 14; 91st percentile) for her age. These scores were combined to yield a *phonological awareness composite* of 112 (79th percentile), which falls in the high average range for her age. Her scores on the phonological memory subtests ranged from below average (*nonword repetition*, 6; 9th percentile) to average (*memory for digits*, 9; 37th percentile), corresponding to a *phonological memory composite* of 85 (16th percentile). This score falls in the low-average range for her age. Her scores on the rapid naming subtests ranged from very poor (*rapid digit naming*, 3; <1st percentile) to below average (*rapid letter naming*, 6; 9th percentile), corresponding to a very depressed *rapid-naming composite* of 55 (<1st percentile). On the rapid naming tests, Gail frequently began to say a number or letter then quickly self-corrected with an accurate response (e.g., if the number was a "3," she would begin to say "7," and then quickly self-correct). Also, there were instances in which she seemed to lose her place when naming the RAN stimuli. Her performance on the CTOPP indicates that her phonological awareness skills are age appropriate, but her phonological memory is somewhat weak, and her rapid naming abilities are depressed for her age.

Reading Testing

The *Test of Word Reading Efficiency* (TOWRE) was used to measure Gail's ability to pronounce printed words in isolation accurately and fluently under timed conditions (refer to Profile 4a). On the *sight word*

TABLE 5-9 Gail's Test Scores

Test	Subtest	Standard Score	Percentile Rank	Descriptive Rating
Clinical Evaluation of Language Fundamentals–4 (CELF-4)				
	Formulating sentences	6	9	depressed
	Understanding spoken paragraphs	6	9	depressed
	Recalling sentences	8	25	lower end of average
Test of Word Reading Efficiency (TOWRE)				
	Sight word efficiency	85	16	below average
	Phonemic decoding efficiency	90	25	lower end of average
	Total Word Reading Efficiency	85	16	below average
Comprehensive Test of Phonological Processes (CTOPP)				
	Elision	10	50	average
	Blending words	14	91	above average
	Phonological Awareness Composite	112	79	higher end of average
	Memory for digits	9	37	average
	Nonword repetition	6*	9	depressed
	Phonological Memory Composite	85	16	below average
	Rapid letter naming	6*	9	depressed
	Rapid digit naming	3*	<1	very depressed
	Rapid Naming Composite	56*	<1	very depressed
Gray Oral Reading Test–4th Edition (GORT-4)				
	Rate	3*	1	very depressed
	Accuracy	7*	16	below average
	Fluency (rate + accuracy)	5*	5	depressed
	Passage comprehension	9	36	average
	Oral Reading Quotient	82*	12	below average
Woodcock Johnson Tests of Achievement–3rd Edition (WJ III ACH)				
	Letter-word identification	97	43	average
	Reading fluency	86	18	low average
	Spelling	101	52	average
	Writing fluency	94	35	average
	Writing samples	90	26	lower end of average
	Word attack	115	83	above average
	Passage comprehension	96	39	average
Woodcock Johnson Tests of Cognitive Abilities–3rd EDITION (WJ III COG)				
	Verbal comprehension	77*	7	below average
	Concept formation	87	20	lower end of average
	Visual matching	79*	8	below average
	Brief Intellectual Ability	78*	7	below average

*score is at or below one standard deviation of the mean.

efficiency subtest, she read 34 words correctly in 45 seconds, corresponding to a standard score of 85 (16th percentile). Examples of her errors included reading "fin" for *fine* and "keen" for *kind*. On the *phonemic decoding efficiency* subtest, she read 14 words correctly in 45 seconds, corresponding to a standard score of 90 (25th percentile). Gail's *total word reading efficiency* score of 85 (16th percentile) is in the low average range for her age.

The *Gray Oral Reading Test–4* is used to assess *reading rate, accuracy, fluency,* and *comprehension* (refer to Profile 4a). Gail's reading rate score (3; 1st percentile) was very depressed while her accuracy score (7; 16th percentile) was below average. The rate and accuracy scores combined yielded a depressed fluency score (5; 5th percentile). In contrast, Gail's *reading comprehension* score (9; 36th percentile) fell within the average range. Her oral reading quotient of 82 is in the low average range (12th percentile).

As noted by her depressed fluency score, Gail's reading of the GORT-4 paragraphs was extremely slow. As she read the paragraphs out loud, she frequently read words over and over correctly before she moved to the next word. Her reading accuracy was better than her rate but still below the level expected for her age. Examples of her word reading errors are: "go" for *goes*, "sad" for *said*, "own" for *one*, and "pill" for *pile*. In spite of her depressed fluency and borderline accuracy scores, Gail showed average reading comprehension.

Academic Achievement Testing

Eight subtests from the *Woodcock-Johnson III Test of Achievement* (WJ III ACH) were used

to measure Gail's academic achievement in the domains of reading, spelling, and writing (refer to Profiles 4a and 4b). Gail performed above average on the *word-attack* (115; 83rd percentile) subtest and in the average range on the *passage comprehension* (96; 39th percentile), *spelling* (101; 52nd percentile), *writing samples* (90; 25th percentile), *writing fluency* (94; 35th percentile), *editing* (90; 26th percentile), and *letter-word identification* (97; 43rd percentile) subtests. Consistent with her performance on the GORT-4, she showed the most difficulty on the *reading fluency* (86; 18th percentile) subtest, for which her score was in the low average range for her age. Gail's overall performance on the WJ III ACH tests showed a strength in decoding and a weakness in reading fluency. An unexpected pattern was observed in that Gail's reading comprehension scores on the GORT-4 and WJ III ACH tests were much higher than her verbal comprehension score on the WJ III COG. This discrepancy between verbal comprehension and reading comprehension may be due to test format differences. The verbal comprehension test measures lexical knowledge without context whereas both comprehension measures, although different from each other in format, measure reading in context.

Spontaneous Writing Sample

The *Writing Evaluation Scale* from the WJ III ACH was used to analyze a writing sample in which Gail was asked to write a paragraph about things that were fun to her. The scoring system is a 4-point Likert scale in which 0 represents very poor performance and 4 represents very good performance for nine writing skills: handwriting, spelling, punctuation and capitalization, vocabulary, syntax/usage, narrative text structure, expository or event text structure, sense of audience, and affect.

Gail received an overall score of 1 on these components, which corresponds to a poor rating for her age. Her writing contained no elements of a cohesive text structure. Her sentences were not linked together; they were simply five descriptive sentences about things that she likes. Her sentences were all similar in form (e.g., "I like . . .") and written in a list-like format. Further testing is required to assess her ability to write text because it is unclear whether this sample reflects her knowledge of written text structure. It is possible that Gail did not understand the directive to write a paragraph.

Examples of her spelling errors include: "qucoot" for *cute*, "yello" for *yellow*, and "charly" for *Charlie*. According to Mrs. Gomez, the word "sgumale" in the handwriting sample shown in Figure 5-9 is a made-up word for one of her toys. Gail spelled most regularly spelled words correctly, but had difficulty with irregularly spelled words. Although Gail placed periods at the end of each idea, in most instances she failed to connect independent clauses with a conjunction or use a period to separate independent clauses.

Using the *Handwriting Legibility Scale*, from the WJ III ACH, Gail's handwriting on the writing samples subtest and on her spontaneous writing sample was analyzed. This analysis was based on the following six elements that affect handwriting quality: slant, spacing, size, horizontal alignment, letter formation, and line quality. The scale ranges from 100 (artistic) to 0 (illegible) in 10-point increments. She received a rating of 50, which is considered satisfactory. Gail's handwriting was characterized by consistent slant, letter size and letter formation. However, her horizontal alignment of the letters on the line and spacing were inconsistent.

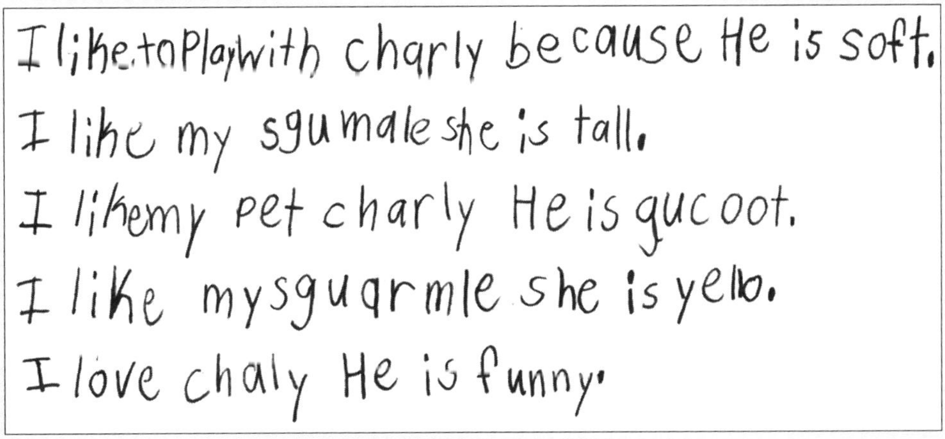

FIGURE 5-9 Gail's Writing Sample

Spoken Language Testing

Three subtests from the *Clinical Evaluation of Language Fundamentals–4* (CELF-4) were used to measure Gail's receptive and expressive oral language skills. The following three subtests were administered: *formulating sentences* measures vocabulary and grammar by having the student use a given word in a sentence about a picture provided; *recalling sentences* measures auditory comprehension, syntax, and vocabulary of increasing length and complexity by having the student repeat sentences provided by the examiner; and *understanding spoken paragraphs* measures the auditory comprehension of paragraphs of increasing length and complexity by having the student answer questions about a paragraph that has been read by the examiner.

Gail received a standard score of 6 (9th percentile) on both the formulating sentences and understanding spoken paragraphs subtests, which is in the depressed range for her age. On the recalling sentences subtest, she scored 8 (25th percentile), which falls at the lower end of the average range for her age. Her performance on these subtests indicates depressed receptive and expressive oral language. These scores are consistent with her depressed verbal comprehension score on the WJ III COG.

Observations

Gail appeared to have difficulty staying on task and needed constant reminders to focus and attend to tasks. She seemed very sleepy and tired, even though she was given several breaks throughout the testing session. Examples of her behavior included not listening to questions, putting her head down on the table on several occasions, and not paying attention to subtest directions. Although Gail demonstrated these focusing difficulties, she was able to redirect her attention and focus on the testing stimuli when given prompts or repetition of directions, which was done several times during the testing session. Although it is possible that her lack of energy/focus could have affected her scores on these tests, her scores are generally considered to be an accurate representation of her abilities. It is interesting to note that her ability to focus on the testing stimuli greatly improved after the examiner told her that she was almost finished for the day. In addition, she seemed to have much more energy when she was out of the testing room on breaks or leaving for lunch.

Evaluation Summary

Gail Gomez, an 8-year, 8-month-old female, was evaluated for her reading and reading-related abilities in the domains of phonological awareness, phonological memory, rapid naming, word recognition, word decoding, spelling, reading comprehension, writing, reading fluency, and oral language. On this battery of tests, she demonstrated weaknesses in both her written (reading) and oral language skills. Her profile is consistent with the diagnoses of reading disability, unspecified (315.00), and mixed receptive and expressive language disability (315.32). The test results show strengths in phonological awareness, word decoding, reading fluency, and spelling, and weaknesses in rapid naming, verbal comprehension, working memory, and processing speed. Gail's scores for

TABLE 5-10   Summary of Gail's Primary Areas of Strength and Weakness

	Processing Speed	Working Memory	Phonological Awareness	Decoding	Rapid Naming	Fluency	Language Concepts	Writing Composition	Writing Mechanics
Weakness	✓	✓			✓	✓	✓	✓	
Strength			✓	✓					✓

© Cengage Learning 2012

all tests administered are shown in Table 5-9. Gail's primary areas of strength and weakness are shown in Table 5-10.

Recommendations

Based on Gail Gomez's performance on this battery of tests, and in conjunction with parental report and school performance, it is recommended that:

1. Gail be evaluated by a medical specialist who diagnoses and treats children with attention deficit disorder and other neurodevelopmental disorders.

2. Gail receive language intervention that targets word meanings in the context of listening comprehension activities.

3. Gail be given a more complete oral language evaluation in the context of diagnostic therapy. Because of her attentional problems, it was difficult to obtain a comprehensive profile of Gail's spoken language skills. A structured language sample along with an assessment of Gail's use of discourse across modalities (speaking, writing) and genres (narrative, expository) is advised.

4. Gail receive reading intervention that targets strengthening her reading fluency and improving her knowledge of word meanings. Programs such as the *One Minute Reader* (http://www.oneminutereader.com) *and Quick Reads: A Research–Based Fluency Program* (http://www.pearsonlearning.com) are recommended. These programs have been shown to facilitate automatic word reading ability in connected text through repeated, timed readings.

5. Mrs. Gomez share the results of this evaluation with pertinent school personnel. Gail will most likely require additional assistance (e.g., tutoring) for academic coursework, especially as the demands on reading increase with grade.

6. Mrs. Gomez investigate the *Language Tune-Up Kit* at Home Reading Software. This highly effective tool, which is based on the Orton-Gillingham principles, helps individuals from 6 years old through adulthood develop their reading skills at home through the eighth-grade reading level. More information about this software can be found at http://www.jwor.com.

The nature of Gail Gomez's disability creates an impairment that substantially limits several major life activities, including reading and writing, learning and listening.

To meet her educational needs as adequately as a child without these disabilities, Gail will need the following classroom accommodations, which can be provided through a 504 Plan. Some of these accommodations may not be appropriate now, but may be needed in later grades.

The following accommodations are recommended:

1. Gail should be given extended time on tests and other class work. The same accommodation should be provided for all standardized tests.

2. Gail should not be required to learn a foreign language. Because of her language-learning difficulties, this could be a very frustrating and stressful challenge.

3. Gail should be given reduced homework assignments in all of her subjects, as needed.

Suggested Resources for Parents and Teachers

1. Rasinski, T. (2003). *The fluent reader: Oral reading strategies for building word recognition, fluency, and comprehension.* New York: Scholastic Professional Books.

2. QuickReads (http://www.pearsonlearning.com) is a series of educational and interesting texts designed to facilitate vocabulary and fluency through varying levels of text difficulty.

3. Language Tune-Up Kit (http://www.jwor.com). This is an interactive-reading software program based on Orton-Gillingham principles that includes (1) word building, (2) oral reading of sentences, and (3) stories with comprehension questions and oral dictation for typing.

SAMPLE DIAGNOSTIC REPORT FOR PROFILE 6: COMPREHENSION DEFICIT

Statement of Problem

Harry Harper, a 14-year, 8-month-old male, was seen at our university language and literacy clinic on March 18, 2009. Harry was accompanied to the evaluation by his father. Mr. Harper reported that Harry is having difficulty in school, particularly in the area of reading comprehension and comprehension of mathematics problems. Although Harry is doing satisfactory work in school, Mr. Harper states that Harry works very hard at his studies and often becomes frustrated because it takes him much more time than his classmates to complete his in-class work and his homework assignments. Mr. Harper noted that although Harry's grades are satisfactory, he would like Harry to address his learning difficulties now so he can enjoy his high school years and succeed in school without experiencing a great deal of stress. Mr. Harper reported much of the historical information on Harry's development. Harry briefly discussed his frustrations with school and said that he only reads when he needs to find the answer to a question.

Background Information

Developmental and Medical History

Harry lives with his father, stepmother, two younger sisters, and younger brother.

Mr. Harper reported that Harry's early development was normal. He first became aware of Harry's problems between the fourth and fifth grades, when Harry seemed to have difficulty comprehending his school texts. In sixth grade, Harry was diagnosed with attention deficit disorder for which he takes medication daily.

Educational and Family History

Harry is completing eighth grade at First Street Middle School and hopes to begin ninth grade at Second Street High School next fall. He recently took an entrance exam in preparation for beginning high school. He did not do well on the reading comprehension or mathematics portions of the exam. Despite Harry's poor performance on the entrance exams, school officials are willing to admit Harry into the ninth grade. There is no known family history of speech, language, or reading difficulties.

Assessment Procedures

Purpose of Testing and Test Protocol

The purpose of today's visit was to determine if Harry has a language-based learning disability and to recommend strategies to help him succeed in high school. The following diagnostic tools were used:

- Comprehensive Test of Phonological Processing (CTOPP; Wagner, Torgesen, & Rashotte, 1999a)
- Gray Oral Reading Mastery Test–4th Edition (GORT-4); Wiederholt & Bryant, 2001)
- Test of Word Reading Efficiency (TOWRE; Wagner, Torgesen, & Rashotte, 1999b)

- Wide Range Achievement Test–3rd Edition (WRAT-3; Wilkinson, 1993)
- Woodcock Reading Mastery Tests–Revised (WRMT-R; Woodcock & Pines, 1998)
- Clinical Evaluation of Language Fundamentals–4th Edition (CELF-4; Wiig & Secord, 2003)
- Written Language Sample (nonstandardized task)

Phonological Processing, Reading, and Spelling Testing

The *Comprehensive Test of Phonological Processing* (CTOPP) was used to assess Harry's phonological awareness, phonological memory, and rapid-naming skills (see Profile 4a for a complete description of this test). Composite scores were calculated for *phonological awareness*, *phonological memory*, and *rapid naming*. Harry's scores on the phonological-processing subtests ranged from average to high average, with the majority of his scores clustering around the average range. Harry's highest subtest score of 13 was in *rapid letter-naming*, with a standard score of 13, and his lowest subtest score of 7 was on *memory for digits*. Harry's performance showed a clear strength in rapid naming with a high average standard score of 112.

The *Woodcock Reading Mastery Tests–Revised* (WRMT-R) was administered to measure Harry's reading abilities for single word reading, nonsense word decoding, passage comprehension, and word comprehension. The *word identification* subtest measured Harry's ability to read isolated words. The *word attack* subtest was used to measure his ability to apply phonics skills in reading phonetically structured non-words. The *passage comprehension* subtest measured Harry's ability to read a short passage and identify a missing word in that passage. The *word comprehension* subtest measured his reading vocabulary for antonyms, synonyms, and analogies. Harry's subtest scores ranged from a superior score of 139 in word identification to an average score of 96 for passage comprehension. He performed similarly on the test of word comprehension (i.e., knowledge of word meanings) and passage comprehension with average scores of 98 and 96, respectively. In contrast, he performed in the high average range in word decoding with a score of 114 and in the superior range in word recognition with a score of 139. Harry's composite score for *basic skills* (word identification and word decoding) was 127 and his composite score for *reading comprehension* (word comprehension and passage comprehension) was 97. This discrepancy between good word-level reading and comprehension skills is the signature profile of a reading comprehension disorder.

The *Gray Oral Reading Mastery Test–4th Edition* (GORT-4) was used to assess Harry's reading fluency (rate + accuracy), and comprehension (see Profile 4a for a complete description of this test). Harry's reading *fluency* score (12, 75th percentile) was in the high average range and contrasted with his weak *reading comprehension* score (6, 9th percentile). As in the pattern noted on the WRMT-R above, Harry's

profile of poor comprehension and good fluency is the *opposite* of the signature profile of students who have dyslexia. He exhibited a clear weakness in answering reading comprehension questions as demonstrated by his below average scaled score of 6. His *oral reading quotient* fell in the average range and reflects a combination of strong reading accuracy and weak passage comprehension.

The *Test of Word Reading Efficiency* (TOWRE) was used to measure Harry's *sight word efficiency* and *phonemic decoding efficiency* (see Profile 4a for a complete description of this test). His standard score of 111 for phonemic decoding efficiency falls in the high average range and his sight word efficiency score of 106 falls in the average range. Overall, Harry's *total word reading efficiency* score is average.

The *Wide Range Achievement Test–3rd Edition* (WRAT-3) was used to assess Harry's reading and spelling abilities. For the *reading* subtest, he read a series of words that increased in difficulty. For the *spelling* subtest, he spelled to dictation a series of words that increased in difficulty. The mean standard score for these tests is 100 with a standard deviation of ±15. Harry's standard score of 122 on the reading subtest was well above average and his spelling subtest score of 113 fell at the high end of the average range.

Spoken Language Testing

Six subtests from the *Clinical Evaluation of Language Fundamentals–4th Edition* (CELF-4) were used to measure Harry's expressive and receptive language on four types of language tasks. The *recalling sentences* subtest evaluated his ability to (a) listen to spoken sentences of increasing length and complexity; and (b) repeat sentences without changing word meanings, inflections, derivations, or sentence structure. The *formulating sentences* subtest evaluated his ability to formulate semantically and grammatically correct spoken sentences using specific words. The *word class receptive and expressive* subtests evaluated his ability to understand (receptive) and to explain (expressive) logical relationships in the meanings of associated words, respectively. The *word definitions* subtest assessed his ability to define words by describing them as well as referring to class relationships and shared meanings. Harry performed within the average range on all subtests of the CELF-4. His *core language* score was 100 and his subtest scores ranged from 9 to 11.

Written Language Sample

A written language sample was taken to assess Harry's ability to formulate and generate written text. He was given the following prompt: "Write about a memorable moment in your life and include as much detail as you can recall." A transcription of Harry's written sample is shown in Box 5-1.

The sample was examined for syntactic and semantic accuracy, spelling accuracy, punctuation, and story organization and cohesion. His sentences were generally well constructed and the sample was free of spelling errors. Although Harry showed some knowledge of the organizational structure of a story by including a topic and a concluding sentence, he (1) failed to explain the causal factors associated with

BOX 5-1 **Transcription of Harry's Written Language Sample**

My most memorable moment was when I moved to Nevada. The ride there was the worst part because I had to ride in a Uhaul [*sic*] truck with my uncle. When I got there I unpacked my things and put them in my room. The next day I went outside and played baseball with my sisters. Then a couple months later August rolled around and school started, the school was called Middleton School. A few weeks later I started baseball at the league in Las Vegas that some of the kids from the school played at. In conclusion, my move to Nevada was my most memorable moment.

driving with his uncle ("The ride there was the worst part because I had to ride in a Uhaul [sic] truck with my uncle,"), (2) failed to tell why his move to Nevada was one of the most memorable events in his life, (3) failed to provide the reader with enough information to understand his feelings, and (4) failed to tell an integrated and cohesive story; instead he listed a sequence of events.

Evaluation Summary

Harry Harper, a 14-year, 8-month-old male was evaluated for his abilities in reading and reading-related domains including phonological awareness, reading, spelling, writing, and spoken language. He demonstrated a profile of strengths and weaknesses that reflect a specific deficit in reading comprehension, otherwise classified as a nonspecific reading disability (ICD-9-315.00). This type of reading disability is associated with a relative weakness in the semantic domain of language.

Harry performed very well on tests of word decoding, word recognition, and spelling, In contrast, he demonstrated a weaknesses in reading comprehension and written composition. Harry's knowledge of word meanings was in the average range in spite of his superior ability to read words. Harry's test scores are shown in Table 5-11 and a summary of his primary areas of strength and weakness are shown in Table 5-12.

Recommendations

Harry Harper is a bright young man with a specific disability that is negatively impacting his life. He spends more time than the average student on his homework and experiences frustration with his work. However, with the proper intervention his deficit in reading comprehension should not prevent him from succeeding academically. Harry currently approaches reading comprehension questions by looking for the answers in the text without having a solid understanding of what he has read. This is not an efficient way to comprehend text, and as Harry's academic demands increase, this strategy will become less productive. Thus, the following recommendations are made to promote Harry's success in school. Language therapy for Harry should focus on teaching him comprehension strategies that he can implement prior to reading, during reading, and after reading.

It is recommended that:

1. Harry be taught to use graphic organizers to help him synthesize the information he is reading. Graphic organizers include but are not limited to: chronology and sequence, description and enumeration, classification, comparison and contrast, cause and effect, and problem and solution.

2. Harry be taught to use a prereading strategy to help him activate his background knowledge when reading text. This strategy can also help increase his interest in reading text.

3. Harry be taught to use semantic webbing, which can assist him with selecting pertinent information from the reading material that is assigned as part of his school work.

4. Harry be taught how to monitor his comprehension while reading for information. For instance, he can learn to code text with a "+" for information he already knows. He can code with a "!" for information that is new and code text with a "?" for information that is unclear.

5. Harry be taught metacognitive strategies for answering questions. In order for Harry to benefit from this type of strategy, it is important that he practice answering both explicit and implicit questions. It is also important for Harry to be aware of how he answered the questions. For

TABLE 5-11 Harry's Test Scores

Test	Subtest	Standard Score	Percentile Rank	Descriptive Rating
Comprehensive Test of Phonological Processes (CTOPP)				
	Elision	10	50	average
	Blending words	9	37	average
	Memory for digits	7*	16	below average
	Nonword repetition	10	50	average
	Rapid digit naming	11	63	average
	Rapid letter naming	13	84	higher end of average
	Phonological Awareness Composite	97	42	average
	Phonological Memory Composite	91	27	lower end of average
	Rapid Naming Composite	112	79	high average
Woodcock Reading Mastery Tests-Revised (WRMT-R)				
	Word identification	139	99.6	superior
	Word attack	114	82	high average
	Word comprehension	98	45	average
	Passage comprehension	96	40	average
	Basic Skills Cluster	127	96	well above average
	Reading Comprehension Cluster	97	41	average
	Total Reading Cluster	112	79	higher end of average
Gray Oral Reading Test–4th Edition (GORT-4)				
	Rate	10	50	average
	Accuracy	13	84	above average
	Fluency (rate + accuracy)	12	75	higher end of average
	Passage comprehension	6*	9	depressed
	Oral Reading Quotient	94	34	average
Wide Range Achievement Test–3rd Edition (WRAT-3)				
	Reading	122	92	well above average
	Spelling	113	81	higher end of average
Test of Word-Reading Efficiency (TOWRE)				
	Sight word efficiency	99	48	average
	Phonemic decoding efficiency	111	77	higher end of average
	Total Word Reading Efficiency	106	66	average
Clinical Evaluation of Language Fundamentals–4th Edition (CELF-4)				
	Recalling sentences	11	63	average
	Formulating sentences	9	37	average
	Word class receptive	11	63	average
	Word class expressive	11	63	average
	Word classes total	10	50	average
	Word definitions	9	37	average
	Core language score	100	50	average

*Score is at least one standard deviation below the mean.

TABLE 5-12 Summary of Harry's Primary Areas of Strength and Weakness

	Rapid Naming	Short-Term Memory	Word Decoding	Word Recognition	Spelling	Fluency	Word-Level Reading Comprehension	Text-Level Reading Comprehension	Written Composition	Core Language
Weakness		✓					✓	✓	✓	✓
Strength	✓		✓	✓	✓	✓				

© Cengage Learning 2012

example, he might consider asking himself questions such as: (1) Were the answers in the book? (2) Did my knowledge about the topic help me answer the questions? (3) Did I have to think about it before answering?

6. Harry should be introduced to the comprehension skills and strategies in *Making Connections: Explicit Instruction for Comprehension Skills and Strategies* (http://www.epsbooks.com).

7. Harry should be given strategies to improve the organization and cohesion of his written discourse.

8. Harry should be given accommodations in the classroom as needed, including extended time on classroom tasks and tests that require reading comprehension.

CHAPTER SIX

Counseling and Intervention

Rebecca Wiseheart, PhD, CCC-SLP

THIS CHAPTER AIMS TO:

- Equip tho practitioner with tools and tips for diagnostic counseling.
- Review critical factors and principles that need to be considered when transitioning from diagnosis to treatment.
- Outline the seven major component areas of reading that need to be addressed in treatment planning.
- Provide the practitioner with sample treatment plans for four diagnostic profiles described in chapters 4 and 5 under the MAR^{W}R framework.

A fundamental tenet of this book on reading and writing disabilities is that there is not a one-size-fits-all diagnosis. Reading disability affects individuals of all ages, from all walks of life, and varies tremendously in terms of etiology and severity. In addition, the behavioral symptoms of reading disabilities are manifested in many different ways. Some of these symptoms can be completely debilitating while others go virtually unnoticed. Previous chapters in this book have focused on helping the reader understand the complex process of differential diagnosis by using the MAR^wR model as a framework for describing and assessing strengths and weaknesses in spoken and written language. The primary purpose of the diagnostic evaluation is to hone in on the underlying cause of the reading problem and to make appropriate recommendations for instruction/intervention. Thus, the diagnostic process should never be viewed as a means to an end. This chapter focuses on what to do after the testing session is over.

In addition to administering, scoring, and interpreting tests, it is the responsibility of the practitioner to (1) share the results of the evaluation with the learner and his family, (2) explain the diagnosis, and (3) make appropriate recommendations for treatment. For many reasons, these responsibilities are often as challenging as making the diagnosis itself. First and foremost, the practitioner must be able to explain complex psychometric data to the learner and his family in a way that is easily accessible and understandable. Aside from the difficulty of presenting technical terminology in layman's terms, the practitioner's explanation of the evaluation results will often be delivered in an environment that is less than optimal: no matter how simply the diagnostic results are explained, parents' emotions often run high, and this can impede understanding. Finally, the practitioner must make treatment recommendations that are based on scientifically sound conclusions and best practices. Unfortunately, the best-case treatment plan may not be feasible because of lack of financial or provider resources, leaving the practitioner and the family feeling compromised and disappointed. To assist the practitioner in meeting these challenges, this chapter takes a step-by-step approach to addressing the postdiagnostic process, from counseling to implementing a treatment plan.

THE EMOTIONAL ROLLER COASTER OF DIAGNOSTIC COUNSELING

As for how I felt when I was told the kids were dyslexic…. We had been through so much trying to find out why Spencer struggled so much…I think I was scared, but relieved…by that time I knew that if he was ever going to catch up…we had to know what the actual problem was—then we could finally make a plan that might work for him. And you know I called and talked to you, months before we actually met…and that was actually Mom's fault—she was scared about him being "labeled" at school. When in reality finding out about his learning disability and meeting the right person…was the best thing that ever happened to us.

And when Haley came along, it was so evident that she and Spencer learned so much alike—that we were able to get her the help she needed much earlier... making her school life so much easier for her, and she had such good success at an earlier age... So it's scary, but [finally getting the right diagnosis was] the best thing that happened to us.

—LeeAnn B., mother of three, two with dyslexia

Receiving a diagnosis of any kind is often an emotionally charged experience. For some, like Spencer's mother, dyslexia was a looming and scary possibility that was always in the back of her mind. Despite having her son tested numerous times in school and by private educational psychologists, no one could give her a definitive diagnosis. By the time Spencer arrived for his final diagnostic evaluation, he had been retained once and was spending the majority of his fifth-grade school year away from his peers in Exceptional Student Education (ESE) classes. This handsome, well-spoken, talented athlete, who had an IQ bordering on the gifted range, was reading below a second-grade level. After reviewing no less than four diagnostic evaluation reports that his mother had meticulously filed away, it was clear that Spencer's severe deficits in phonological processing, decoding, and fluency—all of the classic markers of dyslexia—had been observed as early as the first grade.

This dismal scenario is, unfortunately, all too common. Accordingly, when learners are finally diagnosed with a specific reading disability, parents experience a range of emotions. Spencer's mom felt a strong sense of relief—the diagnosis of dyslexia validated a hunch she had for a very long time. For others, emotions can be less positive. For example, if a child, like Spencer, had been tested previously but not given a specific diagnosis, and then later received a diagnosis of dyslexia by another professional, the student and her family could be left feeling confused, skeptical, or even angry.

Some parents experience tremendous feelings of guilt for waiting so long to have their child diagnosed. One study found that 44% of parents who notice their child struggling to learn to read wait a year or more before acknowledging their child might have a serious problem (Roper Starch Poll, 2000). After that, the actual diagnosis might still be a year or more away. Most learners are diagnosed with reading disability after third grade.

Debunking the Myths of Dyslexia

Many parents will also be in denial—a reading problem parents will buy, but not dyslexia! More than anything the practitioner can do in counseling, taking the time to explain what dyslexia is and what it is not—will provide parents, struggling readers, and other family members the most relief about the past and the most hope for the future. In *The Source for Dyslexia and Dysgraphia* (1999), Regina Richards provides a comprehensive list of commonly held myths about dyslexia:

1. Dyslexia only affects reading.
2. If a person is able to read, that person cannot have dyslexia.

3. Individuals with dyslexia can learn to read just like anybody but progress at a slower rate. Therefore, standard core reading instruction should be used but presented at a much slower speed.

4. Individuals with dyslexia will never learn to read.

5. Individuals with dyslexia struggle with phonics; therefore, phonics should be avoided with these learners.

6. Mirror writing is a signature feature of dyslexia. Therefore, if a learner does not write backwards, he cannot have dyslexia.

7. All individuals who have dyslexia have very poor writing skills.

8. All individuals who have dyslexia are clumsy, or the converse, all are well coordinated.

9. All individuals with dyslexia have a poor sense of direction, or conversely, all have a superior directional sense.

10. All individuals with dyslexia have a poor memory, or conversely, all have a superior memory.

11. All individuals with dyslexia are left-handed.

12. Many more boys than girls have dyslexia.

13. Since dyslexia is genetic, if a parent is able to read, the child cannot have dyslexia.

14. Individuals with dyslexia cannot go to college.

15. Individuals with dyslexia can be cured.

Maintaining a Positive Relationship with Schools

Because dyslexia and language impairment tend to run in families, many parents have experienced extreme difficulties learning to read themselves. Because of their own negative experiences in school, many parents carry with them an underlying sense of disillusionment and sometimes outright contempt for educational professionals and schools in general. Other parents are incensed, perhaps rightfully so, that many school districts do not recognize dyslexia as an educational diagnosis. All too often, parents spend more time in mediation with schools than they spend seeking intervention for their children. It is unfortunate that many schools are unable to provide the direct, one-to-one treatment that is so effective with learners who have severe reading disabilities, but the greater misfortune occurs when a child's instructional needs are not met at all or are misguided, resulting in prolonging and often exacerbating the learner's daily struggles at school.

EXPLAINING THE DIAGNOSTIC RESULTS

An explanation of the diagnostic results should be thorough and extemporaneous. Using a visual aid to help explain to parents the range of strengths and weaknesses of the child is often very helpful. Plotting the pertinent test results on a simple bell curve will illustrate where the child is functioning relative to his peers and will provide a clear visual representation of where her strengths and weaknesses lie. A simple explanation of "standard scores" and "average range" using a bell curve is usually sufficient for most parents to understand the results of testing. A sample bell curve form with diagnostic codes is included in this chapter (Appendix 6-1).

As the test results are discussed, it is important that the practitioner explain to the parent how the child's performance on the tests are related to the reading and writing behaviors observed at home and at school. For example, if the parent has described the child as "taking forever to finish homework," the practitioner can explain that the child's scores on the *Test of Rapid Automatized Naming* (RAN) and on the *Test of Word Reading Efficiency* (TOWRE) indicate that the child has a very difficult time quickly reading words on a page, even if the child has demonstrated knowledge of the words' pronunciations previously. Slower processing of orthographic patterns (i.e., words' spellings in print) is a common root cause of prolonged time spent on homework for children who have reading disabilities.

After the test results are discussed, the practitioner can explain how the learner's scores reflect a specific diagnostic profile. Some tips for discussing the results of the diagnostic evaluation are shown in Box 6-1. Providing parents with written information on the learner's diagnosis will allow the parents to absorb information in their own time after the counseling session. Finally, treatment options should be discussed. Although a complete therapy plan may not be necessary at this diagnostic session, it is very comforting to the family to receive advice that they can follow immediately, such as (1) providing a list of interventionists in their geographic area, (2) instructing them to

---

| BOX 6-1 | **Tips for Discussing the Results of the Diagnostic Evaluation** |

- Highlight the child's strengths first, then review the weaknesses
- Relate the findings to observable symptoms noted by the parent or patient
- Avoid jargon: use terms that are easily understood
- Use a visual aid to highlight pertinent test results used to inform both the diagnosis and treatment plan
- Be aware of any difficult emotions that might be brewing. Rule of thumb for counseling: listen more than you talk!
- Provide the parent with at least two handouts: one to describe the diagnosis and one with a list of therapy providers
- Allot enough time for questions and make yourself available for questions that may arise later

---

provide a copy of the child's diagnostic report to the school, (3) and providing them with the names of other parents whose children have been diagnosed with a similar disorder and who have agreed to help other families work their way through the process of seeking help within and outside of school, when necessary.

Below are answers to questions frequently asked by parents:

Q: How did you come up with this diagnosis, what does it mean, and what caused this to happen?

A: In the most general terms, a diagnosis is simply a descriptive term that best characterizes the strengths and weaknesses revealed either through formal, historical information, informal observations, and learning trajectories. In no way does it define the child—the child is the same person walking out of the as he was when he arrived. A diagnosis describes a problem or a condition, not a person. Giving this problem a name helps others understand, in very clear terms, the reason for specific behaviors. Saying "Johnny can't read" is shrouded in all kinds of uncertainties: Is it because he is slow? lazy? his parents do not push him? he goes to a low-performing school? he just is not focused? Saying that Johnny has trouble reading because he has dyslexia says to those who know: Johnny can't read well because his brain is wired differently for information processing than his peers who have learned to read with relative ease. To those who do not know what the diagnosis means, they simply hear that there is an underlying cause or condition that keeps Johnny from reading well.

There is no litmus test for reading disability. Reading is a complex skill that requires the integration of a range of subskills along with adequate environmental supports. Therefore, the practitioner should view the assessment process as a time when information from as many sources as possible—test results, school history, preschool development, family history, literacy opportunities, and so on—are explored and used to create a profile of strengths and weaknesses along with a well-grounded hypothesis about the cause(s) of the problem. Taking all of these factors into consideration helps to ensure an accurate and thorough interpretation of the nature of the learner's difficulties and a data-based-driven formulation of treatment goals.

In clear-cut cases of dyslexia or mixed spoken and written language impairment, practitioners can tell parents with a high degree of certainty that there is something very different about the way that the brain is wired to process reading or language. This difference doesn't preclude learning to read well but does require that more intensive and often alternative procedures be adopted for reading and writing instruction. There is also very strong evidence that both dyslexia and language impairment are frequently inherited, and characteristics of similar difficulties are quite readily identified in other family members.

Q: How did you come up with a treatment plan, where do we go for treatment, and how much will it cost?

A: The diagnostic report, along with observations at home and at school, will provide the information needed to determine the focus of intervention. The treatment for reading disability targets the learner's weak areas and takes advantage of the learner's strengths. For example, if a learner can understand the meaning of a word in context but cannot read the word in isolation or spell the word, meaning units within the word (e.g., as in suffixes such as "pre" and "-ful", latin root forms such as "flect" and "grad", and greek root forms such as "bio" and "meta") can be used to access a word's pronunciation and meaning.

While there are a number of different options for treatment, ideally, learners with reading disabilities should receive one-to-one treatment by a professional who has been expertly trained to teach learners who have reading disabilities. Because schools are geared toward teaching "typically developing readers" or children with depressed reading skills associated with a lack of systematic instruction, school is not always the best option for treatment, especially for learners with severe reading disabilities. There are many reading clinics that specialize in treating disabilities and there are often a few tutors in a geographic area that can provide this kind of treatment, as well. The bad news is that private treatment can be quite costly—ranging anywhere from $40 to $120 an hour—and, unfortunately, most insurance companies do not cover it. The good news is that (1) schools are becoming increasingly aware of the specific needs of students who have a reading disability, and (2) properly focused and delivered instruction in schools can have a strong positive impact on the learner's reading and writing achievement.

Q: Realistically, how long will reading therapy take, and will my child get better?

A: The amount of therapy needed depends on a number of factors: the severity of the disability, the age of the child, the strengths the child brings to the table, the approach and intensity of therapy, and the dedication of the learner and his family. It also depends on how well the child is compensating in school. Typically, at least one year of relatively intense therapy is needed to get moderately impaired learners with dyslexia well situated for academic success, though some learners, especially those with mixed spoken and written language disabilities, may continue to need therapy or tutoring support throughout the elementary, middle, and secondary school grades.

Research over the past 30 years has provided us a wealth of knowledge regarding the best ways to teach learners with learning disabilities to read (Hall & Moats, 2002; Shaywitz, 2003). With the right kind of treatment, almost all learners show improved reading skills, and studies with learners who have dyslexia have shown corresponding changes in the areas of the brain known to support reading (Shaywitz, Lyon, & Shaywitz, 2006). Some subskills of reading are easier to remediate than others. For example, numerous studies have demonstrated that learners who struggle with reading words can be taught to decode words quite accurately with systematic instruction. What researchers still do not know—what researchers continue to work on—is how to teach these learners to read quickly and effortlessly. It is likely that for children with dyslexia, automaticity for reading words will always be slower than expected, though their reading may be highly accurate. Accommodations such as allowing extended time on assignments and tests and breaking up large segments of reading into smaller, more manageable sections will help them compensate for their depressed automaticity for word recognition.

Additional Resources for Parents

Whether it takes the form of a support group, educational workshops, or independent research, parents are encouraged to continue educating themselves about their child's specific reading disability. Leading parents to credible, scientifically sound sources of information will help them avoid snake oil and quick fixes, which are, unfortunately, teeming on the Internet. Lists of resources designed specifically for parents are provided in Boxes 6-2 and 6-3.

| BOX 6-2 | List of Parent Resources—Books |

Special Education: One Family's Journey through the Maze of Learning Disabilities, by Dana Buchman

Basic Facts about Dyslexia and Other Reading Problems, by Louisa Cook Moats and Karen E. Dakin

Dyslexia: A Complete Guide for Parents, by Gavin Reid

From ABC to ADHD: What Every Parent Should Know about Dyslexia, by Eric Q. Tridas

Overcoming Dyslexia, by Sally Shaywitz

Parenting a Struggling Reader, by Susan L. Hall and Louisa C. Moats

Straight Talk about Reading: How Parents Can Make a Difference during the Early Years, by Susan L. Hall and Louisa C. Moats

Wright's Law—From Emotions to Advocacy: The Special Education Survival Guide, 2nd Edition, by Pam Wright and Pete Wright

---

| BOX 6-3 | List of Parent Resources—Web Sites |

Florida Center for Reading Research (http://www.fcrr.org)

Reading Rockets (http://www.readingrockets.com)

Learning Disabilities Online (http://www.ldonline.com)

International Dyslexia Association (IDA) (http://www.interdys.org)

Put Reading First: Helping Your Child Learn to Read: A Parent Guide Preschool through Grade 3, National Institute for Literacy (http://www.nifl.gov/nifl/nifl_pubs.html)

INTERVENTION SETTING

The practitioner may be the same person who provides therapy. In such cases, the transition from diagnosis to treatment can be seamless. However, it is often the case that treatment will be provided by someone else. This section provides the reader with an overview of school-based and clinic-based intervention models.

The General Education Setting

In line with procedures described in the reauthorization of the Individuals with Disabilities Education Act of 2004 (IDEA; Public Law 108–446), schools nationwide have instituted a response-to-intervention (RTI) model to ensure that all learners with learning difficulties have access to intervention (Fuchs & Fuchs, 2001; Wright & Wright, 2007). IDEA legislation allows educators to use learners' responsiveness-to-intervention to determine the nature and intensity of the intervention needed rather than relying on other standards, such as performance on a battery of standardized tests, to determine if learners qualify for intervention services. This alternative approach to identifying and treating struggling learners was developed to encourage early intervention and to promote more accurate identification of learners who have learning disabilities (Fuchs & Fuchs, 2001). In educational settings, RTI is a systematic method for improving learners' academic success by identifying those who are not meeting grade-level academic benchmarks, providing more intensive levels of instruction when needed, and carefully monitoring the effectiveness of interventions. This multi-tiered model of reading instruction is typically shown as a triangle that represents different levels of instruction (see Figure 6-1). It is an adaptation of a three-tiered public health framework that has been used for decades to help prevent and treat health conditions under the designations of primary, secondary, and tertiary health care services (Vaughn, Wanzek, & Fletcher, 2007). This tiered educational model of reading represents three sequentially ordered stages of reading intervention. Vaughn, Wanzek, and Fletcher (2007) identified five dimensions of instruction that need to be considered when evaluating the intervention process: (1) screening and ongoing progress monitoring, (2) differentiating instruction through small-group instruction or tutoring, (3) increasing the duration of the intervention, (4) targeting instruction to learners' specific needs, and (5) identifying the content of the instructional approach. Because this model is a conceptual framework designed to be descriptive rather than prescriptive (Stewart,

Benner, Martella, & Marchand-Martella, 2007), the way in which it is implemented varies across school districts and states. In the tier-model system, the learner's intensity of instructional support is determined by his performance on benchmark testing from kindergarten through third grade. *The Dynamic Indicators of Basic Early Literacy Skills* (DIBELS; Good & Kaminski, 2002) and *AIMSweb* (http://www.aimsweb.com/) are examples of commonly used standardized benchmark and progress-monitoring instruments for assessing specific areas of reading (e.g., phonemic awareness, vocabulary, reading fluency) across the grade levels.

Tier 1 refers to the core classroom reading instruction. Approximately 70%–80% of learners will meet the benchmarks for proficiency at Tier 1; 15%–20% will require Tier 2 intervention; and another 5%–10% will require Tier 3 intervention (Marchand-Martella, Ruby, & Martella, 2007). In Tier 1 intervention, all learners are provided with 90 minutes per day of reading instruction from a reading curriculum that is grounded in scientifically based principles and includes five components of reading: phonemic awareness, decoding, fluency, vocabulary, and comprehension (Archer, 2009). A high level of quality instruction at Tier 1 is expected to prevent reading difficulties that could result from too little or inadequate reading instruction. Learners are tested at the beginning, middle, and end of the academic year to determine whether or not they are meeting the designated benchmarks for their grade. Learners who do not meet grade-level benchmarks at Tier 1 are moved into Tier 2.

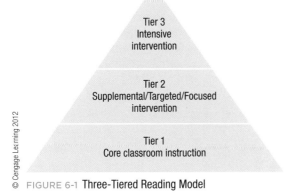

FIGURE 6-1 **Three-Tiered Reading Model**

In Tier 2, learners are given an additional 30–40 minutes of small supplemental group instruction (ratios of 1:3–1:5) daily and their progress is monitored regularly, often weekly. Learners who do not meet grade-level benchmarks after receiving Tier 2 intervention are placed in Tier 3 intervention, the most intensive layer of tiered instruction.

In Tier 3, learners are given a minimum of two 30-minute individual or small-group (1:2 or 1:3) instructional sessions daily in addition to the 90 minutes of core classroom reading instruction. Tier 3 reading instruction is typically accomplished with intensive, explicit, and structured remedial programs (Archer, 2009). Whereas some of these programs target specific aspects of reading, such as word reading and spelling skills (e.g., Wilson Reading System, Alphabetic Phonics, Barton Reading and Spelling System) and fluency skills (e.g., Great Leaps, Reading Naturally), other programs target a broader range of reading skills that include vocabulary and comprehension (e.g., Reading Mastery, Corrective Reading, Language!). Most practitioners who use this book will be working with learners who require Tier 3 intensive intervention.

Though many researchers support the RTI model in theory, it is not without criticism. Many question whether RTI can be implemented with integrity because (1) there remains a general lack of specificity in terms of assessment and intervention (Berkeley, Bender, Peaster, & Saunders, 2009) and (2) teachers are inadequately prepared to meet the curricular and logistical demands of the model (Carreker & Joshi, 2010). The primary purpose of implementing the RTI model was to improve reading outcomes of students by ensuring that all students receive adequately differentiated instruction. Purportedly, this practice should serve a secondary purpose of reducing the number of children identified as learning disabled. In theory, then, RTI should help differentiate children who are struggling to read because of environmental deprivation or poor teaching practices from those who are struggling because of biological factors (e.g., dyslexia) (Carreker & Joshi, 2010). This, however, may not be the case. Although reading outcomes have generally improved, several researchers have pointed out that there is currently no clear evidence that RTI has improved the process of identifying children with learning disabilities (Berkeley et al., 2009; Carreker & Joshi, 2010).

The Special Education Setting

Many struggling readers will already be enrolled in special education or ESE programs. Special education programs are funded at a higher level than general education programs, and this funding is used to provide learners with special needs more intensive, small-group instruction. Currently, the process for being enrolled in special education requires a lengthy RTI process. Learners who do not respond to intervention are referred for further testing. At that point, a team meeting is held to determine whether the learner meets the state eligibility criteria for special education services. Learners with rather severe reading disabilities are most often placed in specific learning disabilities (SLD) programs or sometimes language impaired (LI) programs. Special education services can vary markedly from school to school. The IDEA dictates that learners should be served in the least restrictive environment that meets their needs. In more restrictive service delivery models, the students are "pulled out" of their general education classes to receive differential instruction in a special class. In less restrictive service delivery models, a special education teacher "pushes in" to the general education class to provide support for the students in their particular area(s) of difficulty. Eligibility for ESE services varies from state to state and may or may not employ an aptitude-achievement discrepancy standard.

The Clinical Setting

In most clinical settings, such as university communication disorders clinics, hospital clinics, and private practices, a learner who struggles with reading is evaluated with a comprehensive battery of tests that includes spoken language skills, written language skills, and cognitive processes such as phonological processing, processing speed, and working memory. These skills and procedures for evaluating them are discussed in Chapters 4 and 5. An assessment of this nature should lead to an intervention approach that is designed specifically to identify the learner's profile for weaknesses and strengths in reading and reading-related skills. Frequently, practitioners will use an intervention approach that is phonics based, systematic, repetitive, intensive, and multisensory (e.g., Orton-Gillingham–based approaches) because many of the learners who receive instruction outside of the school environment have a severe reading disability. A list of pros and cons of reading intervention settings is provided in Table 6-1.

TABLE 6-1 Pros and Cons of Reading Intervention Settings

Intervention Setting	Pros	Cons
General education	Eligibility criteria are based on classroom assessments/benchmark testing.	Eligibility criteria (children who compensate well may never get treatment for underlying deficits) Professionals providing intervention may be well trained for teaching reading to typically developing readers but may have little specialized training in reading or language disorders.
Special education	Professionals providing intervention have had at least some specialized training in reading and language disorders.	Students must meet state eligibility criteria to participate. Possible social stigma.
Clinical	Professionals providing intervention have most likely had specialized training in reading and language disorders. 1:1 treatment	Costly and most often not covered by medical insurance.

Intensive one-to-one treatment for learners diagnosed with a reading disability is highly recommended, but in many cases this is simply not practical. It is imperative that practitioners working with learners and their families be knowledgeable about available school programs and creative in helping find reasonable solutions that address the specific needs of their students.

INSTRUCTIONAL PRINCIPLES FOR LITERACY PRACTITIONERS

The professional who provides reading therapy must employ intervention practices that promote the learner's eventual integration and synchronistic use of all component reading skills, leading to grade-level reading achievement. Toward this objective, practitioners should consider the following five principles when prescribing or implementing an intervention plan.

Principle #1: Use Case History, Observational Classroom Data (as much as possible), and Behavioral Data to Determine the Learner's Strengths and Weaknesses in Spoken and Written Language

Practitioners should target directly the learner's component skill deficit when an isolated area of weakness is identified (e.g., word-level reading). If the learner is deficient in more than one component area (e.g., decoding, vocabulary) or across all component areas (i.e., spoken language and written language), it is essential to determine if the learner's oral language skills and foundational emergent literacy skills (see Chapters 3–5) are sufficient to support reading, or if the learner

needs to develop spoken language or emergent literacy skills first.

The majority of emergent literacy learners who are at risk for later reading difficulties can become skilled readers with classroom instruction that employs more *phonemically explicit and comprehensive instruction*, more *intensive or frequent instruction*, and more *practice* learning new skills than is typically provided in the regular classroom (Foorman & Torgesen, 2001). Some learners, typically those with severe reading disabilities, may retain weaknesses in one or more of the component skill areas and will require more intensive, explicit, and structured small-group or one-to-one instruction. Practitioners who have used multisensory structured-language classroom instruction for learners with specific reading disabilities have documented that many of these learners can achieve grade-level reading skills (Henry, 1998). In a recent synthesis on remedial intervention with learners who have dyslexia, Torgesen (2005) notes that sufficient data are available to support the finding that explicit, systematic, and intensive instruction can narrow the gap between the skills of severely reading-impaired learners and their peers, but that there are no sufficient data from long-term instructional studies to suggest how to eliminate this gap altogether.

Principle #2: Consider the Learner's Overall Stage of Literacy Development When Developing Instructional Goals

The practitioner's understanding of the learner's general stage of literacy development is particularly important when evaluating preliterate or emergent-literate learners who are at risk for later reading difficulties. Regarding remedial reading intervention for struggling readers, it is imperative to keep in mind that critical gaps in reading development for learners with dyslexia are considered low-level deficits that are generally learned and mastered during the very early stages of reading instruction (phonological awareness, phoneme-grapheme correspondences, word decoding), but gaps for learners with comprehension deficits involve higher-level aspects of reading, such as summarizing and making inferences. Thus, for those with dyslexia, remediation often needs to begin at the very beginning, with sound-symbol correspondences.

In reference to Chall's (1983) developmental model, discussed in Chapter 1, most practitioners who are working with learners in preschool through the early elementary grades will be addressing skills that develop between Stages 0 and 2. Conversely, most practitioners who are working with middle school through secondary school learners will be addressing the skills that develop between Stages 3 and 4. Providing intervention for adolescents who are struggling with reading is particularly challenging because they display marked gaps between their stage of reading skill, language knowledge, and background knowledge relative to their expected grade-level performance (Deshler, Hock, & Catts, 2006). Through the University of Kansas Center for Research on Learning (http://www.kucrl.org/), Lenz, Ehren, and Deshler (2005) present a framework called *The Content Literacy Continuum* that is de-

signed to guide the development of literacy instruction for secondary school learners. Their framework addresses five levels of instruction: (1) content instruction needed at the secondary level regardless of the learners' level of reading skill, (2) strategies that match the curricular demands, (3) intensive strategy instruction for learners who require more frequent and explicit teaching, (4) intensive basic skill instruction for learners who need the foundational skills that typically develop in grades 1–3, and (5) therapeutic intervention for learners who have underlying language disorders that interfere with their ability to learn curricular content.

Principle #3: Adopt a Scientifically Based and Sequenced Instructional Framework for Developing Treatment Goals

The practitioner should pay particular attention to both the form and content of instruction when teaching learners the foundation skills of reading. For example, Henry (2003, 2010), whose work in reading is based on the Orton-Gillingham approach to reading, spelling, and writing, has created a sequence for teaching decoding and spelling throughout the elementary school years. Table 6-2 shows an adaptation of Henry's (2003) grade-level developmental scheme for word structures and word origins from her book, *Unlocking Literacy: Effective Decoding & Spelling Strategies.* Henry notes that "learners who recognize letter-sound correspondences, syllable patterns, and morpheme patterns in words of Anglo Saxon, Latin, and Greek origin hold the strategies necessary to read and spell most unfamiliar words" (2003, p. 5).

TABLE 6-2 Adapted Version of Henry's (2003) Developmental Scheme for Teaching Word-Level Reading and Spelling

Grade Level	Concepts and Constructs for Decoding and Spelling Training
K	Phonological awareness
1	Alphabet letters and corresponding sounds
2	Anglo-Saxon consonants and vowels
3	Compound words, prefixes and suffixes, syllable types and syllable division patterns
4	Latin roots
5–8	Greek combining forms

© Cengage Learning 2012

Orton-Gillingham (OG) principles have been used since the 1920s to guide the teaching of reading, spelling, and writing to learners with dyslexia (Gillingham & Stillman, 1997). Sheffield (1991) notes that in OG instruction: "A learner is directly taught reading, handwriting, spelling, and expressive writing as part of one logical body of knowledge. He is taught language as a science. The steps of learning are built closely together. His teacher continually teaches small logical pieces of language and then connects them to what the learner already knows" (p. 42). It is these severely reading-impaired learners who will need the assistance of practitioners who are skilled in using the core instructional components of the OG approach. These components are: (1) *multisensory instruction*: training memories for orthographic (i.e., print) patterns across the visual, auditory, and kinesthetic modalities; (2) *phonics-based instruction:* teaching phonemic-orthographic associations and segmenting and blending of these sequences in reading and in spelling; (3) *sequential instruction*: progressing from the phoneme to the text level in each session; (4) *systematic and logical instruction*:

using strategies such as visual and auditory phoneme/grapheme-level drills, letter tracing, and syllable tapping; (5) *fluency instruction*: using drills to practice skills to a level of automaticity; (6) *cumulative instruction*: using previously taught information to teach new information; reviewing previously learned information and introducing a new target structure in the same lesson; (7) *cognitive instruction*: teaching reasoning or "discovery" strategies for approaching novel print patterns by using skills already acquired; and (8) *flexible instruction*: using the fundamental principles in ways that meet the needs of individual learners (Gillingham & Stillman, 1997). There are several OG-based reading programs (e.g., Alphabetic Phonetics; S.P.I.R.E.; Project Read; Slingerland, Wilson Training Program) that differ in format but that adhere to many of the core principles just described.

Principle #4: Adopt a Framework for Individualizing Direct Instructional Practices

Using a framework for direct or explicit instruction (National Reading Panel, 2000;

TABLE 6-3 Five-Step Model of Explicit Text

1. Describe strategy explicitly, including when and how it should be used

2. Model strategy use in action

3. Collaborate with learners in strategy use

4. Provide opportunities for guided practice and gradual release of responsibility

5. Encourage independent strategy use.

Adapted from Duke & Pearson (2002)

© Cengage Learning 2012

NIFL, 2001) facilitates successful learning at various grade levels (Anderson, 1992; Anderson & Roit, 1993; Block, 1993, 1999; Brown, Pressley, Van Meter, & Schuder, 1996; Collins, 1991). Table 6-3 outlines Duke and Pearson's (2002) five-step model of *explicit instruction*. In this model, practitioners provide differentiated instructional support, gradually releasing responsibility as learners become better able to monitor their own reading skills and more competent in strategy use (Pearson & Gallagher, 1983). In the initial stages of instruction, practitioners assume the greatest responsibility for the lesson while describing the strategy and modeling how it is used. Throughout modeling, practitioners may "think aloud," explaining their own implementation of the strategy. The most powerful explanations are not scripted. They arise "on the spot" from practitioners who modify their explanations based on learners' responses. When one or another of these explanations fails to help learners, practitioners must find an alternative method and provide learners with multiple opportunities to apply the strategy in real reading. Some learners require as many as 6 to 10 consecutive applications of a strategy before

mastering it (Block & Duffy, 2008). Through years of practice, observation, and basic trial-and-error strategies, experienced practitioners often develop their own methods for troubleshooting specific areas of difficulty.

At the next stage, practitioners and learners share joint responsibility for implementation of the strategy. Both of them may engage in the task together or alternate responsibility for different aspects of the task. Practitioners may also guide learners' practices by observing their implementation of the strategy, providing feedback, and encouraging continued practices. During the last stage, practitioners release total responsibility for strategy implementation to learners, who now work independently to integrate newly learned skills into their repertoires.

Additional frameworks for explicit instruction include Rasinski and Padak's (2003) four-step framework: (1) formulating a philosophy for instruction, (2) developing instructional goals in general areas of reading instruction, (3) using instructional practices and activities as target instructional goals, and (4) developing a method of evaluating the effectiveness of the intervention plan; and Moore and Lyon's (2005) four-step instructional sequence: (1) explaining and modeling, (2) guided practice, (3) independent practice, and (4) review of previously learned material.

Principle #5: Take into Account the Learner's Motivation to become a More Proficient Reader

The majority of young learners in treatment are quite easily motivated to read and write when given appropriate instruction. In contrast, the majority of older learners, especially those beyond the middle school years, and who have experienced years of failure with written language, are frequently unenthusiastic about participating in instruction that requires them to learn fundamental constructs such as word decoding when their peers are well beyond this initial stage of reading instruction. In such cases, where an older learner requires word-level (decoding, word recognition) instruction and is willing to "give it [therapy] a try," the practitioner should teach decoding skills and use decodable texts written on topics of interest for older learners. Once the learner can decode, reading fluency and comprehension should be taught with the learner's preference for literacy forms (e.g., typing, texting), content (e.g., sci-fi, sports), and contexts (magazines, blogs) in mind.

CORE COMPONENTS OF INSTRUCTION

This section of the chapter systematically and separately addresses each of the seven core instructional goal areas shown in Table 6-4.

TABLE 6-4 Seven Core Components of Reading

Core Instructional Components	
	Oral language instruction
	Phonological awareness instruction
	Print- and letter-knowledge instruction
	Phonics and word-recognition instruction
	Vocabulary instruction
	Fluency instruction
	Text-comprehension instruction

© Cengage Learning 2012

These components of instruction are cited by national reading resources (e.g., National Research Council, National Reading Panel) as the core areas or subskills of both oral and written language that work synchronously to support the acquisition and development of skilled reading. The following sections address each component separately under three headings: (1) a scientifically supported *rationale and support* for its critical role in supporting reading success; (2) suggested *treatment goals* that may be targeted within each of the component areas; and (3) a list of *instructional resources and intervention programs* that include evidence-based practices, strategies, and activities designed to facilitate mastery of these goals. This overview is designed to be used in developing treatment plans for the heterogeneous groups of struggling readers described in earlier chapters.

Spoken Language Instruction

Rationale and Support

Spoken language proficiency provides the foundation for the mastery of written language skills. All areas of spoken language are strongly tied to higher-level literacy skills in reading comprehension and written expression (Scarborough, 2001). Weaknesses in either receptive or expressive spoken language ability will greatly influence the ease with which learners acquire proficiency with written language. Learners with specific language impairment (SLI), in particular, are at high risk for experiencing pervasive reading and writing difficulties, even after deficits in spoken language have been resolved (Bishop & Snowling, 2004; Stothard, Snowling, Bishop,

Chipchase, & Kaplan, 1998). Some evidence-based treatment goals for weaknesses in spoken language are provided in Table 6-5.

Learners with dyslexia generally have relative strengths in grammar and vocabulary. However, subtle syntactic and morphological deficits have been found even among high-achieving college learners with dyslexia. For example, Leikin and Assayag-Bouskila (2004) found that children with dyslexia performed more poorly than typically developing learners on oral language tasks such as grammaticality judgment and word ordering. Furthermore, Wiseheart, Altman, Park, and Lombardino (2009) reported that compensated adults with dyslexia performed more poorly than their peers on language comprehension tasks of complex sentence structures (e.g., relative clauses); however, working memory contributed to these differences.

Suggested Instructional Resources

- Language!
- Handbook of Exercises for Language Processing (HELP)
- CLIP for Morphology
- CLIP for Syntax
- Strategic Learning: Compound and Complex Sentences

Phonological Awareness Instruction

Rationale and Support

Phonological awareness is the explicit knowledge that the continuous flow of oral language actually consists of smaller units. As noted in Chapter 2, this awareness develops in a predictable, hierarchical fashion such that awareness of larger units, like words and syllables, is attained before awareness of small linguistic units, such as rimes

---

TABLE 6-5 Possible Treatment Goals: Spoken Language Instruction

Syntax	Listening, speaking, reading, and writing:
	• Simple sentences
	• Compound sentences
	• Noncanonical constructions (e.g., passives)
	• Negative constructions
	• Question constructions
	• Complex sentences
Morphology	Listening, speaking, reading, and writing:
	• Plurals—regular and irregular
	• Present progressive (*is* + *-ing*)
	• Pronouns (especially subject vs. object pronouns)
	• Past-tense verb forms—regular and irregular
	• Possessive *-s*
	• 3rd-person singular *-s*
	• Subject-verb agreement (especially for *be*, *do*, and *have*)

and individual phonemes. Although learners become aware of large-grain units through exposure to spoken language, awareness of individual phonemes develops in tandem with learning orthographic codes. The development of phonological awareness (PA) has been shown to coincide with formal reading instruction, regardless of the age of the individual (Ziegler & Goswami, 2005). Thus, PA does not develop as a natural progression of spoken language development: it is explicitly acquired in conjunction with learning an alphabetic code (Ramus, 2003; Share, 2008; Ziegler & Goswami, 2005). PA can be taught, and learners who receive PA training improve their reading and spelling skills (National Reading Panel, 2000). Sample treatment goals for phonological awareness instruction can be found in Table 6-6.

Suggested Instructional Resources

- Developmental Reading Disabilities: A Language-Based Treatment Approach
- Sounds Abound Storybook Activities
- Sounds Abound: Multisensory Phonological Awareness
- Sounds Abound: Listening, Rhyming, and Reading
- Phonological Awareness Kit
- Phonological Awareness in Words and Sentences (PAWS)
- More than Words: Activities for Phonological Awareness and Comprehension
- More Story Making: Using Predictable Literature to Develop Communication

TABLE 6-6 Possible Treatment Goals: Phonological Awareness Instruction

Word-Level Awareness	• Detecting word boundaries in spoken language
Syllable-Level Awareness	• Counting or tapping syllables • Blending and deleting syllables in compound words • Blending and deleting syllables in multisyllabic words with weak syllables
Rime-Level Awareness	• Detecting rimes • Producing rimes • "Odd man out" • Blending onset-rime
Phoneme-Level Awareness	• Matching phonemes in initial, medial, and final word positions • Blending phonemes • Counting or marking phonemes • Deleting phonemes • Substituting phonemes • Transposing phonemes (e.g., Pig Latin)

- Once Upon a Sound: Literature-Based Phonological Activities
- Earobics interactive software
- Lexercise interactive software (for children who are receiving Orton-Gillingham–based intervention)
- Lindamood Individualized Phoneme Sequencing Program (LiPS) (for children who need intensive phonemic awareness instruction by a professionally trained instructor)

Print- and Letter-Knowledge Instruction

Rationale and Support

Before formal reading instruction begins, learners are developing a host of reading-related preliteracy skills. As young learners are exposed to printed materials, concepts of print are being implicitly acquired. For example, young learners who are read to come to understand very early on that books have a beginning and end, that words and sentences are read from left to right, that pages are turned, and that pictures are related to the story. Later the learners de-velop an understanding that letters are different from pictures, that printed words represent spoken language, and, eventually, that the sounds of spoken language are systematically related to individual letters and letter sequences. These important emergent literacy skills are highly predictive of later reading achievement (refer to Chapter 2). Knowledge of letter names and letter-sound knowledge have been shown to be the two best predictors of later reading achievement (Scarborough, 2002). Sample treatment goals for print- and letter-knowledge instruction can be found in Table 6-7.

Suggested Instructional Resources

- Learning about Print in Preschool
- Handwriting without Tears
- Phono-Graphix
- Road to the Code
- Explode the Code
- Earobics interactive software
- Lexercise interactive software (for children who are receiving Orton-Gillingham–based intervention)

TABLE 6-7 Possible Treatment Goals: Print- and Letter-Knowledge Instruction

Print Skills	• Identify the parts of a book • Identify word boundaries in a book • Use picture cues to support text • Finger-point read • "Read" words in environmental print
Letter-Knowledge Skills	• Match letters • Match uppercase and lowercase letters • Name letters, when presented out of order • Write letters, when dictated out of order

© Cengage Learning 2012

Phonics and Word-Recognition Instruction

Rationale and Support

Phonics is a method of teaching reading that emphasizes the connection between letter-sound correspondences and regular spelling patterns. Weak or deficient skills in phonics underlie the majority of reading and spelling difficulties among struggling readers. Learners with poor phonological processing skills have a particularly difficult time mastering phonics rules when reading and spelling are taught in a traditional way. Learners fail to develop automatic word recognition if they lack the alphabetic basis for amalgamating letter-sound sequences into words that they can recognize automatically (refer to Chapter 2). When phonics rules are taught systematically and explicitly (i.e., in a planned sequence), learners with reading disabilities can and do learn to read using phonics.

Acquiring phoneme-grapheme correspondences serves to organize the continuous flow of oral language into well-defined "phonological prototypes" (i.e., phonemes) that can be more easily managed, remembered, and manipulated. This "augmented" phonological form (Share, 2008) supports performance on written language tasks (reading and spelling) and on spoken language tasks (PA) that require explicit awareness of phonemic boundaries (Carroll, Snowling, Hulme, & Stevenson, 2003). Thus, the importance of explicit phonics instruction cannot be overemphasized for learners with dyslexia or other phonologically based reading disabilities. Sample treatment goals for phonics and word recognition instruction can be found in Table 6-8.

Suggested Instructional Resources

Primary Instructional Resource

- O-G Programs: Barton, Wilson Reading and Spelling, Slingerland

Supplementary Instructional Resources

- Phono-Graphix
- Road to the Code

TABLE 6-8 Possible Treatment Goals: Phonics and Word Recognition Instruction

Phonics	Identify letter-sound correspondences
	Read and spell:
	• simple syllables with short vowel sounds
	• complex syllables with short vowel sounds
	• words with vowel pairs
	• words with "silent *e*"
	• words with *r*-vowels
Word Identification	• Read and spell high-frequency phonetically regular words
	• Read and spell phonetically irregular words

© Cengage Learning 2012

- Explode the Code
- Seeing Stars: Symbol Imagery for Fluency, Orthography, Sight Words & Spelling
- Seeing Stars Decoding Workbooks
- Word Journeys
- Teaching Word Recognition
- Earobics interactive software
- Lexercise interactive software (for children who are receiving Orton-Gillingham–based intervention)

Vocabulary Instruction

Rationale and Support

Because much of a child's vocabulary is learned through either reading or being read to, learners with reading disabilities may have weak vocabularies. Vocabulary encompasses a range of component skills, from knowing the definition of a word, to understanding how words are related, classified, and used in various contexts. The most efficacious vocabulary-building programs provide formal definitions combined with the use of context cues and incorporate repeated exposure of target words across various contexts. Sample treatment goals for vocabulary instruction can be found in Table 6-9.

Suggested Instructional Resources

- Bringing Words to Life
- Wordly Wise 3000
- Words Their Way
- Word Journeys 100% Concepts
- 100% Vocabulary

Fluency Instruction

Rationale and Support

Fluent reading refers to efficient and automatic word identification. When learners read automatically (without consciously thinking), cognitive resources are available for comprehension. Learners demonstrate fluency by reading rapidly, accurately, and with appropriate expression or prosody. Deficits in fluency have detrimental effects on reading comprehension. Guided oral reading (with feedback from a skilled instructor) has the greatest impact on reading accuracy and prosody, and repeated reading improves reading speed, word recognition, and text comprehension (Rasinski, 2003). Sample treatment goals for fluency instruction can be found in Table 6-10.

Suggested Instructional Resources

- Quick Reads
- Read Naturally
- Great Leaps
- RAVE-O (for young readers who require a comprehensive and highly structured curriculum for reading fluency and comprehension with supplementary phonics instruction).

Text-Comprehension Instruction

Rationale and Support

Text comprehension, of course, is the purpose of reading. The National Reading Panel (National Reading Panel, 2000) has identified the following strategies as being most effective for improving text comprehension: comprehension monitoring, cooperative learning,

TABLE 6-9 Possible Treatment Goals: Vocabulary Instruction

Specific Vocabulary	Identify, define, and use: • Content-area vocabulary (e.g., words specific to math, science, history, etc.) • Literature-based vocabulary
Basic Concepts	Identify, define, and use concepts of: • space/location • time/order/sequence • number/frequency • size
Semantic Relationships	Identify, define, and use: • Associations (e.g., bread/butter; sock/shoe) • Classifications (e.g., animals; things that are hot) • Antonyms • Synonyms • Homophones • Multiple-meaning words
Metalinguistic Concepts	Identify, define, and use: • Analogies • Similes • Metaphors • Idioms • Proverbs

© Cengage Learning 2012

TABLE 6-10 Possible Treatment Goals: Fluency Instruction

Oral Reading Fluency	• Improve the number of words read correctly within a specific time frame (correct words per minute—cwpm—is often used). • Improve spoken expression or prosody when reading aloud.

© Cengage Learning 2012

graphic organizers, story structure, question answering, question generating, and summarization. Reading comprehension is a complex process because it requires the learner to move beyond the meaning of individual words ". . . to understand the ideas and the relationships between ideas conveyed in the text" (McNamara, 2007, xi). The edited book *Reading Comprehension Strategies* (McNamara, 2007) provides a rich resource of comprehension interventions for the practitioner.

Sample treatment goals for text-comprehension instruction can be found in Table 6-11.

TABLE 6-11 Possible Treatment Goals: Text-Comprehension Instruction

Literal Text Comprehension	• Answer "wh" questions
	• Identify beginning, middle, and end
	• Describe order of events
	• Understand stated causal relationships
Inferential Text Comprehension	• Identify main idea
	• Identify author's purpose
	• Predict outcomes and events
	• Understand inferred causal relationships
	• Identify the mental states/emotions of characters

© Cengage Learning 2012

Suggested Instructional Resources

- More than Words: Activities for Phonological Awareness and Comprehension

- More Story Making: Using Predictable Literature to Develop Communication

- Peer Assisted Learning Strategies (PALS)

- POSSE (Predict, Organize, Search, Summarize, and Evaluate)

- Questioning the Author

- Close Analysis of Texts with Structure (CATS)

- Visualizing-Verbalizing

SAMPLE TREATMENT PLANS

Table 6-12 shows a general overview of the components of instruction that need to be targeted for each of the following profiles: emergent reading deficit ("Carlos Calas"), dyslexia ("Evan Edsen"), mixed language and reading disorder ("Gail Gomez"), and comprehension

disorder ("Harry Harper"). The full evaluation reports for these profiles were presented in Chapters 4 and 5. Obviously, individualized treatment plans will vary according to the needs and ages of learners and the service delivery model that is chosen. The following examples are provided to give the practitioner an idea of how to follow up with a treatment plan that is diagnostically informed and targets the learner's specific areas of weakness.

Treatment Plan for Emergent Literacy Deficit Profile: Carlos Calas

Carlos is at risk for expressing a reading disability. Along with a strong family history of dyslexia and failure to meet kindergarten reading benchmarks, his depressed score on the phonological-orthographic composite of the *Assessment of Literacy and Language* (ALL) indicates that Carlos is having extreme difficulty making the connection between oral and written language forms. Although his phonological awareness score is in the average range at this time, Carlos did not meet the criterion for his age on the concept-of-word subtest, a

TABLE 6-12 Instructional Focus Guidelines for MAR^WR Profiles

Instructional Focus	Profile 2 Emergent Literacy Deficit	Profile 4a Dyslexia	Profile 5 Mixed Language and Reading Disorder	Profile 6 Comprehension Deficit
Oral language			✓	
Phonological awareness	✓	✓		
Print and letter knowledge	✓			
Phonics and word recognition	✓	✓	✓*	
Vocabulary			✓	✓
Fluency		✓	✓	
Comprehension			✓	✓
Writing	NA	✓	✓	✓

* See treatment plan for Profile 5 for an explanation.

© Cengage Learning 2012

measure of word awareness in text. This score, taken together with his poor performance on the letter-knowledge, phonics-knowledge, and invented-spelling subtests, indicates that Carlos is showing difficulty developing the *alphabetic principle.*

Accordingly, therapy should begin with helping Carlos develop an understanding of the relationship between spoken language and written language. Some learners simply need to hear someone say "Stories are just like talking but instead of saying the words, we write them down." It is easy to forget that what is implicitly understood by skilled readers must be taught explicitly to struggling readers. It is quite common to hear learners in reading intervention exclaim: "Oh! Why didn't somebody just tell me?"

Many activities are available in phonological awareness programs to help a child develop spoken-word awareness, and this is where therapy should begin. To help a child

understand the concept of a *written* word, the practitioner should begin by pointing out not the words themselves, but the *spaces* between words. Using a large-print board book, the practitioner can show the child how to stick a small piece of Play-Doh in those spaces. This provides a clear visual marker for word boundaries. From here the practitioner can have the child count or point to each of the words. Finally, as the child moves his finger from one word to the next, the practitioner can read the words. This gives the child a very explicit understanding that each "clump" of letters corresponds to a single word that "comes out of your mouth." This concept of separate words in print takes only one or two sessions to establish, but is a critical and often overlooked cornerstone to phonological awareness therapy and understanding the alphabetic principle. This activity of "finger-point reading" can be easily practiced at home. Using books with simple phonetically regular words, the child can begin "pretend" reading a memorized story while pointing to each word.

The practitioner should follow a hierarchy of phonological awareness activities, using other visual manipulatives to scaffold his understanding of segmenting units from words to syllables and rhymes. Once the child is ready to begin activities focused at the level of individual phonemes, introduction to letters and letter sounds should begin, using an explicit, systematic scope and sequence of instruction, such as an Orton-Gillingham–based program. During the beginning stages of phonics instruction, the practitioner should also incorporate phonemic awareness activities, but only for the sounds that have been introduced. This approach, pairing phonics and phonemic awareness instruction, leads to much better outcomes than if either is used alone. Carlos appears to have difficulty making visual-verbal connections and may need additional support in establishing symbol-sound correspondences. A supplementary phonics program that emphasizes the visual-spatial orientation of letters and letter formation may be helpful (e.g., Explode the Code or Phono-Graphix, Handwriting without Tears). Though spoken language and vocabulary appear to be within normal limits for Carlos, these areas can be informally facilitated by using phonological awareness programs that incorporate the use of storybook materials. *Sounds Abound Storybook Activities* are examples of well-orchestrated lessons that take learners step by step through the phonological awareness hierarchy.

Suggested Therapy Resources

- Phonological awareness program (e.g., *Sounds Abound Storybook Activities*)
- Supplementary software programs for home practice (e.g., Earobics, Lexercise, Dr. Seuss ABC's)
- Explicit and comprehensive Orton-based reading programs (e.g., Barton, Wilson, Slingerland)
- Supplementary support materials (e.g., *Explode the Code, Phono-Graphix, Handwriting without Tears*)

Long-Term Goals (6 months)

Print- and Letter-Knowledge Goals

Carlos will:
- Identify word boundaries in a book with 90% accuracy.
- Use picture cues to support text with 90% accuracy.
- Match and copy uppercase and lowercase letters with 100% accuracy.
- Name letters, when presented out of order, with 100% accuracy.
- Write letters, when dictated out of order, with 100% accuracy.

Phonological Awareness Goals

Carlos will:
- Demonstrate awareness of word and syllable boundaries in spoken language with 90% accuracy.
- Demonstrate awareness of rimes in spoken language with 90% accuracy.

- Match words with the same beginning or ending sounds with 90% accuracy.

- Delete or substitute initial consonants in simple syllables with 90% accuracy.

- Analyze and blend sounds in simple syllables with 90% accuracy.

Phonics and Word-Identification Goals

Carlos will:
- Identify sounds of 18 consonants and 5 vowels with 100% accuracy.

- Read and spell consonant-vowel-consonant (CVC) words using manipulatives with 80% accuracy.

- Read and spell CVC words using manipulatives with 80% accuracy.

- Read sentences consisting of high-frequency or phonetically regular CVC words with 80% accuracy.

Treatment Plan for Dyslexia Profile: Evan Edsen

Evan's profile is the "classic" picture of a learner with dyslexia. He shows primary deficits in phonological processing, decoding, and reading fluency and relative strengths in comprehension and spoken language. Despite intensive treatment, his oral reading continues to be extremely slow, labored, and also inaccurate.

Therapy for Evan should focus on building accurate decoding skills through explicit, systematic phonics instruction. Because several of his reading and spelling errors are indicative of deficits in morphological

awareness, this area should also be targeted. In addition, as Evan is approaching middle school and will be encountering many multisyllabic words in content areas such as science and social studies, therapy should also incorporate direct instruction in the syllable patterns and morphemic patterns (prefixes, suffixes, root words) that are common in more complex words across his curriculum.

Learners who begin intervention with strengths in comprehension are often very resistant to using phonics strategies for decoding. This is especially apparent when they are reading connected text. Learners like Evan often use context cues, background knowledge, and a few sounds to guess words that may logically fit in a sentence but are, nonetheless, inaccurate. Several strategies can be used to override Evan's natural reliance on using his strengths to compensate for weaknesses in decoding accuracy. First, the practitioner should increase the number of pseudo-words practiced at each lesson. Because pseudo-words have no semantic representation, the learner is forced to rely on phonics, rather than context, to arrive at the word's pronunciation. The practitioner should also create absurd or unpredictable sentences using targeted phonemes and syllable types to minimize the impact of context while practicing newly learned words (e.g., The sloth perched at the edge of the slum and slithered down the sidewalk).

Intervention goals should also target oral reading fluency using repeated timed readings that Evan can read with 95% accuracy.

At this point in Evan's treatment, the emphasis should be on accuracy of reading over fluency, though fluency should also be charted. During practice and guided rereadings of each passage, Evan should not be timed, so accuracy can be established first. For each and every miscue, Evan should be instructed to use a phonics strategy using the phrase "touch and say." This explicit prompt draws the learner's attention to the fact that every letter matters—not just the beginning and ending ones. Once accuracy is established for the miscue, Evan should be instructed to practice reading the word in its context, starting at the beginning of the sentence. To generalize morphological awareness instruction to reading connected text, it is often helpful to have the learner simply circle or highlight "endings" and "beginnings" directly on the page. These morphological markers are often omitted during reading; marking them focuses the learner's attention directly to the problem. Although guided reading techniques of this nature are a bit time consuming, they are typically very effective. Over time, Evan will begin to self-monitor his own miscues and the practitioner can begin to minimize the number of prompts needed.

Suggested Therapy Resources

- Explicit phonics programs (e.g., Barton, Wilson, Slingerland)
- Syllabification programs (e.g., Megawords)
- Fluency programs (e.g., QuickReads, Read Naturally, Great Leaps)

Long-Term Goals (6 months)

Phonological Awareness Goals:

Evan will:

- Blend phonemes in known words of up to three syllables in length with 90% accuracy.
- Delete phonemes in CCVC, CVCC, and CCVCC syllables with 90% accuracy.

Phonics and Word-Recognition Goals:

Evan will:

- Read and spell CVC, CCVC, CVCC, CVCe and *r*-controlled syllables (words and pseudo-words) with 90% accuracy at the single-word level.
- Read and spell CVC, CCVC, CVCC, CVCe and *r*-controlled syllables (words and pseudo-words) with 90% accuracy in sentences.
- Read and spell CVC, CCVC, CVCC, CVCe and *r*-controlled syllables (words and pseudo-words) with 90% accuracy in paragraphs.
- Read and spell compound words with 90% accuracy at the single-word level.
- Read multisyallabic words with closed (CVC/CVC) and open (CV/CVC) syllables with 90% accuracy at the single-word level.
- Identify, read, and spell morphological markers (e.g., grammatical endings, prefixes, and suffixes) with 90% accuracy in words and sentences.

Fluency Goals

Evan will:

- Improve current oral reading fluency of connected text by 20 correct words per minute.
- Accurately read 60 multisyllabic words in one minute.

Treatment Plan for Mixed Language and Reading Deficit Profile: Gail Gomez

Gail presents with a mixed language and reading disorder. A review of Gail's profile shows that her scores fell below the 10th percentile on two of the three CELF-4 subtests, on the CTOPP tests of rapid naming, and on the GORT-4 fluency composite. Such significant and broad-based deficits are likely to severely impact academic achievement across all subject areas and will require ongoing support, especially as curricular demands increase beyond third grade.

With a more specific reading disability, such as dyslexia, it is easy to pinpoint the focus of treatment. However, when a learner is struggling in both the spoken and written modalities of language, it is often difficult to determine the initial instructional targets for intervention. One strategy is to begin with the child's area of strength. Gail's reading comprehension, while below the average range, is an area of relative strength compared to her reading accuracy. Thus, improving Gail's decoding skills and helping her generalize this skill to connected text through extensive guided reading practice will likely have dramatic effects on her overall reading fluency and comprehension.

Suggested Instructional Resources

- Comprehensive language programs with an explicit phonics component (e.g., Language!)
- Passages for guided reading (e.g., QuickReads; Read Naturally)

Long-Term Goals (6 months)

Phonological Awareness Goals

Gail will:

- Blend phonemes in known words of up to two syllables in length with 90% accuracy.
- Delete phonemes in CCVC, CVCC, and CCVCC syllables with 90% accuracy.

Phonics and Word-Identification Goals

Gail will:

- Read and spell CVC, CCVC, CVCC, CVCe, and r-controlled syllables with 90% accuracy at the single-word level.
- Read and spell CVC, CCVC, CVCC, CVCe, and r-controlled syllables (words and pseudo-words) with 90% accuracy in sentences.
- Read and spell CVC, CCVC, CVCC, CVCe, and r-controlled syllables with 90% accuracy in paragraphs.
- Read and spell compound words with 90% accuracy at the single-word level.
- Identify, read, and spell morphological markers (e.g., grammatical endings, prefixes, and suffixes) with 90% accuracy in words and sentences.

Fluency Goals

Gail will:

- Improve current oral reading fluency of connected text by 20 correct words per minute.

Listening and Text Comprehension Goals

After reading or listening to a story, Gail will:

- Answer literal comprehension questions (who, what, where).
- Describe the sequence of events.
- Understand stated causal relationships.

Treatment Plan for Comprehension Deficit Profile: Harry Harper

Harry presents with a specific deficit in reading comprehension. Many learners have comprehension deficits that are secondary to poor word-reading skills and/or oral language weakness (Cain & Oakhill, 2007). A review of his diagnostic profile reveals weakness in three areas, reading comprehension, written language comprehension, and short-term verbal memory; and strengths in word recognition, word decoding, and rapid word naming. Futhermore, Harry has a previous diagnosis for attention deficit disorder.

While many of Harry's scores fell well within the average range, there was a discrepancy between his high word-level reading scores in untimed conditions and his (a) average phonological awareness and memory scores, (b) average spoken language scores, (c) depressed word- and text-level comprehension scores, and (d) below-average written composition sample. The most apparent weaknesses in his narrative writing sample were seen in its overall simplicity, its lack of cohesive markers for connecting ideas, and the lack of overall coherence for a well-educated 13-year-old student. Additional language testing of higher-level language skills such as comprehension monitoring, depth of word meanings, and understanding of inferences and story structures (Oakhill & Cain, 2007) would likely have uncovered areas of weakness that were not identified on the CELF-4. It is likely that Harry's depressed comprehension is secondary to subtle weakness in higher-level language, memory, and executive function processes.

Rapp, van den Broek, McMaster, Kendeou, and Espin (2007) note that processing capacity is a major source of comprehension difficulty. As such, therapy for Harry should focus on helping him develop reading strategies that make reading comprehension more efficient in terms of cognitive load. In order to comprehend connected text, readers must construct a coherent mental representation of the ideas and concepts that are conveyed. This process may be very taxing because it relies heavily on working memory resources. The process of creating coherence requires the reader to make meaningful connections over long distances. For example, pertinent details and concepts presented at the beginning of a passage must be held in working memory so that these details can be integrated with information revealed later in the text. The process of establishing coherence over long distances also requires the reader to selectively allocate and reallocate attention to pertinent details and to let go of irrelevant or extraneous information. Additionally, the reader must make immediate decisions as to whether or not background information or prior knowledge stored in long-term memory is relevant to the text that is being read. This complex balancing act of shifting, inhibiting, and self-monitoring requires the use of the cognitive processes referred to as executive functions.

Rapp et al. (2007) have identified several sources of difficulty that can affect text comprehension:

- Lack of background knowledge
- Inefficient activation of background knowledge
- Over-reliance on background knowledge
- Inability to construct inferences
- Inability to self-monitor (e.g., repair comprehension breakdowns)
- Inability to make use of the structure or organization of text

Therapy for Harry should begin by trying to pinpoint the types of difficulties experienced and focus on the types of comprehension breakdowns exhibited. An instructional method that has been proven effective for improving comprehension is reciprocal teaching (Palincsar & Brown, 1984). This method involves interactive questioning, summarizing, and predicting during the process of reading, which helps the reader learn to focus on the pertinent information in the text.

Learners with reading comprehension deficits often derive little pleasure from reading and avoid it at all cost. This difficulty is captured in the statement of a 13-year-old boy who, when asked what is hard about reading, responded

> It's not hard, I just hate it. You'll be reading about one thing and then all of a sudden you're reading about some random thing that has nothing to do with the first part. It just doesn't make any sense. That's why I hate reading.

Because reading itself is a hard sell—especially to struggling adolescent boys—and because employing all kinds of comprehension strategies is frankly quite effortful, it is extremely important that the practitioner begin the therapy process by selecting reading material that is both interesting and familiar to the learner. Research has shown that personal interest and extensive background knowledge can significantly improve comprehension.

Many texts are not particularly well structured (Rapp et al., 2007), making it necessary for practitioners to pay special attention to the organization of the texts learners choose. The Close Analysis of Texts with Structure (CATS) program provides short, well-structured passages that highlight causal chains, which are integral to understanding inferences. Tying achievement to short-term external rewards (e.g., computer time, video-game time) will also keep learners motivated in the short term, before they experience the long-term benefits of the comprehension strategies.

Suggested Therapy Resources

- Supplementary comprehension programs with a reciprocal teaching component (e.g., *POSSE, Questioning the Author, CATS*)
- High-Interest Reading Material
- Short, leveled passages (e.g., QuickReads, Read Naturally)
- www.Booksforboys.com
- www.Guysread.com

Long-Term Goals (6 months)

Harry will:

- Construct stated inferences with minimal cues with 90% accuracy.
- Construct implied inferences with minimal cues with 80% accuracy.
- Construct inferences requiring integration of background knowledge with minimal cues with 80% accuracy.
- Identify component structures of various types of text and genres with 80% accuracy.

SUMMARY

After a comprehensive assessment that profiles the child's strengths and weaknesses, there are many factors to consider for getting the child on the optimal path for reading intervention. Simply naming the problem is not enough. Indeed, most parents know that their child has a reading disability before stepping foot in your office! What parents and educators working with the child need are specifics: specific answers to the questions *why, who*, and, perhaps most importantly, *what now?* MAR^{w}R, as presented in this book, is designed to be utilized both as a starting point for diagnostic counseling and as a framework for prescribing treatment goals that are specifically focused to meet the individual needs of each child. Keeping in mind that receiving a diagnosis of any kind is often an emotionally charged experience, and taking the time to ensure that parents thoroughly understand the intricate relationship between diagnosis and treatment, will give families strength and confidence as they begin weighing their therapy options and pursuing the intervention path that is most beneficial for their child.

Appendix 6-1

A Sample Bell Curve for Reporting Assessment Results

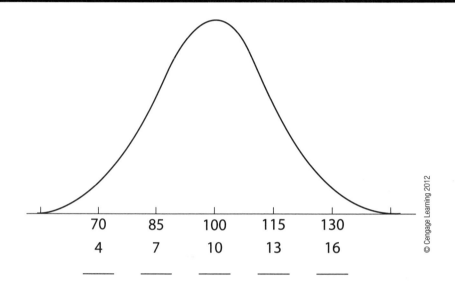

70   85   100   115   130

4   7   10   13   16

____ ____ ____ ____ ____

© Cengage Learning 2012

Name: _____ Date of Evaluation: _____

Results from this assessment reveal a pattern of strengths and weaknesses that are consistent with a diagnosis of:

_____ Reading Disorder, unspecified (315.00)

_____ Developmental Dyslexia (315.02)

_____ Receptive-Expressive Language Disorder (315.32)

Test and subtest scores that support this diagnosis:

_____   _____   _____

_____   _____   _____

_____   _____   _____

Comments

_____   _____   _____

_____   _____   _____

_____   _____   _____

Checklist of Accommodations Recommended to Facilitate the Learner's Academic Success

	Test Modifications
	Should be given extended time on tests that require reading or writing
	Should be provided with a reader for written tests whenever necessary
	Should be permitted to provide oral responses in many or all testing situations
	Should be permitted to take tests in segments to allow for extended time to read and to minimize fatigue
	Should be able to mark answers directly on the exam rather than on a bubble sheet
	Should be permitted to highlight sections on the exam to facilitate memory
	Should be given a formula sheet for equations and other sequences that are expected to be memorized
	Should have a proofreader to ensure that mistakes, such as reversals of numbers, can be identified and corrected
	Auxiliary Aids
	Should be provided with textbooks on CD-ROM, when needed
	Should be permitted to use a calculator for math assignments and exams, if needed
	Should be permitted to use a computer for writing assignments and spell-checking, if needed
	Should have access to word recognition software for writing assignments, if needed
	Should have access to text-to-speech software for reading textbooks, if needed
	Curriculum Modifications
	Should be seated in front of the class so that classroom assignments can be carefully monitored
	Should not be required to read aloud if this causes stress and embarrassment for the student
	Should be permitted to tape-record lectures, when necessary
	Should be provided with a tutor who has knowledge of alternative techniques needed for teaching reading to students with learning disabilities, if needed
	Should be permitted to substitute a course for a foreign language requirement if it is clear that learning a second language will be extraordinarily time consuming and difficult
	Should be permitted to take a reduced course load, if necessary
	Should be permitted to withdraw from a course without being penalized if student is failing in spite of extraordinary effort
	Should be permitted to substitute a course of interest (e.g., music) for a course that may very difficult and does not coincide with the older student's plans for the future

References

Aaron, P. G. (1997). The impending demise of the discrepancy formula. *Review of Educational Research, 67,* 461–502.

Aaron, P. G., & Joshi, R. M. (1992). *Reading problems: Consultation and remediation.* New York: Guilford Press.

Aaron, P. G., Joshi, R. M., Boulware-Gooden, R., & Bentum, K. (2008). Diagnosis and treatment of reading disabilities based on the component model of reading: An alternative to the discrepancy model of learning disabilities. *Journal of Learning Disabilities, 41,* 67–84.

Aaron, P. G., Joshi, R. M., & Quatroche, D. (2008). *Becoming a professional reading teacher.* Baltimore: Brookes.

Aaron, P. G., Joshi, R. M., & Williams, K. A. (1999). Not all reading disabilities are alike. *Journal of Learning Disabilities, 32,* 120–137.

Abedi, J. (2008). Measuring students' level of English proficiency. Educational significance and assessment requirements. *Educational Assessment, 13,* 193–214.

Adams, M. J. (1990). *Beginning to read: Thinking and learning about print.* Cambridge, MA: MIT Press.

Adams, M. J. (2002). Alphabetic anxiety and explicit, systematic phonics instruction: A cognitive science perspective. In S. B. Neuman & D. K. Dickinson (Eds.), *Handbook of early literacy research* (pp. 97–125). New York: Guilford Press.

Adams, M. J., Foorman, B. R., Lundberg, I., & Beeler, T. (1998). *Phonemic awareness in young children. A classroom curriculum.* Baltimore: Brookes.

Al Otaiba, S., Puranik, C. S., Rouby, D. A., Greulich, L., Sidler, J. F., & Lee, J. (2010). Predicting kindergarteners' end-of-year spelling ability based on their reading, phonological awareness skills, as well as prior literacy experiences. *Learning Disability Quarterly, 33,* 171–183.

Allington, R. (1983). Fluency: The most neglected goal in reading instruction. *Reading Teacher, 36,* 556–561.

Alphabetic Phonics. (n.d.). Retrieved August 17, 2011, http://www.eps.schoolspecialty.com.

Anderson, V. (1992). A teacher development project in transactional strategy instruction for teachers of severely reading- disabled adolescents. *Teaching & Teacher Education, 8,* 391–403.

Anderson, V., & Roit, M. (1993). Planning and implementing collaborative strategy instruction for delayed readers in grades 6–10. *Elementary School Journal, 94,* 121–137.

Anglin, J. M. (1993). Vocabulary development: A morphological analysis. *Monographs of the Society for Research in Child Development, 58* (10, Serial No. 238), 1–165.

ANSI. (1996). *Determination of occupational noise exposure and estimation of noise-induced hearing impairment.* New York: American National Standards Institute. Standard S 3.44–1996.

Apel, K., Masterson, J. J., & Niessen, N. L. (2004). Spelling assessment frameworks. In A. Stone, E. R. Silliman, B. Ehren, & K. Apel (Eds.), *Handbook of language and literacy: Development and disorders* (pp. 644–660). New York: Guilford Press.

Applebee, A. (1978). *The child's concept of story: Ages two to ten.* Chicago: University of Chicago Press.

Aram, D., & Nation, J. (1982). *Child Language Disorders,* C.V. Mosby Co., St. Louis.

Archer, A. (2009). *Big ideas: Tier II and Tier III interventions.* Retrieved April 25, 2009, from www.updc.org/assets/files/. . .by. . ./**archer**/. . . **2009**/RTIIRevisedNov.ppt

Artiles, A. J., & Ortiz, A. A. (Eds.). (2002). *English language learners with special education needs: Identification, assessment, and instruction.* Washington, DC: Center for Applied Linguistics and Delta Systems.

Atkinson, R., & Shiffrin, R. (1968). Human memory: A proposed system and its control processes. In K. Spence & J. Spence (Eds.), *The psychology of learning and motivation: Advances in research and theory* (Vol. 2). New York: Academic Press.

August, D., Francis, D., Hsu, H.-Y. A., & Snow, C. (2006). Assessing reading comprehension in bilinguals. In R. Gersten (Ed.), Instructional research on English learners [Special issue]. *Elementary School Journal, 107*(2), 221–238.

August, D., & Hakuta, K. (Eds.). (1997). *Improving schooling for language-minority children: A research agenda.* Washington, DC: National Academy Press.

Baddeley, A. (1986). *Working memory.* Oxford, UK: Oxford University Press.

Baddeley, A. (2000). The episodic buffer: A new component of working memory? *Trends in Cognitive Studies, 4*(11), 417–423.

Baddeley, A. (2003). Working memory and language: An overview. *Journal of Communication Disorders, 36,* 189–208.

Badian, N. (1982). The prediction of good and poor reading before kindergarten entry: A 4-year follow-up. *The Journal of Special Education, 16,* 309–318.

Badian, N. (1994). Preschool prediction: Orthographic and phonological skills, and reading. *Annals of Dyslexia, 44,* 3–25.

Badian, N. (1995). Predicting reading ability over the long term: The changing roles of letter naming, phonological awareness and orthographic processing. *Annals of Dyslexia, 45,* 79–96.

Badian, N. (1998). A validation of the role of preschool phonological and orthographic skills in the prediction of reading. *Journal of Learning Disabilities, 31,* 472–481.

Ball, E. W. (1993). Phonological awareness: What's important and to whom? *Reading and Writing: An Interdisciplinary Journal, 5,* 141–159.

Barton, S. (2000). *Barton reading and spelling system.* San Jose, CA: Author.

The Barton Reading & Spelling System: http://www.bartonreading.com/

Bear, D., Invernizzi, M., Templeton, S., & Johnston, F. (2004). *Words their way: Word study for vocabulary, phonics, and spelling instruction* (3rd ed.). Upper Saddle River, NJ: Pearson.

Beck, I. L. (2006). *Making sense of phonics.* New York: Guilford Press.

Beck, I. L., McKeown, M. G., & Kucan, L. (2002). *Bringing words to life: Robust vocabulary instruction.* New York: Guilford Press.

Bereiter, C., & Scardamalia, M. (1987). *The psychology of written composition.* Hillsdale, NJ: Erlbaum.

Berkeley, S., Bender, W. N., Peaster, L. G., & Saunders, L. (2009). Implementation of response to intervention. *Journal of Learning Disabilities, 42,* 85–95.

Berninger, V. (1999). Coordinating transcription and text generation in working memory during composing: Automatic and Constructive Processes. *Learning Disability Quarterly, 22,* 99–112.

Berninger, V. (2001). *Process assessment of the learner—Test battery for reading and writing, PAL-RW.* San Antonio, TX: The Psychological Corporation.

Berninger, V. (2007). *Process assessment of the learner II user's guide (CD formatted book).* San Antonio, TX: Pearson (formerly Harcourt/The Psychological Corporation).

Berninger, V. (2008). Defining and differentiating dysgraphia, dyslexia, and language learning disability within a working memory model. In M. Mody & E. R. Silliman (Eds.), *Brain, behavior, and learning in language and reading disorders* (pp. 103–134). New York: Guilford Press.

Berninger, V., Abbott, R. D., Billlngsley, F., & Nagy, W. (2001). Process underlying timing and fluency of reading: Efficiency, automaticity, coordination, and morphological awareness. In M. Wolf (Ed.), *Dyslexia, fluency and the brain.* Timonium, MD: York Press (pp. 383–414).

Berninger, V., Abbott, R. D., Thomson, J. B., & Raskind, W. H. (2001). Language phenotype for reading and writing disability: A family approach. *Scientific Studies of Reading, 5*(1), 59–106.

Berninger, V., Abbott, R. D., Thomson, J., Wagner, R., Swanson, H. L., Wijsman, E., et al. (2006). Modeling developmental phonological core deficits within a working-memory architecture in children and adults with developmental dyslexia. *Scientific Studies in Reading, 10,* 165–198.

Berninger, V., Fuller, F., & Whitaker, D. (1996). A process model of writing development across the life span. *Educational Psychology Review, 8,* 193–218.

Berninger, V., O'Donnell, L., & Holdnack, J. (2008). Research-supported differential diagnosis of specific learning disabilities and implications for instruction and response to instruction (RTI). In A. Prifitera, D. Saklofske, & L. Weiss (Eds.), *WISC-IV clinical assessment and intervention* (2nd ed., pp. 69–108). San Diego, CA: Academic Press.

Berninger, V., & Swanson, H. L. (1994). Modifying Hayes & Flower's model of skilled writing to explain beginning and developing writing. In E. Butterfield (Ed.), *Children's writings: Toward a process theory of development of skilled writing* (pp. 57–81). Greenwich, CT: JAI Press.

Berninger, V., Vaughan, K., Abbott, R., Brooks, A., Begay, K., Curtin, G., et al. (2000). Language-based spelling instruction: Teaching children to make multiple connections between spoken and written words. *Learning Disability Quarterly, 23,* 117–135.

Berninger, V., & Wolf, B. J. (2009). *Teaching students with dyslexia and dysgraphia: Lessons from teaching and science.* Baltimore: Brookes.

Berninger, V., Yates, C., Cartwright, A., Rutberg, J., Remy, E., & Abbot, R. (1992). Lower-level developmental skills in beginning writing. *Reading and Writing: An Interdisciplinary Journal, 4,* 257–280.

Bicmiller, A. (2003). Oral comprehension sets the ceiling on reading comprehension. *American Educator, 27,* 23–44.

Biemiller, A. (2005). Size and sequence in vocabulary development: Implications for choosing words for primary grade vocabulary instruction. In E. H. Hiebert & M. Kamil (Eds.), *Teaching and learning vocabulary: Bringing research to practice* (pp. 223–245). Mahwah, NJ: Erlbaum.

Biemiller, A. (2006). Vocabulary development and instruction: A prerequisite for school learning. In S. B. Neuman & D. K. Dickson (Eds.), *Handbook of early literacy research* (pp. 41–51). New York: Guilford Press.

Biemiller, A., & Boote, C. (2006). An effective method for building meaning vocabulary in the primary grades. *Journal of Educational Psychology, 98*, 44–62.

Biemiller, A., & Slonim, N. (2001). Estimating root word vocabulary growth in normative and advantaged populations: Evidence for a common sequence of vocabulary acquisition. *Journal of Educational Psychology, 93*, 498–520.

Bishop, D. V. M. (2001). Genetic influences on language impairment and literacy problems in children: Same or different. *Journal of Child Psychology and Psychiatry and Allied Disciplines, 42*, 189–198.

Bishop, D. V. M. (2008). Specific language impairment, dyslexia, and autism: Using genetics to unravel their relationship. In C. F. Norbury, J. B., Tomblin, & D. V. M. Bishop (Eds.), *Understanding developmental language disorders: From theory to practice* (pp. 67–78). New York: Psychology Press.

Bishop, D. V. M., & Adams, C. (1990). A prospective study of the relationship between specific language impairment, phonological disorders and reading retardation. *Journal of Child Psychology and Psychiatry, 31*, 1027–1105.

Bishop, D. V. M., & Clarkson, B. (2003). Written languages as a window into residual language deficits: A study of children wih persistent and residual speech and language impairments. *Cortex, 39*, 215–237.

Bishop, D. V. M., & Edmundson, A. (1987). Language-impaired four-year-olds: Distinguishing transient from persistent impairment. *Journal of Speech and Hearing Disorders, 52*, 156–173.

Bishop, D. V. M., & Snowling, M. J. (2004). Developmental dyslexia and specific language impairment: Same or different? *Psychological Bulletin, 130*, 858–888.

Blachman, B. (1997). *Foundations of reading acquisition and dyslexia: Implications for early intervention.* Mahwah, NJ: Erlbaum.

Blaiklock, K. (2004). The importance of letter knowledge in the relationship between phonological awareness and reading. *Journal of Research in Reading, 27*, 36–57.

Blair, C. (2006). How similar are fluid cognition and general intelligence? A developmental neuroscience perspective on fluid cognition as an aspect of human cognitive ability. *Behavioral and Brain Sciences, 29*, 109–160.

Block, C. C. (1993). Strategy instruction in a student-centered classroom. *Elementary School Journal, 94*(2), 137–153.

Block, C. C. (1999). The case for exemplary teaching, especially for students who begin first grade without the precursors for literacy success. In T. Shanahan (Ed.), *49th yearbook of the National Reading Conference* (pp. 71–85). Chicago: National Reading Conference.

Block, C., & Duffy, G. (2008). Research on teaching comprehension: Where we've been and where we're going. In C. Block & S. Paris (Eds.), *Comprehension instruction: Research-based best practices* (2nd ed., pp. 19–37). New York: Guilford Press.

Bosse, M. L., Tainturier, M. J., & Valdois, S. (2007). Developmental dyslexia: The visual attention span deficit hypothesis. *Cognition, 104*(2), 198–230.

Botting, N. (2007). Comprehension difficulties in children with specific language impairment and pragmatic language impairment. In K. Cain & J. Oakhill (Eds.), *Children's comprehension problems in oral and written language: A cognitive perspective* (pp. 81–103). New York: Guilford Press.

Boudreau, D. (2008). Narrative abilities: Advances in research and implications for clinical practice. *Topics in Language Disorders, 28*, 99–114.

Boudreau, D., & Hedberg, N. (1999). A comparison of early literacy skills in children with specific language impairment and their typically developing peers. *American Journal of Speech-Language Pathology, 8*, 249–260.

Bowers, P., & Swanson, L. (1991). Naming speed deficits in reading disability: Multiple measures of a single process. *Journal of Experimental Psychology, 51*, 195–219.

Bowers, P., & Wolf, M. (1993). Theoretical links among naming speed, precise timing mechanisms and orthographic skill in dyslexia. *Reading and Writing: An Interdisciplinary Journal, 5*, 69–85.

Bowey, J. A. (1986a). Syntactic awareness and verbal performance from preschool to fifth grade. *Journal of Psycholinguistic Research, 15*, 285–306.

Bowey, J. A. (1986b). Syntactic awareness in relation to reading skill and ongoing comprehension monitoring. *Journal of Experimental Child Psychology, 41*, 282–299.

Bowey, J. A. (1996). Grammatical priming of visual word recognition in fourth-grade children. *Quarterly Journal of Experimental Psychology: Human Experimental Psychology, 49A*, 1005–1023.

Bowey, J. A. (2005). Predicting individual differences in learning to read. In M. J. Snowling & C. Hulme (Eds.), *The science of reading: A handbook* (pp. 155–172). Oxford, UK: Blackwell.

Breznitz, Z. (2006). *Fluency in reading: Synchronization of processes.* Mahwah, NJ: Erlbaum.

Breznitz, Z. (2008). The origins of dyslexia: The Asynchrony phenomenon. In G. Reid, A. A. Fawcett, F. Manis, & L. Siegel (Eds.), *The Sage handboook of dyslexia* (pp. 11–20). Los Angeles: Sage.

Brinton, B., & Fujiki, M. (1989). *Conversational management with language-impaired children: Pragmatic assessment and intervention.* Rockville, MD: Aspen.

Brown, R., Pressley, M., Van Meter, P., & Schuder, T. (1996). A quasi-experimental validation of transactional strategies instruction with low-achieving second grade readers. *Journal of Educational Psychology, 88*, 18–37.

Bruck, M. (1993). Component spelling skills of college students with childhood diagnoses of dyslexia. *Learning Disability Quarterly, 16*, 171–184.

Bruck, M., & Waters, G. S. (1988). An analysis of the spelling errors of children who differ in their reading and spelling skills. *Applied Psycholinguistics, 9*, 77–92.

Burgess, S. R., & Lonigan, C. J. (1998). Bidirectional relations of phonological sensitivity and prereading abilities: Evidence from a preschool sample. *Journal of Experimental Child Psychology, 70*, 117–141.

Burns, J. M., & Richgels, D. J. (1989) An investigation of task requirements associated with the invented spelling of 4-year-olds with above average intelligence. *Journal of Reading Behavior, 21*, 1–14.

Bus, A., van Ijzendoorn, M., & Pellegrini, A. (1995). Joint book reading makes for success in learning to read: A meta-analysis on intergenerational transmission of literacy. *Review of Educational Research, 65*, 1–21.

Byrne, B., Wadsworth, S., Corley, R., Samuelsson, S., Quain, P., DeFries, J. C., et al. (2005). Longitudinal twin study of early literacy development: Preschool and kindergarten phases. *Scientific Studies of Reading, 9*, 219–235.

Cain, K. (2007). Syntactic awareness and reading ability: Is there any evidence for a special relationship? *Applied Psycholinguistics, 28*, 679–694.

Cain, K., & Oakhill, J. (2006). Profiles of children with specific reading comprehension difficulties. *British Journal of Educational Psychology, 76*, 683–696.

Cain, K., & Oakhill, J. (2007a). *Children's comprehension problems in oral and written language: A cognitive perspective.* New York: Guilford Press.

Cain, K., & Oakhill, J. (2007b). Reading comprehension difficulties: Correlates, causes, and consequences. In K. Cain & J. Oakhill (Eds.), *Children's comprehension problems in oral and written language: A cognitive perspective.* New York: Guilford Press.

Cain, K., Oakhill, J., & Bryant, P. (2004). Children's reading comprehension ability: Concurrent prediction by working memory, verbal ability, and component skills. *Journal of Educational Psychology, 96*, 31–42.

Caravolas, M. (2005). The nature and causes of dyslexia in different languages. In M. J. Snowling & C. Hulme (Eds.), *Science of reading: A handbook*

(pp. 336–357). Malden, MA: Blackwell Publishing.

Caravolas, M., Hulme, C., & Snowling, M. J. (2001). The foundations of spelling ability: Evidence from a 3-year longitudinal study. *Journal of Memory and Language, 45*, 751–774.

Carlisle, J. F. (2000). Awareness of the structure and meaning of morphologically complex words: Impact on reading. *Reading and Writing: An Interdisciplinary Journal, 12*(3), 169–190.

Carlisle, J. F. (2003). Morphology matters in learning to read: A commentary. *Reading Psychology, 24*, 291–322.

Carreker, S., & Joshi, R. M. (2010). Response to intervention: Are the emperor's clothes really new? *Psichothema, 22*, 943–948.

Carroll, J. M., Snowling, M. J., Hulme, C., & Stevenson, J. (2003). The development of phonological awareness in preschool children. *Developmental Psychology, 39*, 913–923.

Carrow-Woolfolk, E. (1999). *Comprehensive Assessment of Spoken Language, CASL.* Circle Pines, MN: American Guidance Service.

Carver, R. P. (1997). Reading for one second, one minute, or one year from the perspective of rauding theory. *Scientific Studies of Reading, 1*, 3–43.

Carver, R. P. (2000). *The causes of high and low reading achievement.* Mahwah, NJ: Erlbaum.

Carver, R. P., & Clark, S. W. (1998). Investigating reading disabilities using the rauding diagnostic system. *Journal of Learning Disabilities, 31*(5), 143–174.

Carver, R. P., & David, A. H. (2001). Investigating reading achievement using a causal model. *Scientific Studies of Reading, 5*, 107–140.

Cassar, M., & Treiman, R. (2004). Developmental variations in spelling: Comparing typical and poor spellers. In C. A. Stone, E. R. Silliman, B. Ehren, & K. Apel (Eds.), *Handbook of language and literacy: Development and disorders.* New York: Guilford Press.

Cassar, M., Treiman, R., Moats, L., Pollo, T. C., & Kessler, B. (2005). How do the spellings of children with dyslexia compare with those of nondyslexic children? *Reading and Writing: An Interdisciplinary Journal, 18,* 27–49.

Castles, A., Datta, H., Gayán, J., & Olson, R. K. (1999). Varieties of developmental reading disorder: Genetic and environmental influences. *Journal of Experimental Child Psychology, 72,* 73–94.

Catell, R. B., & Horn, J. L. (1978). A check on the theory of fluid and crystallized intelligence with description of new subtest design. *Journal of Educational Measurement, 15,* 139–164.

Catts, H. (1993). The relationship between speech language impairments and reading disabilities. *Journal of Speech and Hearing Research, 36,* 948–958.

Catts, H., Adlof, S. M., & Weismer, S. E. (2006). Language deficits in poor comprehenders: A case for the simple view of reading. *Journal of Speech, Language, and Hearing Research, 49,* 278–293.

Catts, H., Fey, M., Tomblin, J., & Zhang, X. (2002). A longitudinal investigation of reading outcomes in children with language impairments. *Journal of Speech, Language, and Hearing Research, 45,* 1142–1157.

Catts, H., Fey, M., Zhang, X., & Tomblin, J. (1999). Language basis of reading and reading disabilities: Evidence from a longitudinal investigation. *Scientific Study of Reading, 3,* 331–336.

Catts, H., Fey, M. F., Zhang, X., & Tomblin, J. B. (2001). Estimating the risk of future reading difficulties in kindergarten children: A research-based model and its clinical implementation. *Language, Speech, and Hearing Services in Schools, 32,* 38–50.

Catts, H., Gillispie, M., Leonard, L. B., Kail, R. V., & Miller, C. A. (2002). The role of speed of processing, rapid naming, and phonological awareness in reading achievement. *Journal of Learning Disabilities, 35*(6), 510–525.

Catts, H., Hogan, T. P., & Fey, M. (2003). Subgrouping poor readers on the basis of reading-related abilities. *Journal of Learning Disabilities, 36,* 151–164.

Catts, H., & Kamhi, A. G. (2003). *The connections between language and reading disabilities.* Mahwah, NJ: Erlbaum.

Catts, H., & Kamhi, A. G. (2005). *Language and reading disabilities.* Boston: Pearson.

Chall, J. S. (1967). *Learning to read: The great debate; an inquiry into the science, art, and ideology of old and new methods of teaching children to read.* New York: McGraw Hill.

Chall, J. S. (1979). The great debate: Ten years later, with a modest proposal for reading stages. In L. Resnick & P. A. Weaver (Eds.), *Theory and practice of early reading* (Vol. 1, pp. 29–55). Hillsdale, NJ: Erlbaum.

Chall, J. S. (1983). *Stages of reading development.* New York: McGraw Hill.

Clay, M. (1979). *The early detection of reading difficulties: A diagnostic survey with recovery procedures.* London: Heinemann.

Collins, C. (1991). Reading instruction that increases thinking abilities. *Journal of Reading, 34,* 510–516.

Compton, D., & Catts, H. (2009). *Examining the behavioral profiles of children with late-emerging reading disabilities (LERD)*. Paper presented at the sixteenth annual meeting of the Society for the Scientific Study of Reading, Boston, MA.

Conti-Ramsden, G., & Botting, N. (1999). Classification of children with specific language impairment. Longitudinal considerations. *Journal of Speech, Language, and Hearing Research, 42,* 1205–1219.

Conti-Ramsden, G., Crutchley, A., & Botting, N. (1997). The extent to which psychometric tests differentiate subgroups of children with SLI. *Journal of Speech, Language, and Hearing Research, 40,* 765–777.

Cossu, G. (1999). Biological constraints on literacy acquisition. *Reading and Writing: An Interdisciplinary Journal, 11,* 213–237.

Coyne, M. D., Simmons, D. C., & Kame'enui, E. J. (2004). Vocabulary instruction for young children at risk of experiencing reading difficulties: Teaching word meanings during shared storybook readings. In J. F. Baumann & E. J. Kame'enui (Eds.), *Vocabulary instruction: Research to practice* (pp. 41–58). New York: Guilford Press.

Crosson, B., Rao, S. M., Woodley, S. J., Rosen, A. C., Bobholz, J. A., Mayer, A., et al. (1999). Mapping of semantic, phonological, and orthographic verbal working memory in normal adults with functional magnetic resonance imaging. *Neuropsychology, 13,* 171–187.

Cunningham, A., & Stanovich, K. (1997). Early reading acquisition and its relation to reading experience and ability 10 years later. *Developmental Psychology, 33,* 934–945.

Cunningham, A., & Stanovich, K. (1998). The impact of print exposure on word recognition. In J. L. Metsala & L. C. Ehri (Eds.), *Word recognition in beginning reading* (pp. 235–262). Mahwah, NJ: Erlbaum.

Cutting, L. E., & Scarborough, H. S. (2006). Prediction of reading comprehension: Relative contributions of word recognition, language proficiency, and other cognitive skills can depend on how comprehension is measured. *Scientific Studies of Reading, 10*(3), 277–299.

Davies, P., Shanks, B., & Davies, K. (2004). Improving narrative skills in young children with delayed language development. *Educational Review, 56,* 271–286.

Dawson, J., Stout, C., & Eyer, J. (2003). *Structured Photographic Expressive Language Test (SPELT-3)* (3rd ed.). Sandwich, IL: Janelle.

de Jong, P. F. (1998). Working memory deficits of reading disabled children. *Journal of Experimental Child Psychology, 70,* 75–96.

de Jong, P. F., & van der Leij, A. (2002). Effects of phonological abilities and linguistic comprehension on the development of reading. *Scientific Studies of Reading, 6,* 51–77.

Deacon, S. H., & Kirby, J. R. (2004). Morphological awareness: Just "more phonological"? The roles of morphological and phonological awareness in reading development. *Applied Psycholinguistics, 25,* 223–238.

Deane, P., Sheehan, K. M., Sabatini, J., Futagi, Y., & Kostin, I. (2006). Differences in text structure and its implications for assessment of struggling readers. *Scientific Studies of Reading, 10*(3), 257–275.

Denckla, M. B., & Cutting, L. E. (1999). History and significance of rapid automatized naming. *Annals of Dyslexia, 49,* 29–42.

Denckla, M. B., & Rudel, R. G. (1972). Color-naming in dyslexic boys. *Cortex, 8,* 164–176.

Denckla, M. B., & Rudel, R. G. (1974). Rapid "automatized" naming of pictured objects, colors, letters, and numbers by normal children. *Cortex, 10,* 186–202.

Denckla, M. B., & Rudel, R. G. (1976). Naming of objects by dyslexic and other learning-disabled children. *Brain and Language, 3,* 1–15.

Deshler, D. D., Hock, M. F., & Catts, H. (2006). Enhancing outcomes for struggling adolescent readers. *IDA Perspectives, 10*(2), 21–26.

Dickinson, D. K., & Neuman, S. B. (2006). *Handbook of early literacy research* (Vol. 2). New York: Guilford Press.

Dickinson, D. K., & Sprague, K. (2002). The nature and impact of early childhood care environments on the language and early literacy development of children from low-income families. In S. Neuman & D. K. Dickinson (Eds.), *Handbook of early literacy* (pp. 263–292). New York: Guilford Press.

Difino, S., Johnson, B., & Lombardino, L. (2008). The role of the SLP in assisting college students with dyslexia in fulfilling foreign language requirements: A case study. *Contemporary Issues in Communication Disorders, 35,* 54–64.

Difino, S., & Lombardino, L. (2004). Language learning disabilities: The ultimate foreign language challenge. *Foreign Language Annals, 37,* 390–400.

Dockrell, J. E., Lindsay, G., & Connelly, V. (2009). The impact of specific language impairment on adolescents' written text. *Exceptional Children, 75,* 427–446.

Duke, N., & Pearson, D. (2002). Effective practices for developing reading comprehension. In A. Farstrup & S. J. Samuels (Eds.), *What research has to say about reading instruction*

(3rd ed., pp. 205–242). Newark, DE: International Reading Association.

Dyslexia software with human sounding voices— Natural Reader. (n.d.). Retrieved January 29, 2011, from http://www.confidentreader.com/

Echols, L. D., West, R. F., Stanovich, K. E., & Zehr, K. S. (1996). Using children's literacy activities to predict growth in verbal cognitive skills: A longitudinal investigation. *Journal of Educational Psychology, 88,* 296–304.

Eckert, M., Lombardino, L., & Leonard, C. (2001). Planar asymmetry tips the phonological playground and environment raises the bar. *Child Development, 72,* 988–1002.

Eden, G. F., Stein, J. F., Wood, H. M., & Wood, F. B. (1994). Differences in eye movements and reading problems in dyslexic and normal children. *Vision Research, 34*(10), 1345–1358.

Ehri, L. C. (1983). A critique of five studies related to letter name knowledge and learning to read. In L. M. Gentile, M. L. Kamil, & J. S. Blanchard (Eds.), Reading research revisited (pp. 143–153). Columbus, OH: Merrill.

Ehri, L. C. (1991). Learning to read and spell words. In L. Rieben & C. Perfetti (Eds.), *Learning to read: Basic research and its implications* (pp. 57–73). Hillsdale, NJ: Erlbaum.

Ehri, L. C. (1992). Reconceptualizing the development of sight word reading and its relationship to recoding. In P. B. Gough, L. C. Ehri, & R. Treiman (Eds.), *Reading acquisition* (pp. 107–143). Hillsdale, NJ: Erlbaum.

Ehri, L. C. (1995). Phases of development in learning to read words by sight. *Journal of Research in Reading, 18*(2), 116–125.

Ehri, L. C. (2005). Development of sight word reading: Phases and findings. In M. Snowling &

C. Hulme (Eds.), *The science of reading, a handbook* (pp. 135–154). Malden, MA Blackwell.

Ehri, L. C., & Roberts, T. (2006). The roots of learning to read and write: Acquisition of letters and phonemic awareness. In D. K. Dickinson & S. B. Neuman (Eds.), *Handbook of early literacy research* (Vol. 2, pp. 113–131). New York: Guilford Press.

Ehri, L. C., & Rosenthal, J. (2007). Spellings of words: A neglected facilitator of vocabulary learning. *Journal of Literacy Research, 39,* 389–409.

Ehri, L. C., & Soffer, A. G. (1999). Graphophonemic awareness: Development in elementary students. *Scientific Studies of Reading, 3,* 1–30.

Ehri, L. C., & Wilce, L. (1987). Cipher versus cue reading: An experiment in decoding acquisition. *Journal of Educational Psychology, 79,* 3–13.

Elbaum, B., & Vaughn, S. (2003). Self-concept and students with learning disabilities. In H. L. Swanson, K. R. Harris, & S. Graham (Eds.), *Handbook of learning disabilities* (pp. 229–241). New York: Guilford Press.

Ellis-Weismer, S., Evans, J., & Hesketh, L. (1999). An examination of verbal working memory capacity in children with specific language impairment. *Journal of Speech, Language and Hearing Research, 42,* 1249–1260.

Evans, M. A., Williamson, K., & Pursoo, T. (2008). Preschoolers' attention to print during shared book reading. *Scientific Studies of Reading, 12,* 106–129.

Ezell, H. K., & Justice, L. M. (2000). Increasing the print focus of adult-child shared book reading through observational learning. *American Journal of Speech-Language Pathology, 9,* 36–47.

Felton, R. H., Naylor, C. E., & Wood, F. B. (1990). Neuropsychological profile of adult dyslexics. *Brain and Language, 39,* 485–497.

Fey, M. (1986). *Language intervention with young children.* San Diego, CA: College Hill Press.

Fitzgerald, J., & Shanahan, T. (2000). Reading and writing relations and their development. *Educational Pscyhologist, 35,* 39–50.

Fletcher, J. M. (2009). Dyslexia: The evolution of a scientific concept. *Journal of the International Neuropsychological Society, 15,* 501–508.

Fletcher, J. M., Coulter, W. A., Reschly, D. J., & Vaughn, S. (2004). Alternative approaches to the definition and identification of learning disabilities: Some questions and answers. *Annals of Dyslexia, 54,* 304–331.

Fletcher, J. M., & Lyon, G. R. (2008). Dyslexia: Why precise definitions are important and how we have achieved them. *Perspectives on Language and Literacy, 34,* 27–31.

Fletcher, J. M., Lyon, G. R., Fuchs, L. S., & Barnes, M. A. (2007). *Learning disabilities: From identification to intervention.* New York: Guilford Press.

Fletcher, J. M., Morris, R. D., & Lyon, G. R. (2003). Classification and definition of learning disabilities: An integrative perspective. In H. L. Swanson, K. R. Harris, & S. Graham (Eds.), *Handbook of learning disabilities* (pp. 30–56). New York: Guilford Press.

Fletcher, J. M., Shaywitz, S. A., Shankweiler, D. P., Katz, L., Liberman, I. Y., Stuebing, K. K.,et al. (1994). Cognitive profiles of reading disability: Comparisons of discrepancy and low achievement definitions. *Journal of Educational Psychology, 86,* 6–23.

The Florida Center for Reading Research. (n.d.). Retrieved January 29, 2011, from http://www .fcrr.org/

Foorman, B. R. (2008). *Florida assessments for instruction in reading.* Tallahassee, FL: Florida Center for Reading Research and Florida Department of Education.

Foorman, B. R., Francis, D. J., Shaywitz, S. E., Shaywitz, B. A., & Fletcher, J. M. (1997). The case for early reading interventions. In B. Blachman (Ed.), *Foundations of reading acquisition and dyslexia: Implications for early intervention* (pp. 243–264). Mahwah, NJ: Erlbaum.

Foorman, B. R., & Torgesen, J. K. (2001). Critical elements of classroom and small-group instruction promote reading success in all children. *Learning Disabilities Research and Practice, 16,* 203–212.

Francis, D., Shaywitz, S., Stuebing, K., Shaywitz, B., & Fletcher, J. (1996). Developmental lag versus deficit models of reading disability: A longitudinal, individual growth curves analysis. *Journal of Educational Psychology, 88,* 3–17.

Friend, A., DeFries, J. C., & Olson, R. K. (2008). Parental education moderates genetic influences on reading disability. *Psychological Science, 16,* 1124–1130.

Friend, A., DeFries, J. C., Wadsworth, S. J., & Olson, R. K. (2006). Developmental differences in the genetic etiology of reading and spelling disabilities (Abst.). *Behavior Genetics, 36,* 964.

Friend, A., DeFries, J. C., Wadsworth, S. J., & Olson, R. K. (2007). Genetic and environmental influences on word recognition and spelling deficits as a function of age. *Behavior Genetics, 37,* 477–486.

Frijters, J. C., Barron, R. W., & Brunello, M. (2000). Direct and mediated influences of home literacy and literacy interest on prereaders' oral vocabulary and early written language skill. *Journal of Educational Psychology, 92,* 466–477.

Frith, U. (1980). *Cognitive processes in spelling.* New York: Academic Press.

Frith, U. (1985). Beneath the surface of developmental dyslexia. In K. E. Patterson, J. C. Marshall, & M. Coltheart (Eds.), *Surface dyslexia: Neuropsychological and cognitive studies of phonological reading* (pp. 301–330). London: Erlbaum.

Fuchs, D., & Fuchs, L. S. (2001). Responsiveness-to-intervention: A blueprint for practitioners, policymakers, and parents. *Teaching Exceptional Children, 38,* 57–61.

Fuchs, L. S., Fuchs, D., Hosp, M. K., & Jenkins, J. R. (2001). Oral reading fluency as an indicator of reading competence: A theoretical, empirical, and historical analysis. *Scientific Studies of Reading, 5,* 239–256.

Fuchs, L. S., Fuchs, D., & Kazdan, S. (1999). Effects of peer assisted learning strategies on high school students with serious reading problems. *Remedial and Special Education, 20,* 309–318.

Fuchs, L. S., Fuchs, D., & Maxwell, L. (1988). The validity of informal measures of reading comprehension. *Remedial and Special Education, 9,* 20–28.

Gaab, N., Chang, M., Lee, M., Buechler, R., & Raschle, N. (2009). *Neural pre-markers of developmental dyslexia in the pre-reading brain: An fMRI investigation.* Paper presented at the sixteenth annual meeting of the Society for the Scientific Study of Reading, Boston, MA.

Gaab, N., Gabrieli, J. D. E., Deutsch, G. K., Tallal, P., & Temple, E. (2007). Neural correlates of rapid auditory processing are disrupted in children with training: An fMRI study. *Restorative Neurology and Neuroscience, 25,* 295–310.

Ganske, K. (2000). *Word journeys: Assessment-guided phonics, spelling, and vocabulary instruction.* NY: Guilford Press.

Ganske, K., Monroe, J. K., & Strickland, D. S. (2003). Questions teachers asks about struggling readers and writers. *The Reading Teacher, 57,* 118–128.

Garner, J. K., & Bochna, C. R. (2004). Transfer of a listening comprehension strategy to independent reading in first-grade students. *Early Childhood Education Journal, 32*(2), 69–74.

Gathercole, S. E., Alloway, T. P., Willis, C., & Adams, A. (2006). Working memory in children with reading disabilities. *Journal of Experimental Child Psychology, 93,* 265–281.

Gathercole, S. E., & Baddeley, A. D. (1990). Phonological memory deficits in language disordered children: Is there a causal connection? *Journal of Memory & Language, 29,* 336–360.

Gathercole, S. E., Hitch, G. J., Service, E., & Martin, A. J. (1997). Phonological short-term memory and new word learning in children. *Developmental Psychology, 33,* 966–979.

Gathercole, S. E., Tiffany, C., Briscoe, J., Thorn, A., & The ALSPAC Team. (2005). Developmental consequences of poor phonological short-term memory function in childhood: A longitudinal study. *Journal of Child Psychology and Psychiatry, 46,* 598–611.

Gauger, L. M., Lombardino, L. J., & Leonard, C. M. (1997). Brain morphology in children with specific language impairment. *Journal of Speech and Language Research, 40,* 1272–1284.

Gayán, J., & Olson, R. K. (2001). Genetic and environmental influences on orthographic and phonological skills in children with reading disabilities. *Developmental Neuropsychology, 20*(2), 487–511.

Gayán, J. & Olson, R. K. (2003). Genetic and environmental influences on individual differences in printed word recognition, *J. Experimental Child Psychology, 84,* 97–123.

Gentry, J. R. (1982). An analysis of developmental spelling in GNYS AT WRK. *Reading Teacher, 36,* 192–200.

Gentry, J. R. (2000). A retrospective on invented spelling and a look forward. *Reading Teacher, 54,* 318–332.

Georgiou, K., Torppa, M., Manotitsis, G., Lyytinen, H., & Parrila, R. (2010). Longitudinal predictors of reading and spelling across language varying in orthographic consistency. *Reading and Writing.* doi:10.1007/s11145-010-9271-x

German, D. J. (1984). Diagnosis of word-finding disorders in children with learning disabilities. *Journal of Learning Disabilities, 17,* 353–358.

German, D. J. (1990). *Test of Adolescent/Adult Word Finding, TAWF.* Austin, TX: Pro-Ed.

German, D. J. (2000). *Test of Word Finding, TWF-2* (2nd ed.). Austin, TX: Pro-Ed.

German, D. J., & Newman, R. S. (2007). Oral reading skills of children with oral language (word finding difficulties). *Reading Psychology, 28*(5), 397–442.

Gibson, E. J., & Levin, H. (1975). *The psychology of reading.* Cambridge: Massachusetts Institute of Technology Press.

Gilger, J. W., Pennington, B. F., & Defries, J. C. (1992). A twin study of the etiology of comorbidity: Attention-deficit hyperactivity disorder and dyslexia. *Journal of the American Academy of Child and Adolescent Psychiatry, 31,* 343–348.

Gillam, R. B., & Johnston, J. R. (1992). Spoken and written language relationships in language/learning impaired and normally achieving school age children. *Journal of Speech and Hearing Research, 35,* 1303–1315.

Gillam, R. B., & Pearson, N. (2004). *Test of narrative language.* Austin, TX: Pro-Ed.

Gillingham, A., & Stillman, B. W. (1997). *The Gillingham manual: Remedial training for students with specific disability in reading, spelling, and penmanship.* Cambridge, MA: Educators Publishing Service.

Ginger Software. (n.d.). *Ginger Software.* Retrieved January 30, 2011, from http://www.gingersoftware.com

Good, R. H., & Kaminski, R. A. (Eds.). (2002). *Dynamic indicators of basic early literacy skills* (6th ed.). Eugene, OR: Institute for the Development of Educational Achievement.

Goswami, U. (2002). Early phonological development and acquisition of literacy. In S. B. Neuman & D. K. Dickson (Eds.), *Handbook of early literacy research* (pp. 111–125). New York: Guilford Press.

Goswami, U., & Bryant, P. (1990). *Phonological skills and learning to read.* Mahwah, NJ: Erlbaum.

Gough, P. B., Juel, C., & Griffith, P. L. (1992). Reading, spelling, and the orthographic cipher. In P. B. Gough, L. C. Ehri, & R. Treiman (Eds.), *Reading acquisition* (pp. 35–48). Hillsdale, NJ: Erlbaum.

Gough, P. B., & Tunmer, W. E. (1986). Decoding, reading, and reading disability. *Remedial and Special Education, 7,* 6–10.

Graham, S., Berninger, V., Abbott, R., Abbott, S., & Whitaker, D. (1997). The role of mechanics in composing of elementary school students: A new methodological approach. *Journal of Educational Psychology, 89,* 170–182.

Graham, S., & Harris, S. (1997). It can be taught, but does not develop naturally: Myths and realities in writing instruction. *School Psychology Review, 26,* 414–24.

Graham, S., Harris, K., & Fink, B. (2000). Is handwriting causally related to learning to write? Treatment of handwriting problems in beginning writers. *Journal of Educational Psychology, 92,* 620–633.

Great leaps! Building fluency, phonics and motivation. (n.d.). Retrieved January 29, 2011, from http://www.greatleaps.com/

Grigg, W., Donahue, P., and Dion, G. (2007). *The Nation's Report Card: 12th-Grade Reading and Mathematics 2005* (NCES 2007-468). U.S. Department of Education, National Center for Education Statistics. Washington, DC: U.S. Government Printing Office.

Grigorenko, E. L., Klin, A., & Volkmar, F. (2003). Annotation: Hyperlexia: disability or superability? *Journal of Child Psychology and Psychiatry, 44*(8), 1079–1091.

Habib, M. (2000). The neurological basis of developmental dyslexia: An overview and working hypothesis. *Brain, 123,* 2373–2399.

Hall, S. L., & Moats, L. C. (2002). *Parenting a struggling reader.* New York: Broadway Books.

Hammer, C. S., Scarpino, S., & Davison, M. D. (2011). Beginning with language: Spanish-English bilingual preschoolers' early literacy development. In S. B. Neuman & D. K. Dickinson (Eds.), *Handbook of early literacy research* (Vol. 3, pp. 118–135). New York: Guilford Press.

Hammill, D. D., Brown, V. L., Larsen, S. C., & Wiederholt, J. L. (2007). *Test of Adolescent and Adult Language–Fourth Edition (TOAL-4).* Austin, TX: Pro-Ed.

Hammill, D. D., Mather, N., & Roberts, R. (2001). *Illinois Test of Psycholinguistic Abilities ITPA-3* (3rd ed.). Austin, TX: Pro-Ed.

Hammill, D. D., & Newcomer, P. L. (1997). *Test of Oral Language Development-Preschool 3, TOLD-P:3* (3rd ed.). Austin, TX: Pro-Ed.

Hammill, D. D., Pearson, N. A., & Wiederholt, J. L. (1997). *Comprehensive Test of Nonverbal Intelligence: Manual.* Austin, TX: Pro–Ed.

Hannon, B., & Daneman, M. (2001). A new tool for understanding individual differences in the component processes reading comprehension. *Journal of Educational Psychology, 93*, 103–128.

Hart, B., & Risley, T. (1995). *Meaningful differences in the everyday experience of young American children.* Baltimore: Brookes.

Hasbrouck, J., & Tindal, G. A. (2006, April). Oral Reading Fluency Norms: A Valuable Assessment Tool for Reading Teachers. *The Reading Teacher, 59*(7), 636-644.

Hayes, J. R. (1996). A new framework for understanding cognition and affect in writing. In C. M. Levy & S. Randell (Eds.), *The science of writing: Theories, methods, individual differences, and application* (pp. 1–27). Mahwah, NJ: Erlbaum.

Hayes, J. R., & Flower, L. S. (1980). Identifying the organization of writing processes. In L. Gregg & E. Steinberg (Eds.), *Cognitive processes in writing: An interdisciplinary approach* (pp. 3–30). Hillsdale, NJ: Erlbaum.

Hayes, J. R., & Flower, L. S. (1987). On the structure of the writing process. *Topics in Language Disorders, 7,* 19–30.

Hedberg, N. L., & Westby, C. E. (1993). *Analyzing story-telling skills: Theory to practice.* Tucson, AZ: Communication Skill Builders.

Henderson, E. H. (1981). *Learning to read and spell: The child's knowledge of words.* DeKalb, IL: Northern Illinois University Press.

Henderson, E. H., & Beers, J. (Eds.). (1980). *Developmental and cognitive aspects of learning*

to spell. Newark, DE: International Reading Association.

Henry, M. (1989). Children's word structure knowledge: Implications for decoding and spelling instruction. *Reading and Writing: An Interdisciplinary Journal, 2,* 135–152.

Henry, M. (1998). Structured, sequential, multisensory teaching: The Orton legacy. *Annals of Dyslexia, 48,* 3–26.

Henry, M. (2003). *Unlocking literacy instruction: Effective decoding and spelling instruction.* Baltimore: Brookes.

Henry, M. (2010). *Unlocking literacy: Effective decoding and spelling instruction.* Baltimore: Brookes.

Herman, R. (1993). *The Herman method for reversing reading failure.* Sherman Oaks, CA: Herman Method Institute.

Hoffman, L. M., & Gillam, R. B. (2004). Verbal and spatial information processing constraints in children with specific language impairment. *Journal of Speech, Language, and Hearing Research, 47,* 114–125.

Hoover, W., & Gough, P. (1990). The simple view of reading. *Reading and Writing: An Interdisciplinary Journal, 2,* 127–160.

Hudson, R. F., Pullen, P. C., Lane, H. B., & Torgesen, J. K. (2009). The complex nature of reading fluency: A multidimensional view. *Reading and Writing Quarterly, 25,* 4–32.

Hudson, J., & Shapiro, I. (1991). From knowing to telling: The development of scripts, stories, and personal narratives. In A. McCabe & C. Peterson (Eds.), *Developing narrative structure* (pp. 89–136). Hillsdale, NJ: Erlbaum.

Individuals with Disabilities Education Improvement Act of 2004. (2004). *Public Law 108-446.* Retrieved May 11, 2011, from http://idea.ed.gov/explore/view/p/%2Croot%2Cstatute%2C

The International Dyslexia Association: Promoting literacy through research, education and advocacy. (n.d.). Retrieved January 29, 2011, from http://www.interdys.org/

Invernizzi, M. (1992). The vowel and what follows: A phonological frame of orthographic analysis. In S. Templeton & D. R. Bear (Eds.), *Development of orthographic knowledge and the foundations of literacy: A memorial Festschrift for Edmund H. Henderson* (pp. 105–136). Hillsdale, NJ: Erlbaum.

Jenkins, J. R. M., & Jewell, M. (1993). Examining the validity of two measures for formative teaching: Reading aloud and maze. *Exceptional Children, 59*, 321–342.

Joanisse, M. F. (2004). Specific language impairments in children: Phonology, semantics, and the English past tense. *Current Directions in Psychological Science August, 13*(4), 156–160.

Johns, J. L., & Berglund, R. L. (2006). *Fluency strategies and assessments* (3rd ed.). Newark, DE: International Reading Association.

Johnson, C. J. (1995). Expanding norms for narration. *Language, Speech, and Hearing Services in the Schools, 26*, 326–341.

Johnson, D., & Myklebust, H. (1967). *Learning disabilities: Educational principles and practices.* New York: Grune & Stratton.

Johnston, J. (1982). Narratives: A new look at communication problems in older language-disordered children. *Language, Speech, and Hearing Services in the Schools, 13*, 114–155.

Johnston, J. (2008). Narratives twenty-five years later. *Topics in Language Disorders, 28*, 93–98.

Jordan, R. R., Kirk, D. J., & King, K. (2005). *Early diagnostic reading assessment* (2nd ed.) San Antonio, TX: Harcourt Assessment.

Joshi, R. M., & Aaron, P. G. (2008). Assessment of literacy performance based on the componential model of reading. In G. Reid, A. A. Fawcett, F. Manis, & L. Siegel (Eds.), *The Sage handbook of dyslexia* (pp. 268–289). Los Angeles: Sage.

Juel, C. (2006). The impact of early school experience on initial reading. In D. K. Dickinson & S. B. Neuman (Eds.), *The handbook of early literacy research* (Vol. 2, pp. 410–426). NY: Guilford Press.

Just, M. A., & Carpenter, P. A. (1992). A capacity theory of comprehension. Individual differences in working memory. *Psychological Review, 99*, 122–149.

Justice, L., & Ezell, H. (2001). Descriptive analysis of written language awareness in children from low income households. *Communication Disorders Quarterly, 22*, 123–134.

Justice, L., & Ezell, H. (2002). Use of storybook reading to increase print awareness in at-risk children. *American Journal of Speech-Language Pathology, 11*, 17–29.

Kame'enui, E., & Simmons, D. C. (2001). Introduction to this special issue: The DNA of reading fluency. *Scientific Studies of Reading, 5*, 203–210.

Kame'enui, E., Simmons, D., Good, R., & Harn, B. (2001). The use of fluency-based measures in early identification and evaluation of intervention efficacy in schools. In M. Wolf (Ed.), *Dyslexia, fluency and the brain* (pp. 308–331). Timonium, MD: York Press

Katzir, T., Kim, Y., Wolf, M., O'Brien, B., Kennedy, B., Lovett, M., et al. (2006). Reading fluency: the whole is more than the parts. *Annals of Dyslexia, 56*(1), 51–82.

Keenan, J. M., Betjemann, R. S., & Olson, R. K. (2008). Reading comprehension tests vary in the skills they assess: Differential dependence on decoding and oral comprehension. *Scientific Studies of Reading, 12*(3), 281–300.

Keenan, J. M., Betjemann, R. S., Wadsworth, S. J., DeFries, J. C., & Olson, R. K. (2006). Genetic and environmental influences on reading and listening comprehension. *Journal of Research in Reading, 29*(1), 75–91.

Kendeou, P., Lynch, J. S., van den Broek, P., Espin, C., White, M., & Kremer, K. E. (2006). Developing successful readers: Building early narrative comprehension skills through television viewing and listening. *Early Childhood Educational Journal, 33*, 91–98.

Kendeou, P., van den Broek, P., White, M. J., & Lynch, J. (2007). Comprehension in preschool and early elementary children: Skill development and strategy intervention. In D. S. MacNamara (Ed.), *Reading comprehension strategies: Theories, intervention, and technologies.* Mahwah, NJ: Erlbaum.

King, W., Giess, S., & Lombardino, L. (2007). Subtyping of persons with developmental dyslexia via bootstrap aggregated clustering and the gap statistic: Comparison with the double-deficit hypothesis. *International Journal of Communication Disorders, 42*, 77–95.

Kintsch, W., & Rawson, K. A. (2005). Comprehension. In M. J. Snowling & C. Hulme (Eds.), *The science of reading: A handbook* (pp. 209–226). Oxford, UK: Blackwell.

Kirby, J. R., Desrochers, A., Roth, L., & Lai, S. S. V. (2008). Longitudinal predictors of word reading development. *Canadian Psychology, 49*, 103–110.

Laasonen, M., Lahti-Nuuttila, P., & Virsu, V. (2002). Developmentally impaired processing speed decreases more than normally with age. *Cognitive Neuroscience and Neuropsychology, 13*(9), 1111–1113.

LaBerge, D., & Samuels, A. (1974). Toward a theory of automatic information processing in reading. *Cognitive Psychology, 6*, 293–323.

Landi, N., Frost, S. J., Mencl, W. E., Sandak, R., & Pugh, K. R. (in press). Neurobiological bases of reading comprehension: Insights from neuroimaging studies of word level and text level processing in skilled and impaired readers. *Reading and Writing Quarterly.*

Language Tune-up Kit Software. (n.d.). Retrieved January 29, 2011, from http://www.jwor.com/

Learning Ally: Accessible materials for individuals with visual and learning disabilities. (n.d.). Retrieved January 29, 2011, from http://www.learningally.org/

Leikin, M., & Assayag-Bouskila, O. (2004). Expression of syntactic complexity in sentence comprehension: A comparison between dyslexic and regular readers. *Reading and Writing: An Interdisciplinary Journal, 17*, 801–821.

Lenhard, W., Lenhard, A., & Breitenbach, E. (2005). *The neurobiological basis of developmental dyslexia–Current findings and areas of future research.* In H. D. Tobias (Ed.), *Trends in dyslexia research* (pp. 223–244). New York, Haupage: Nova-Science.

Lenz, B. K., Ehren, B. J., & Deshler, D. D. (2005). The content literacy continuum: A school reform framework for improving adolescent literacy for all students. *Teaching Exceptional Children, 37*(6), 60–63.

Leonard, C. M. (2011). Anatomical risk factors for reading comprehension. In A. A. Benasich & R. H. Fitch (Eds.), *Developmental dyslexia: Early precursors, neurobehavioral markers and biological substrates* (The Extraordinary Brain Series). Baltimore: Brookes Publishing.

Leonard, C. M., & Eckert, M. (2008). Asymmetry and Dyslexia. *Developmental Neuropsychology, 33*(6),663–681.

Leonard, C. M., Eckert, M., Given, B., Berninger, V., & Eden, G. (2006). Individual differences in anatomy predict reading and oral language impairments in children. *Brain*, 129, 3329–3342.

Leonard, C. M., Lombardino, L. J., Giess, S. A., & King, W. M. (2005). Behavioral and anatomical distinctions between dyslexia and SLI. In H. W. Catts and A. G. Kamhi (Eds.), *The connections between language and reading disabilities* (pp. 155–172). Mahwah, NJ: Erlbaum.

Leonard, C. M., Lombardino, L. J., Walsh, K., Eckert, M. A., Mockler, J. L., Rowe, L. A., et al. (2002). Anatomical risk factors that distinguish dyslexia from SLI predict reading skill in normal children. *Journal of Communication Disorders, 35*, 501–531.

Leonard, C. M., Low, P., Jonczak, E., Schmutz, K., Siegel, L., & Beaulieu, C. (in press). Brain anatomy, processing speed, and reading in school children. *Developmental Neuropsychology*.

Leonard, L. B. (1998). *Children with specific language impairment*. Cambridge, MA: MIT Press.

Lerner, J. (1989). Educational interventions in learning disabilities. *Journal of the American Academy of Child Adolescent Psychiatry, 28*, 326–331.

Leslie, L., & Caldwell, J. (2001). *Qualitative reading inventory-3*. NJ: Addison Wesley Longman.

Leslie, L., & Caldwell, J. (2006). *Qualitative reading inventory* (3rd ed.). Boston: Pearson Education.

Lexercise. (n.d.). Retrieved January 29, 2011, from http://www.lexercise.com/

Liberman, A. M., Cooper, F. S., Shankweiler, D., & Studdert-Kennedy, M. (1967). Perception of the speech code. *Psychological Review, 74*, 431–461.

Liberman, A. M., Mattingly, I. G., & Shankweiler, D. (1980). Orthography and the beginning reader. In J. F. Kavanagh & R. L. Venezky (Eds.), *Orthography, reading, and dyslexia* (pp. 137–153). Baltimore: University Park Press.

Liberman, I. Y., & Liberman, A. M. (1990). Whole language vs. code emphasis: Underlying assumptions and their implications for reading instruction. *Annals of Dyslexia, 40*, 51–74.

Liberman, I. Y., Shankweiler, D., Fischer, F. W., & Carter, B. (1974). Explicit syllable and phoneme segmentation in the young child. *Journal of Experimental Child Psychology, 18*, 201–212.

Lindamood Bell Learning Processes. (2005). *Phonemic awarenes for reading, spelling, and speech*. Retrieved from http://www.lblp.com/

Lindamood, C., & Lindamood, P. (1998). *The Lindamood phoneme sequencing program for reading, spelling, and speech*. San Luis Obispo, CA: Gander.

Logan, G. D. (1988). Toward an instant theory of automatization. *Psychological Review, 95*, 492–527.

Logan, G. D. (1997). Automaticity and reading: Perspectives from the instance theory of automatization, *Reading and Writing Quarterly, 13*, 123–146.

Lombardino, L., Lieberman, J., & Brown, J. (2005). *Assessment of Literacy and Language, ALL*. San Antonio, TX: The Psychological Corporation.

Lombardino, L., Riccio, C. A., Hynd, G. W., & Pinheiro, S. B. (1997). Linguistic deficits in children with reading disabilities. *American Journal of Speech-Language Pathology, 6*(3), 71–78.

Lonigan, C. (2006). Conceptualizing phonological processing skills in prereaders. In S. B. Neuman & D. K. Dickson (Eds.), *Handbook of early literacy research* (pp. 77–89). New York: Guilford Press.

Lonigan, C., Burgess, S. R., Anthony, J. L., & Barker, T. A. (1998). Development of phonological sensitivity in two-to five-year-old children. *Journal of Educational Psychology, 90*, 294–311.

Lonigan, C., Wagner, R., & Torgesen, J. (2007). *Test of Preschool Early Literacy, TOPEL.* Austin, TX: Pro-Ed.

Lovett, M. (1987). A developmental approach to reading disability: Accuracy and speed criteria of normal and deficient reading skill. *Child Development, 58*, 234–260.

Lyon, G. R. (1995). Toward a definition of dyslexia. *Annals of Dyslexia, 45*, 3–27.

Lyon, G. R., Shaywitz, S. E., & Shaywitz, B. A. (2003). Defining dyslexia, comorbidity, teachers' knowledge of language and reading: A definition of dyslexia. *Annals of Dyslexia, 53*, 1–14.

Marchand-Martella, N. E., Ruby, S. F., & Martella, R. C. (2007). Intensifying reading instruction for students within a three–tier model: Standard-protocol and problem solving approaches within a response-to-intervention (RTI) system. *Teaching Exceptional Children Plus, 3*(5). Retrieved May 4, 2009, from http://escholarship.bc.edu/education/tecplus/vol3/iss5/art2

Masterson, J. J., Apel, K., & Wasowicz, J. (2003). *SPELL model of assessment.* Evanston, IL: Learning by Design.

Masterson, J. J., Apel, K., & Wasowicz, J. (2006). SPELL-2 Spelling Performance Evaluation for Language and Literacy (2nd ed.) [Computer software]. Evanston, IL: Learning By Design.

McArthur, G. M., Hogben, J. H., Edwards, V. T., Heath, S. M., & Mengler, F. D. (2000). On the "specifics" of specific reading disability and specific language impairment. *Journal of Child Psychology and Psychiatry and Allied Disciplines, 41*, 869–874.

McCabe, A., & Rollins, P. (1994). Assessment of preschool narrative skills. *American Journal of Speech-Language Pathology, 1*, 45–56.

McCutchen, D. (1996). A capacity theory of writing: Working memory in composition. *Educational Psychology Review, 8*, 299–325.

McGuinness, D. (2005). *Language development and learning to read: The scientific study of how language development affects reading skill.* Cambridge, MA: MIT Press.

McNamara, D. S. (Ed.). *Reading comprehension strategies: Theories, interventions, and technologies.* New York: Lawrence Erlbaum Associates.

Meyer, M. S., & Felton, R. H. (1999). Repeated reading to enhance fluency: Old approaches and new directions. *Annals of Dyslexia, 49*, 283–306.

Miller, W. H. (1995). *Alternative assessment techniques for reading and writing.* Somerset, NJ: John Wiley & Sons.

Moats, L. (1983). A comparison of the spelling errors of older dyslexic and normal second grade children. *Annals of Dyslexia, 33*, 121–140.

Moats, L. (1995). *Spelling: Development, disabilities, and instruction.* Baltimore: York Press.

Moats, L. (2000). *Speech to print: Language essentials for teachers.* Baltimore: Brookes.

Moats, L., & Dakin, K. E. (2008). *Basic facts about dyslexia and other reading problems.* Baltimore: The International Dyslexia Association.

Mody, M., & Silliman, E. R. (Eds.). (2008). *Brain, behavior, and learning in language and reading disorders.* New York: Guilford Press.

Montgomery, J. (1995). Sentence comprehension in children with specific language impairment: The role of phonological working memory. *Journal of Speech and Hearing Research, 38,* 187–199.

Montgomery, J. (1995). Examination of phonological working memory in specifically language-impaired children. *Applied Psycholinguistics, 16,* 355–378.

Montgomery, J. (2000). Relation of working memory to off-line and real-time sentence processing in children with specific language impairment. *Allied Psycholinguistics, 21,* 117–148.

Moore, P., & Lyon, A. (2005). *New essentials for teaching reading in pre-K–2.* New York: Scholastic Professional Books.

Morais, J. (2003). Levels of phonological representation in skilled reading and in learning to read. *Reading and Writing: An Interdisciplinary Journal, 16,* 123–151.

Morris, D. (1981). Concept of word: A developmental phenomenon in the beginning reading and writing process. *Language Arts, 58,* 659–668.

Morris, D. (1983). Concept of word and phoneme awareness in the beginning reader. *Research in the Teaching of English, 17,* 359–373.

Morris, D. (1993). The relationship between children's concept of word in text and phoneme awareness in learning to read: A longitudinal study. *Research in the Teaching of English, 27,* 133–154.

Morris, D., Nelson, L., & Perney, J. (1986). Exploring the concept of "spelling instructional level" through the analysis of error-types. *Elementary School Journal, 87,* 181–200.

Muter, V., Hulme, C., Snowling, M. J., & Stevenson, J. (2004). Phonemes, rimes and language skills as foundations of early reading development: Evidence from a longitudinal study. *Developmental Psychology, 40,* 663–681.

Nagy, W., Berninger, V. W., & Abbott, R. D. (2006). Contributions of morphology beyond phonology to literacy outcomes of upper elementary and middle-school students. *Journal of Educational Psychology, 98*(1), 134–147.

Nagy, W., Berninger, V., Abbott, R., Vaughan, K., & Vermeulen, K. (2003). Relationship of morphology and other language skills to literacy skills in at-risk second-grade readers and at-risk fourth-grade writers. *Journal of Educational Psychology, 95,* 730–742.

Nagy, W. E., & Scott, J. A. (2000). Vocabulary processes. In M. L. Kamil, P. Mosenthal, P. D. Pearson, & R. Barr (Eds.), *Handbook of reading research* (Vol. 3, pp. 269–284). Mahwah, NJ: Erlbaum.

Nation, K. (2005a). Connections between reading and language in children with poor reading comprehension. In H. Catts & A. Kamhi (Eds.), *Connections between reading and language* (pp. 41–54). Erlbaum.

Nation, K. (2005b). Reading comprehension difficulties. In M. J. Snowling & C. Hulme (Eds.),

The science of reading (pp. 248–265). Oxford, UK: Blackwell.

Nation, K., Adams, J. W., Bowyer-Crane, C. A., & Snowling, M. J. (1999). Working memory deficits in poor comprehenders reflect underlying language impairments. *Journal of Experimental Child Psychology, 73*, 139–158.

Nation, K., Clarke, P., Marshall, C. M., & Durand, M. (2004). Hidden language impairments in children: Parallels between poor reading comprehension and specific language impairment. *Journal of Speech, Language, and Hearing Research, 47*, 199–211.

Nation, K., Cocksey, J., Taylor, J. S. H., & Bishop, D. V. M. (in press). A longitudinal investigation of the early reading and language skills in children with poor reading comprehension. *Journal of Child Psychology and Psychiatry*.

Nation, K., & Hulme, C. (1997). Phonemic segmentation, not onset-rime segmentation, predicts early reading and spelling skills. *Reading Research Quarterly, 32*, 154–167.

Nation, K., Marshall, C. M., & Snowling, M. J. (2001). Phonological and semantic contributions to children's picture naming skill: Evidence from children with developmental reading disorders. *Language and Cognitive Processes, 16*(2–3), 241–259.

Nation, K., & Snowling, M. J. (1997). Assessing reading difficulties: The validity and utility of current measures of reading skill. *British Journal of Educational Psychology, 67*, 359–370.

Nation, K., & Snowling, M. J. (1999). Developmental differences in sensitivity to semantic relations along good and poor comprehenders: Evidence from semantic priming. *Cognition, 70*, B1–B13.

Nation, K., & Snowling, M. J. (2000). Factors influencing syntactic awareness in normal readers and poor comprehenders. *Applied Psycholinguistics, 21*, 229–241.

Nation, K., Snowling, M. J., Clarke, P. (2007). Dissecting the relationship between language skills and learning to read: Semantic and phonological contributions to new vocabulary learning in children with poor reading comprehension. *Advances in Speech-Language Pathology, 9*, 131–139.

National Center for Educational Statistics. (2009). *The condition of education*. Washington, DC: U.S. Government Printing Office.

National Institute of Child Health and Human Development. (2000). *Report of the National Reading Panel. Teaching Children to Read: An Evidence-Based Assessment of the Scientific Research Literature on Reading and its Implications for Reading Instruction*. Washington, DC: U.S. Government Printing Office.

National Reading Panel. (2000). *Teaching children to read: An evidence-based assessment of the scientific research literature on reading and its implications for reading instruction: Reports of the subgroups* (NIH Publication No. 00-4754). Washington, DC: National Institute of Child Health and Human Development.

Nelson, N. (2010). *Language and literacy disorders: Infancy through adolescence*. Boston: Allyn & Bacon.

Nelson, N., Bahr, C., & Van Meter, A. (2004). *The writing lab approach to language instruction and intervention*. Baltimore: Brookes.

Neuman, S. R., & Dickinson, D. K. (2002). Introduction. In S. B. Neuman & D. K. Dickson (Eds.), *Handbook of early literacy research* (pp. 3–10). New York: Guilford Press.

NICHD Early Child Care Research Network. (2005). Early child care and children's development in the primary grades: Results from the NICHD Study of Early Child Care. *American Educational Research Journal, 43,* 537–570.

Nippold, M. A. (2007). *Later language development: The school-age and adolescent years.* Austin, TX: Pro-Ed.

Oakhill, J., & Cain, K. (2007a). Introduction to comprehension development. In K. Cain & J. Oakhill (Eds.), *Children's comprehension problems in oral and written language: A cognitive perspective* (pp. 3–40). New York: Guilford Press.

Oakhill, J., & Cain, K. (2007b). Issues of causality in children's reading comprehension. In D. S. McNamara (Ed.), *Reading comprehension strategies: Theories, interventions, and technologies* (pp. 47–71). Mahwah, NJ: Erlbaum.

Oakhill, J., Cain, K., & Bryant, P. E. (2003). The dissociation of word reading and text comprehension: Evidence from component skills. *Language and Cognitive Processes, 18,* 143–468.

O'Connor, R. E. (2007). *Teaching word recognition: Effective strategies for students with learning difficulties.* New York: Guilford Press.

O'Connor, R. E., & Jenkins, J. R. (1995). Improving the generalization of sound/symbol knowledge: Teaching spelling to kindergarten children with disabilities. *Journal of Special Education, 29,* 255–275.

Oller, D. K., & Eilers, R. E. (2002). *Language and literacy in bilingual children.* Tonawanda, NY: Multilingual Matters.

Olson, R. K. (2002). Dyslexia: Nature and nurture. *Dyslexia, 8,* 143–159.

Olson, R. K. (2004). SSSR, Environment, and Genes. *Society for the Scientific Study of Reading, 8,* 111–124.

Olson, R. K. (2006). Genes, environment, and dyslexia: The 2005 Norman Geschwind memorial lecture. *Annals of Dyslexia, 56,* 205–238.

Olson R. K., & Gáyan, J. (2001). Brains, Genes, and Environment in Reading Development. In S. Neuman & D. Dickinson (Eds.), *Handbook of early literacy research* (pp. 81–94). New York: Guilford Press.

Olson, R. K., Gillis, J. J., Rack, J. P., DeFries, J. C., & Fulker, D. W. (1991). Confirmatory factor analysis of word recognition and process measures in the Colorado Reading Project. *Reading and Writing: An Interdisciplinary Journal, 3,* 235–248. Re-published in B. F. Pennington (Ed.). (1992). *Reading disabilities: Genetic and neurological influences* (pp. 47–60). Dordrecht, The Netherlands: Kluwer Academic Publishers.

One Minute Reader—Read naturally's home reading program. (n.d.). Retrieved January 30, 2011, from http://oneminutereader.com/

Ouellette, G. (2006). What's meaning got to do with it: The role of vocabulary in word reading and reading comprehension. *Journal of Educational Psychology, 98*(3), 554–566.

Palincsar, A. S., & Brown, A. L. (1984). Reciprocal Teaching of Comprehension-Fostering and Comprehension-Monitoring Activities. *Cognition and Instruction, 1,* 117–175.

Paris, A., & Paris, S. (2003). Assessing narrative comprehension in young children. *Reading Research Quarterly. 38*(1), 36–76.

Park, H., Kim, S., & Lombardino, L. J. (2009, November). *A comparison on cognitive skills in developmental dyslexia and language learning disability.* Poster session presented at the sixtieth annual conference of the International Dyslexia Association, Lake Buena Vista, FL.

Park, H., Kim, S., & Lombardino, L. (2010). *Differentiating students with developmental dyslexia and language-learning disability.* Poster session presented at the Annual Convention of the American Speech-Language-Hearing Association (ASHA), Philadelphia, PA.

Park, H., Lombardino, L., & Altmann, L. (2010). *Processing speed deficits in young adults with developmental dyslexia.* Poster session presented at the Annual Convention of the American Speech-Language-Hearing Association (ASHA), Philadelphia, PA.

Park, H., Lombardino, L., DiPietro, K., Magdales, D., Schoepski, D., Martin, K., & Altmann, L. (2011). *Processing Speed in Young Adults with Developmental Dyslexia: A Domain-General or Domain-Specific Deficit?* Poster presented at the 2011 Society for the Scientific Study of Reading (SSSR) Conference, St. Pete Beach, FL.

Paul, R. (2006). *Language disorders from infancy through adolescence: Assessment and intervention* (3rd ed.). St. Louis, MO: Mosby Press.

Pavlak, S. (1985). *Informal tests for diagnosing specific reading problems.* New York: Parker.

Pearson, P. D., & Gallagher, M. (1983). The instruction of reading comprehension. *Contemporary Educational Psychology, 8,* 317–344.

PearsonSchool.com. (n.d.). *QuickReads (2006) and QReads. (2008).* Retrieved January 30, 2011, from http://www.pearsonschool.com/index.cfm?locator=PSZu6g&PMDbSiteId=2781&PMDbSolutionId=6724&PMDbSubSolutionId=&PMDbCategoryId=814&PMDbSubCategoryId=&PMDbSubjectAreaId=&PMDbProgramId=33822

Pennington, B. F. (2006). From single to multiple deficit models of developmental disorders. *Cognition, 101,* 385–413.

Pennington, B. F. (2009). *Diagnosing learning disorders: A neuropsychological framework.* New York: Guilford Press.

Pennington, B. F., & Bishop, D. V. M. (2009). Relations among speech, language, and reading disorders. *Annual Review of Psychology, 60,* 283–306.

Pennington, B. F., McGrath, L. M., Rosenberg, J., Barnard, H., Smith, S. D., Willcutt, E. G., et al. (2009). Gene × environment interactions in reading disability and attention-deficit/hyperactivity disorder. *Developmental Psychology, 45,* 77–89.

Pennington, B. F., & Olson, R. (2005). Genetics of dyslexia. In M. Snowling & C. Hulme (Eds.), *The science of reading: A handbook* (pp. 453–472). Oxford: Blackwell Publishing.

Perfetti, C. (1985). *Reading ability.* New York: Oxford University Press.

Perfetti, C. (2007). Reading ability: Lexical quality to comprehension. *Scientific Study of Reading, 11,* 357–383.

Perfetti, C., Beck, I., Bell, L., & Hughes, C. (1987). Phonemic knowledge and learning to read are reciprocal: A longitudinal study. *Merrill-Palmer Quarterly, 33,* 283–319.

Perfetti, C., & Hart, L. (2001). The lexical basis of comprehension skill. In D. Gorfein (Ed.), *The consequences of meaning selection* (pp. 67–86).

Washington, DC: American Psychological Association.

Perfetti, C., Landi, N., & Oakhill, J. (2005). *The acquisition of reading comprehension.* Oxford, UK: Blackwell.

Perie, M., Grigg, W., & Donahue, P. (2005). The *Nation's Report Card: Reading 2005. (NCES 2006-451).* Washington, DC: U.S. Department of Education.

Perlmutter, B. F., & Parus, M. V. (1983). Identifying children with learning disabilities: A comparison of diagnostic procedures across school district. *Learning Disability Quarterly, 6,* 321–328.

Petersen, D. B., Gillam, S. L., & Gillam, R. B. (2008). Emerging procedures in narrative assessment: The index of narrative complexity. *Topics in language disorders, 28,* 115–130.

Pickering, S. J., & Gathercole, S. E. (2001). *Working Memory Test Battery for Children, WMTB-C.* London: Psychological Corporation Europe.

Pikulski, J. J., & Chard, D. J. (2005, March). Fluency: Bridge between decoding and reading comprehension. *Reading Teacher, 58*(6), 510–519.

Pinnell, G. S., & Fountas, I. C. (2007). *The continuum of literacy learning (Grades K–2): A guide to teaching.* Portsmouth, NH: Heinemann.

Pollo, T. C., Treiman, R., & Kessler, B. (2008a). Preschoolers use partial letter names to select spellings: Evidence from Portuguese. *Applied Psycholinguistics, 29,* 1–18.

Pollo, T. C., Treiman, R., & Kessler, B. (2008b). Three perspectives on spelling development. In E. L. Grigorenko & A. J. Naples (Eds.), *Single-word reading: Behavioral and biological perspectives* (pp. 175–189). New York: Erlbaum.

Prado, C., Dubois, M., & Valdois, S. (2007). The eye movements of dyslexia children during reading and visual search: Impact of the visual attention span. *Vision Research, 47,* 2521–2530.

Pugh, K. R., Mencl, W. E., Jenner, A. J., Katz, L., Lee, J. R., Shaywitz, S. E., et al. (2000). Functional neuroimaging studies of reading and reading disability (developmental dyslexia). *Mental Retardation and Developmental Disabilities Research Reviews, 6,* 207–213.

Pugh, K. R., Mencl, W. E., Jenner, A. R., Lee, J. R., Katz, L., Frost, S. J., et al. (2001). Neuroimaging studies of reading development and reading disability. *Learning Disabilities Research and Practice, 16*(4), 240–249.

Puranik, C., & Lombardino, L. (2006). An assessment paradigm for speech-language pathologists working with reading disabilities. *Contemporary Issues in Communication Science and Disorders, 33,* 101–112.

Puranik, C., Lombardino, L., & Altmann, L. (2008). Assessing the microstructure of written language using a retelling paradigm. *American Journal of Speech-Language Pathology, 17,* 107–120.

Puranik, C. S., Lonigan, C. J., & Kim, Y. (2011). Contributions of emergent literacy skills to name writing, letter writing, and spelling in preschool children. *Early Childhood Research Quarterly.* http://dx.doi.org/10.1016/j.ecresq.2011.03.002

Rack, J. (1997). Issues in the assessment of developmental dyslexia in adults: Theoretical and applied perspectives. *Journal of Research in Reading, 20,* 66–76.

Rack, J., & Olson, R. K. (1993). Phonological deficits, IQ and individual differences in reading disability: Genetic and environmental influences. *Developmental Review, 13,* 269–278.

Rack, J., Snowling, M. J., & Olson, R. K. (1992). The nonword reading deficit in developmental dyslexia: A review. *Reading Research Quarterly, 27*(1), 28–53.

Ramus, F. (2003). Developmental dyslexia: Specific phonological deficit or general sensorimotor dysfunction? *Current Opinion in Neurobiology, 13*(2), 212–218.

Rapp, D. N., van den Broek, P., McMaster, K. L., Kendeou, P., & Espin, C. A. (2007). Higher-order comprehension processes in struggling readers: A perspective for research and intervention. *Scientific Studies of Reading, 11,* 289–312.

Rasinksi, T. (2003). *The fluent reader: Oral reading strategies for building word recognition, fluency, and comprehension.* New York: Scholastic Professional Books.

Rasinski, T., & Hoffman, T. (2003). Theory and research into practice: Oral reading in the school literacy curriculum. *Reading Research Quarterly, 38,* 510–522.

Rasinski, T., & Padak, N. (2003). Effective Reading Strategies: Teaching Children who find Reading Difficult (3rd). Columbus, OH: Merrill/Prentice Hall.

Read Naturally—Better Tools. Better Readers. Brighter Futures. (n.d.). Retrieved January 29, 2011, from http://www.readnaturally.com/

Read, C. (1971). Preschool children's knowledge of English phonology. *Harvard Educational Review, 41,* 1–34.

Reid, D. K., Hresko, W. P., & Hammill, D. D. (2001). *Test of Early Reading Ability, TERA-3* (3rd ed.). Austin, TX: Pro-Ed.

Reid, G., Fawcett, A., Manis, F., & Siegel, L. (2008). *The Sage handbook of dyslexia.* Los Angeles: Sage.

Richards, R. G. (1999). *The source for dyslexia and dysgraphia.* East Moline, IL: LinguiSystems, Riverside, CA.

Richards, T., Aylward, E., Berninger, V., Field, K., Parsons, A., Richards, A., et al. (2006). Individual fMRI activation in orthographic mapping and morpheme mapping after orthographic or morphological spelling treatment in child dyslexia. *Journal of Neurolinguistics, 19,* 56–86.

Richgels, D. J. (2002). Invented spelling, phonemic awareness, and Reading and Writing Instruction. In S. B. Neuman & D. K. Dickinson (Eds.), *Handbook of early literacy research* (pp. 142–155). New York: Guilford Press.

Ripich, D. N., & Griffith, P. L. (1988). Narrative abilities of children with learning disabilities and nondisabled children: Story structure, cohesion, and propositions. *Journal of Learning Disabilities, 21,* 165–173.

Rispens, J. E., Roeleven, S., & Koster, C. (2004). Sensitivity to subject-verb agreement in spoken language in children with developmental dyslexia. *Journal of Neurolinguistics, 17,* 333–347.

Roper Starch Poll: Measuring Progress in Public and Parental Understanding of Learning Disabilities, 2000.

Rosner, J. (1979). *Helping children overcome learning difficulties.* New York: Walker.

Roswell, F. G., Chall, J. S., Curtis, M. E., & Kearns, G. (2010). *Diagnostic assessments of reading* (2nd ed.). Itasca, IL: Riverside.

Roth, F. P., Speece, D. L., & Cooper, D. H. (2002). A longitudinal analysis of the connection between oral language and early reading. *Journal of Educational Research, 95,* 259–272.

Rumsey, J. M., Horwitz, B., Donohue, B. C., Nace, K., Maisog, J. M., & Andreason, P. (1997). Phonological and orthographic components of word recognition: A PET-rCBF study. *Brain, 120,* 739–759.

Samson, J. F., & Lesaux, N. K. (2009). Language-minority learners in special education: Rates and predictors of identification for services. *Journal of Learning Disabilities, 42,* 248–262.

Savage, R., Lavers, N., & Pillay, V. (2007). Working memory and reading difficulties: What we know and what we don't know about the relationship. *Educational Psychology Review, 19,* 185–22.1.

Scarborough, H. (1990). Very early language deficits in dyslexic children. *Child Development, 61,* 1728–1743.

Scarborough, H. (1998). Early identification of children at-risk for reading disabilities: Phonological awareness and some other promising predictions. In B. Shapiro, J. Accardo, & A. Capute (Eds.), *Specific reading disability: A view of the spectrum* (pp. 75–119). Timonium, MD: York Press.

Scarborough, H. (2001). Connecting early language and literacy to later reading (dis) abilities: Evidence, theory, and practice. In S. Neuman & D. Dickinson (Eds.), *Handbook for research in early literacy* (pp. 97–110). New York: Guilford Press.

Scarborough, H. (2002). Connecting early language and literacy to later reading (dis) abilities: Evidence, theory, and practice. In S. B. Neuman & D. K. Dickinson (Eds.), *Handbook of early literacy research* (pp. 97–125). New York: Guilford Press.

Scarborough, H. (2005). Developmental relationships between language and reading: Reconciling a beautiful hypothese with some ugly facts. In H. W. Catts & A. G. Kamhi (Eds.), *The connections between langauge and reading disabilities* (pp. 3–24). Mahwah, NJ: Erlbaum.

Scarborough, H., & Dobrich, W. (1994). On the efficacy of reading to preschoolers. *Developmental Review, 14,* 245–302.

Scardamalia, M., & Bereiter, C. (1986). Written composition. In M. Wittrock (Ed.), *Handbook of research on teaching* (pp. 778–803). New York: MacMillan.

Schlaggar, B. L., Brown, T. T., Lugar, H. L., Visscher, K. M., Miezin, F. M., & Petersen, S. E. (2002). Functional neuroanatomical differences between adults and school-age children in the processing of single words. *Science, 296,* 1476–1479.

Schlaggar, B. L., & McCandliss, B. D. (2007). Development of neural systems for reading. *Annual Reviews of Neuroscience, 30,* 475–503.

School Specialty—Literacy and Intervention. (n.d.). Retrieved January 29, 2011, from http://www.epsbooks.com/

Scott, C. M. (1989). Problem writers: Nature, assessment, and intervention. In A. Kamhi & H. Catts (Eds.), *Reading disabilities: A developmental language perspective* (pp. 303–344). Boston: Allyn & Bacon.

Scott, C. M. (2005). Learning to write. In H. W. Catts & A. G. Kamhi (Eds.), *Language and reading disabilities* (pp. 233–273). Boston: Allyn & Bacon.

Scott, C. M., & Windsor, J. (2000). General language performance measures in spoken and written narrative and expository discourse of school-age children with language learning disabilities. *Journal of Speech, Language, and Hearing Research, 43,* 324–339.

Seigneuric, A., & Ehrlich, M. (2005). Contribution of working memory capacity to children's reading comprehension: A longitudinal investigation. *Reading and Writing: An Interdisciplinary Journal, 18,* 617–656.

Semel, E., Wiig, E. H., & Secord, W. (2003). *Clinical Evaluation of Language Fundamentals, CELF-4* (4th ed.). San Antonio, TX: The Psychological Corporation.

Semrud-Clikeman, M., Biederman, J., Sprich-Buckminster, S., Lehman, B. K., Faraone, S. V., & Norma, D. (1992). Comorbidity between ADDH and LD: A review and report in a clinically referred sample. *Journal of the American Academy of Child and Adolescent Psychiatry, 31,* 439–448.

Sénéchal, M., & LeFevre, J. (2002). Parental involvement in the development of children's reading skill: A five-year longitudinal study. *Child Development, 73,* 445–460.

Sénéchal, M., LeFevre, J., Thomas, E., & Daley, K. (1998). Differential effects of home literacy experiences on the development of oral and written language. *Reading Research Quarterly, 32,* 96–116.

Sénéchal, M., Ouellette, G., & Rodney, D. (2006). The misunderstood giant: On the predictive role of early vocabulary in future reading. In D. Dickinson & S. B. Neuman (Eds.), *Handbook of early literacy research* (Vol. 2, pp. 173–184). New York: Guilford Press.

Seymour, H. N., Roeper, T. W., de Villiers, J., with contributions by de Villiers, P. A. (2008). *Diagnostic evaluation of language variation (DELV): Norm-referenced.* San Antonio: Pearson.

Shanahan, T., & Lomax, R. G. (1986). An analysis and comparison of theoretical models of the reading-writing relationships: Seven instructional principles. *Reading Teacher, 41,* 636–647.

Shankweiler, D., & Liberman, I. Y. (1989). *Phonology and reading disability: Solving the reading puzzle.* Ann Arbor, MI: University of Michigan Press.

Share, D. L. (2005). Phonological recoding and self-teaching: *Sine qua non* of reading acquisition. *Cognition, 55,* 151–218.

Share, D. L. (2008). Orthographic learning, phonological recoding, and self-teaching. In R. Kail (Ed.). Advances in child development and behavior (vol. 36, pp. 31–82). San Diego: Academic Press.

Shaywitz, B. A., Lyon, G. R., & Shaywitz, S. E. (2006). The role of functional magnetic resonance imaging in understanding reading and dyslexia. *Developmental Neuropsychology, 30,* 613-632.

Shaywitz, B. A., Shaywitz, S. E., Blachman, B., Pugh, K. R., Fulbright, R. K., Skudlarski, P., et al. (2004). Development of left occipito-termporal systems for skilled reading following phonologically-based reading intervention in children. *Biological Psychiatry, 55,* 926–933.

Shaywitz, S. (2003). *Overcoming dyslexia: A new and complete science-based program for reading problems at any level.* New York: Knopf.

Shaywitz, S., Gruen, J. R., & Shaywitz, B. (2008). Dyslexia: A new look at neural substrates. In M. Mody & E. R. Silliman (Eds.), *Brain, behavior, and learning in language and reading disorders* (pp. 209–239). New York, NJ: Guilford Press.

Shaywitz, S., Mody, M., & Shaywitz, B. (2006). Neural mechanisms in dyslexia. *Current Directions in Psychological Science, 15*(6), 278–281.

Shaywitz, S., Morris, R., & Shaywitz, B. A. (2008). The education of dyslexic children from childhood to young adulthood. *Annual Review of Psychology, 59,* 451–475.

Shaywitz, S., Shaywitz, B., Fulbright, R., Skudarski, P., Mence, W., Constable, R., et al. (2003). Neural systems for compensation and persistence: Young adult outcome of childhood reading disability. *Biological Psychiatry, 54,* 25–33.

Shaywitz, S., & Shaywitz, B. A. (2007, September 04). *The Neurobiology of Reading and Dyslexia.* The ASHA Leader.

Sheffield, B. B. (1991). The structured flexibility of Orton-Gillingham. *Annals of Dyslexia, 41,* 41–54.

Siegel, L. (2003). IQ-dicrepancy definitions and the diagnosis of LD: Introduction to the special issue. *Journal of Leanring Disabilities, 36,* 2–3.

Siegel, L. (2005). Basic cognitive processes and reading disabilities. In H. L. Swanson, K. R. Harris, & S. Graham (Eds.), *Handbook of learning disabilities* (pp. 158–181). New York: Guilford Press.

Siegel, L., & Lipka, O. (2008). The definition of learning disabilities: Who is the individual with learning disabilities? In G. Reid, A. A. Fawcett, F. Manis, & L. Siegel (Eds.), *The Sage handbook of dyslexia* (pp. 268–289). Los Angeles: Sage.

Siegel, L., & Ryan, E. B. (1989). The development of working memory in normally achieving and subtypes of learning disabled children. *Society for Research in Child Development, 60,* 973–980.

Simkin, Z., & Conti-Ramsden, G. (2006). Evidence of reading difficulty in subgroups of children with specific language impairment. *Child language teaching and therapy, 22,* 315–331.

Simos, P. G., Fletcher, J. M., Denton, C., Sarkari, S., Billingsley-Marshall, R., & Papanicolaou, A. C. (2006). Magnetic source imaging studies of dyslexia interventions. *Developmental Neurology, 30,* 591–611.

Singer, B. D., & Bashir, A. S. (2004). Developmental variations in writing composition skills. In C. A. Stone, E. R. Silliman, B. J. Ehren, & K. Apel (Eds.), *Handbook of language and literacy: Development and disorders.* New York: Guilford Press.

Slavin, R. E., & Cheung, A. (2005). A synthesis of research on language of reading instruction for English language learners. *Review of Educational Research, 75,* 247–284. doi: 10.3102/00346543075002247

Slingerland, B. H. (1971). *A multisensory approach to language arts for specific language disability children: A guide for primary teachers.* Cambridge, MA: Educators Publishing Service.

Smith, S., Macaruso, P., Shankwelle, D., & Crain, S. (1989). Syntactic comprehension in young poor readers. *Applied Psycholinguists, 10,* 429–454.

Snow, C. E. (1983). Literacy and language: Relationships during the preschool years. *Harvard Educational Review, 53,* 165–189.

Snow, C. E., Burns, M., & Griffin, P. (1998). *Preventing reading difficulties in young children.* Washington, DC: National Academy Press.

Snow, C. E., & Dickinson, D. K. (1990). Social sources of narrative skills at home and at school. *First Language, 10,* 87–103.

Snowling, M. J. (2000). *Dyslexia.* Oxford, UK: Blackwell.

Snowling, M. J. (2009, June). *Reading risk families and phenotypes.* Presidential address presented at the sixteenth annual meeting of the Society for the Scientific Study of Reading, Boston, MA.

Snowling, M. J., Bishop, D. V. M., & Stothard, S. E. (2000). Is preschool language impairment a risk factor for dyslexia in adolescence? *Journal of Child Psychology and Psychiatry, 41,* 587–600.

Snowling, M. J., & Hayiou-Thomas, M. E. (2006). The dyslexia spectrum: Continuities between reading, speech, and language impairments. *Topics in Language Disorders, 26,* 110–126.

Snowling, M. J., & Hulme, C. (2005). Learning to read with language impairment. In M. J. Snowling & C. Hulme (Eds.), *The science of reading: A handbook* (pp. 397–412). Oxford, UK: Blackwell.

Snowling, M. J., & Hulme, C. (2008). Reading intervention for children with language learning impairments. In C. F. Norbury, J. B. Tomblin, & D. V. M. Bishop (Eds.), *Understanding developmental language disorders in children* (pp. 179–192). Hove, Sussex: Psychology Press.

Snowling, M. J., van Wagtendonk, B., & Stafford, C. (1988). Object-naming deficits in developmental dyslexia. *Journal of Research in Reading, 11,* 67–85.

Spear-Swerling, L. (2006). Children's reading comprehension and oral reading fluency in easy text. *Reading and Writing, 19,* 199–220.

Spear-Swerling, L., & Sternberg, R. J. (1996). *Off track: When poor readers become "learning disabled."* Boulder, CO: Westview Press.

Specialized Program Individualizing Reading Excellence (S.P.I.R.E): http://www.esp .schoolspecialty.com

Spector, J. E. (1995). Phonemic awareness training: Application of principles of direct instruction. *Reading and Writing Quarterly: Overcoming Learning Difficulties, 11*(1), 37–52. EJ 496 026

Spence, L. K. (2010). Discerning writing assessment: Insights into an analytic rubric. *Language Arts, 87,* 337–352.

Stadler, M., & Ward, G. (2005). Supporting the narrative development of young children. *Early Childhood Education Journal, 33*(2), 73–80.

Stahl, S., & Murray, B. A. (1994). Defining phonological awareness and its relationship to early reading. *Journal of Educational Psychology, 86,* 2221–2249.

Stahl, S., & Nagy, W. (2006). *Teaching word meanings.* Mahwah, NJ: Erlbaum.

Stanovich, K. E. (1980). Toward an interactive-compensatory model of individual differences in the development of reading fluency. *Reading Research Quarterly, 16,* 32–71.

Stanovich, K. E. (1986). Matthew effects in reading: Some consequences of individual differences in the acquisition of literacy. *Reading Research Quarterly, 21,* 360–406.

Stanovich, K. E. (1988a). Explaining the difference between the dyslexic and the garden-variety poor reader: The phonological-core variable-difference model. *Journal of Learning Disabilities, 21,* 590–612.

Stanovich, K. E. (1988b). The right and wrong places to look for the cognitive locus of reading disability. *Annals of Dyslexia, 38,* 154–177.

Stanovich, K. E. (1990). Concepts in developmental theories of reading skills: Cognitive resources, automaticity, and modularity. *Developmental Review, 10*, 72–100.

Stanovich, K. E. (1991). Word recognition: Changing perspectives. In R. Barr, M. Kamil, P. Mosenthal, & P. Pearson (Eds.), *Handbook of reading research* (Vol. 2, pp. 418–452). New York: Longman.

Stanovich, K. E. (1992). Speculations on the causes and consequences of individual differences in early reading acquisition. In P. Gough, L. Ehri, & R. Treiman (Eds.), *Reading acquisition* (pp. 307–342). Hillsdale, NJ: Erlbaum.

Stanovich, K. E. (2000). *Progress in understanding reading: Scientific foundations and new frontiers.* New York: Guilford Press.

Stanovich, K. E., Siegel, L. S., & Gottardo, A. (1997). Converging evidence for phonological and surface subtypes of reading disability. *Journal of Educational Psychology, 89*, 114–127.

Stein, N., & Glenn, C. (1979). An analysis of story comprehension in elementary school children. In R. D. Freedle (Ed.), *Advances in discourse processes: Vol. 2. New directions in discourse processing* (pp. 53–119). Norwood, NJ: Albex.

Stephenson, K. A., Parrila, R. K., Georgiou, G. K., & Kirby, J. R. (2008). Effects of home literacy, parents' beliefs, and children's task-focused behavior on emergent literacy and word reading skills. *Scientific Studies of Reading, 12*, 24–50.

Stewart, R. M., Benner, G. J., Martella, R. C., & Marchand-Martella, N. E. (2007). Three-tier models of reading and behavior: A research review. *Journal of Positive Behavior Interventions, 9*, 239–253.

Stone, B., & Brady, S. (1995). Evidence for deficits in basic phonological processes in less-skilled readers. *Annals of Dyslexia, 45*, 51–78.

Stone, C. A., Silliman, E. R., Ehren, B. J., & Apel, K. (Eds.). (2006). *Handbook of Language and Literacy: Development and Disorders.* New York: Guilford Press.

Stoodley, C. J., & Stein, J. F. (2006). A processing speed deficit in dyslexic adults? Evidence from a peg-moving task. *Neuroscience Letters, 399*, 264–267.

Storch, S., & Whitehurst, G. (2002). Oral language and code-related precursors to reading: Evidence from a longitudinal structural model. *Developmental Psychology, 38*, 934–947.

Stothard, S. E., Snowling, M. J., Bishop, D. V. M., Chipchase, B., & Kaplan, C. (1998). Language impaired pre-schoolers: A follow-up in adolescence. *Journal of Speech, Language, and Hearing Research, 41*, 407–418.

Strong, C. J. (1998). *The Strong narrative assessment procedure.* Eau Claire, WI: Thinking Publications.

Stuart, M., Stainthorp, R., & Snowling, M. (2008). Literacy as a complex activity: Deconstructing the simple view of reading. *Literacy, 42*, 59–66.

Sulzby, E., Teale, W. H., & Kamberelis, G. (1989). Emergent writing in the classroom: Home and school connections. In D. S. Strickland & L. M. Morrow (Eds.), *Emerging literacy: Young children learn to read and write.* Newark, DE: International Reading Association.

Swan, D., & Goswami, U. (1997). Picture naming deficits in developmental dyslexia. The phonological representation hypothesis. *Brain and Language, 56*, 334–353.

Swanson, H. K. (1999). Reading comprehension and working memory in skilled readers: Is the phonological loop more important than the executive system? *Journal of Experimental Child Psychology, 72*, 1–31.

Swanson, H. L. (1993). Working memory in learning disability subgroups. *Journal of Experimental Child Psychology, 56*, 87–114.

Swanson, H. L. (1994). Short-term memory and working memory: Do both contribute to our understanding of academic achievement in children and adults with learning disabilities. *Journal of Learning Disabilities, 27*, 34–50.

Swanson, H. L., & Ashbaker, M. (2000). Working memory, short-term memory, articulation speed, word recognition, and reading comprehension in learning disabled readers: Executive and/or articulatory system? *Intelligence, 28*, 1–30.

Swanson, H. L., & Berninger, V. W. (1995). The role of working memory in skilled and less skilled readers' word comprehension. *Intelligence, 21*, 83–108.

Swanson, H. L., & O'Connor, R. (2009). The role of working memory and fluency practice on the reading comprehension of students who are dysfluent readers. *Journal of Learning Disability, 42*, 548–575.

Swanson, H. L., & Siegel, L. S. (2001). Learning disabilities as a working memory deficit. *Issues in Education, 7*(1–48), 127–154.

Swanson, H. L., Zheng, X., & Jerman, O. (2009). Working memory, short term memory, and reading disabilities. *Journal of Learning Disabilities, 42*, 260–287.

Sylvan Learning. (n.d.). *Read, click and win with BookAdventure!*. Retrieved January 29, 2011, from http://www.bookadventure.org

Tabors, P. O., & Snow, C. E. (2002). In S. B. Neuman & D. K. Dickinson (Eds.), *Handbook of early literacy research* (pp. 159–178). New York: Guilford Press.

Tallal, P., Miller, S., & Fitch, R. H. (1993). Neurobiological basis of speech—A case for the preeminence of temporal processing. *Annals of the New York Academy of Sciences, 682*, 27–47.

Tangel, D., & Blachman, B. A. (1995). Effect of phoneme awareness instruction on kindergarten children's invented spelling. *Journal of Reading Behavior, 24*, 233–261.

Tannenbaum, K. R., Torgesen, J. K., & Wagner, R. K. (2006). Relationships between word knowledge and reading comprehension in third-grade children. *Scientific Studies of Reading, 10*(4), 381–398.

Teale, W., & Sulzby, E. (1986). *Emergent literacy: Writing and reading*. Norwood, NJ: Ablex.

Temple, C., Nathan, R., Burris, N., & Temple, F. (1992). *The beginnings of writing* (3rd ed.). Needham Heights, MA: Allyn & Bacon.

Tomblin, J. B. (2008). Validating diagnostic standards for specific language impairment using adolescent outcomes. In C. F. Norbury, J. B. Tomblin, & D. V. M. Bishop (Eds.), *Understanding developmental language disorders: From Theory to Practice* (pp. 93–114). New York: Psychology Press.

Torgesen, J. (2004). Conceptual, historical and research aspects of learning disabilities. In B. Y. L. Wong (Ed.), *Learning about learning disabilities* (3rd ed., pp. 3–40). San Diego, CA: Elsevier Academic Press.

Torgesen, J. (2005). Recent discoveries from the research on remedial interventions for children with dyslexia. In M. Snowling & C. Hulme (Eds.), *The science of reading* (pp. 521–537). Oxford, UK: Blackwell.

Torgesen, J., & Burgess, S. R. (1998). Consistency of reading-related phonological processes throughout early childhood: Evidence from longitudinal-correlational and instructional studies. In J. Metsala & L. Ehri (Eds.), *Word recognition in beginning reading* (pp. 161–188). Hillsdale, NJ: Erlbaum.

Torgesen, J., Wagner, R. K., Rashotte, C. A., Burgess, S., & Hecht, S. (1997). Contributions of phonological awareness and rapid automatic naming ability to the growth of word-reading skills in second- to fifth-grade children. *Scientific Studies of Reading, 1,* 161–185.

Treiman, R. (1993). *Beginning to spell.* New York: Oxford University Press.

Treiman, R. (1998). Why spelling? The benefits of incorporating spelling into beginning reading instruction. In J. L. Metsala & L. C. Ehri (Eds.), *Word recognition in beginning literacy* (pp. 289–313). Mahwah, NJ: Erlbaum.

Treiman, R., & Broderick, V. (1998). What's in a name: Children's knowledge about the letters in their own name. *Journal of Experimental Child Psychology, 70,* 97 116.

Understanding dysgraphia. (n.d.). Retrieved January 30, 2011, from http://www.interdys.org/ewebeditpro5/upload/Understanding Dysgraphia.pdf

U.S. Department of Education, 71 Fed. Reg. (pt. 2) 46,540. (2006). Assistance to states for the education of children with disabilities and preschool grants for children with disabilities; final rule (to be codified at 34 C.F.R. pts. 300 & 301).

U.S. Department of Health and Human Services, Centers for Disease Control and Prevention, and the Centers for Medicare and Medicaid Services. (2009–2010). *International Classification of Diseases, Ninth Revision, Clinical Modification (ICD-9-CM), Sixth Edition.* Hyattsville, MD: Author. Retreived from http://hdl.handle.net/1902.29/CD-0177, Odum Institute [Distributor], V1 [Version].

United States Office of Education, 42 Fed. Reg G1082 (1977). Assistance to states for education for handicapped children: Procedures for evaluating specific learning disabilities.

van den Broek, P., & Kremer, K. E. (1999). The mind in action. What it means to comprehend during reading? In B. Taylor, M. Graves, & P. van den Broek (Eds.), *Reading for meaning* (pp. 1–31). New York: Teachers College Press.

van der Ley, H. K. J., & Ullman, M. T. (2001). Past tense morphology in specifically language impaired and normally developing children. *Language and Cognitive Processes, 16,* 177–217.

Van Kleeck, A., & Schuele, C. M. (1987). Precursors to literacy: Normal development. *Topics in Language Disorders, 7,* 13–31.

Vasilyeva, M., & Waterfall, H. (2011). Variability in language development: Relations to socioeconomic status and environmental input. In S. B. Neuman & D. K. Dickinson (Eds.), *Handbook of early literacy research* (Vol. 3, pp. 36–48). New York: Guilford Press.

Vaughn, S., Wanzek, J., & Fletcher, J. M (2007). Multiple tiers of intervention: A framework for prevention and identification of students with reading/learning disabilities. In B. M. Taylor & J. E. Ysseldyke (Eds.), *Effective instruction for struggling readers, K–6* (pp. 173–195). New York: Teacher's College Press.

Vaughn, S., Wanzek, J., Woodruff, A. L., & Linan-Thompson, S. (2007). Prevention and early identification of students with reading disabilities. In D. Haager, J. Klinger, & S. Vaughn

(Eds.), *Evidence-based reading practices for response to intervention* (pp. 11–27). Baltimore: Brookes.

Vellutino, F. R., & Fletcher, J. M. (2005). Developmental dyslexia. In M. J. Snowling & C. Hulme (Eds.), *The science of reading: A handbook* (pp. 362–378). Oxford, UK: Blackwell.

Vellutino, F. R., Fletcher, J. M., Snowling, M. J., & Scanlon, D. M. (2004). Specific reading disability (dyslexia): What have we learned in the past four decades? *Journal of Child Psychiatry, 45,* 2–40.

Vellutino, F. R., Scanlon, D. M., & Spearing, D. (1995). Semantic and phonological decoding in poor and normal readers. *Journal of Experimental Psychology, 59,* 76–123.

Verhoeven, L., & van Balkom, H. (Eds.). (2004). *Classification of developmental language disorders: Theoretical issues and clinical implications.* Mahwah, NJ: Erlbaum.

Vernon-Feagans, L., Hammer, C. S., Miccio, A., & Manlove, E. (2002). Early language and literacy skills in low-income African American and Hispanic children. In S. B. Neuman & D. K. Dickinson (Eds.), *Handbook of Early Literacy Research* (pp. 192–210). New York: Guilford Press.

Vogel, S. (1977). Morphological ability in normal and dyslexic children. *Journal of Learning Disabilities, 10,* 292–299.

Vukovic, R. K., & Siegel, L. S. (2006). The double-deficit hypothesis: A comprehensive analysis of the evidence. *Journal of Learning Disabilities, 39,* 25–47.

Wadsworth, S. J., Olson, R. K., Pennington, B. F., & DeFries, J. C. (2000). Differential genetic etiology of reading disability as a function of IQ. *Journal of Learning Disabilities, 33,* 192–199.

Wagner, R., & Ridgewell, C. (2009). A large-scale study of specific reading comprehension disability. *Perspectives on Language and Literacy, 35,* 27–31.

Wagner, R., & Torgesen, J. (1987). The nature of phonological processing and its causal role in the acquisition of reading skills. *Psychological Bulletin, 101,* 192–212.

Wagner, R., Torgesen, J., & Rashotte, C. (1994). Development of reading-related phonological processing abilities: New evidence of bidirectional causality from a latent variable longitudinal study. *Developmental Psychology, 30,* 73–87.

Wagner, R., Torgesen, J., & Rashotte, C. (1999a). *Comprehensive Test of Phonological Processing, CTOPP.* Austin, TX: Pro-Ed.

Wagner, R., Torgesen, J., & Rashotte, C. (1999b). *Test of word reading efficiency, TOWRE.* Austin, TX: Pro-Ed.

Wagner, R., Torgesen, J., Rashotte, C., Hecht, S., Barker, T., Burgess, S., et al. (1997). Changing relations between phonological processing abilities and word-level reading as children develop from beginning to skilled readers: A five-year longitudinal study. *Developmental Psychology, 33,* 468–479.

Walsh, D. J., Price, G. G., & Gillingham, M. G. (1988). The critical but transitory importance of letter naming. *Reading Research Quarterly 23,* pp. 108–122.

Watkins, M. W. (2005). Diagnostic validity of Wechsler subtest scatter. *Learning Disabilities: A Contemporary Journal, 3,* 20–29.

Wechsler, D. (2003). *Wechsler Intelligence Scale for Children–Fourth Edition.* San Antonio, TX: Pearson/The Psychological Corporation.

Wechsler, D. (2009). *Wechsler individual achievement test-third edition (WIAT-III).* San Antonio, TX: The Psychological Corporation.

Welcome to Touch Math, Multisensory Teaching, Learning Math Tools Make Math Fun! (n.d.). Retrieved January 30, 2011, from http://www .touchmath.com/

Westby, C. (1991). Learning to talk-talking to learn: Oral-literate language differences. In C. S. Simon (Ed.), *Communication skills and classroom success* (pp. 181–218). San Diego, CA: College Hill Press.

Westby, C. E. (1984). Development of narrative abilities. In G. Wallach & K. Butler (Eds.), *Language learning disabilities in school age children* (pp. 103–127). Baltimore: Williams & Wilkins.

Westby, C. E. (2005). Assessing and remediating text comprehension. In H. W. Catts & A. G. Kamhi (Eds.), *Language and reading disabilities.* Boston: Pearson.

Westby, C. E., & Clauser, P. S. (2006). The right stuff for writing: Assessing and facilitating written language. In A. Kamhi & H. Catts (Eds.), *Language and reading disabilities* (pp. 274–348). Boston: Allyn & Bacon.

Whitehurst, G. J., & Lonigan, C. J. (1998). Child development and emergent literacy. *Child Development, 69,* 848–872.

Whitehurst, G. L., & Lonigan, C. L. (2002). Emergent literacy: Development from prereaders to readers. In S. B. Neuman & D. K. Dickinson (Eds.), *Handbook of early literacy research* (pp. 11–29). New York: Guilford Press.

Wiederholt, J. L., & Bryant, B. R. (2001). *Gray oral reading test, GORT-4* (4th ed.). Austin, TX: Pro-Ed.

Wiig, E. H., & Secord, W. A. (2006). *Emerging literacy & language assessment, ELLA.* Greenville, SC: Super Duper.

Wiig, E. H., Secord, W. A., & Semel, E. (2004). *Clinical evaluation of language fundamentals— Preschool* (2nd ed.). San Antonio, TX: The Psychological Corporation/A Harcourt Assessment Company.

Wiig, E. H., & Semel, E. M. (1984). *Language assessment and intervention for the learning disabled* (2nd ed.). Columbus, OH: Charles E. Merrill.

Wilkinson, G. S. (1993). *The wide range achievement test: Manual* (3rd ed.). Wilmington, DE: Wide Range.

Wilkinson, G. S., & Robertson, G. J. (2006). *Wide Range Achievement Test, WRAT-4* (4th ed.). Odessa, FL: Psychological Assessment Resources.

Willcutt, E. G., & Pennington, B. F. (2000). Comorbidity of reading disability and attention-deficit/hyperactivity disorder. *Journal of Learning Disabilities, 33,* 179–191.

Wilson, V. L., & Rupley, W. H. (1997). A structural equation model for reading comprehension based on background, phonemic, and strategy knowledge. *Scientific Studies of Reading, 1,* 45–63.

Wiseheart, R., Altmann, L. J. P., Park, H., & Lombardino, L. J. (2009). Sentence comprehension in young adults with developmental dyslexia. *Annals of Dyslexia, 59*(2), 151-167.

Wolf, M. (1999). What time may tell: Towards a new conceptualization of developmental dyslexia. *Annals of Dyslexia, 49,* 1–28.

Wolf, M., Bally, H., & Morris, E. (1986). Automaticity, retrieval processes, and reading: A longitudinal study in average and impaired readers. *Child Development, 57,* 988–1005.

Wolf, M., & Bowers, P. (1999). The "double-deficit hypothesis" for the developmental dyslexias. *Journal of Educational Psychology, 91*(3), 1–24.

Wolf, M., & Denkla, M. B. (2005). *Rapid automatized naming and rapid alternating stimulus tests (RAN/RAS).* Austin, TX: Pro-Ed.

Wolf, M., Goldberg O'Rourke, A., Gidney, C., Lovett, M., Cirino, P., & Morris, R. (2002). The second deficit: An investigation of the independence of phonological and naming-speed deficits in developmental dyslexia. *Reading and Writing, 15,* 43–72.

Wolf, M., & Goodglass, H. (1986). Dyslexia, dysnomia, and lexical retrieval—a longitudinal investigation. *Brain and Language, 28,* 154–168.

Wolf, M., & Katzir-Cohen, T. (2001). Reading fluency and its intervention. *Scientific Studies of Reading, 5*(3), 211–239.

Wolff, P. H. (2000). Impaired temporal resolution in developmental dyslexia. *Annals of the New York Academy of Sciences, 682,* 87–103.

Wolff, P. H., Michel, G. F., & Ovrut, M. (1990). Rate variables and automatized naming in developmental dyslexia. *Brain and Language, 39,* 556–575.

Woodcock, R. W., Mather, N., & Schrank, F. A. (2004). *Woodcock Johnson III Diagnostic Reading Battery, WJ III DRB.* Itasca, IL: Riverside.

Woodcock, R. W., McGrew, K. S., & Mather, N. (2001a). *Woodcock Johnson III Tests of Achievement, WJ III ACH.* Itasca, IL: Riverside.

Woodcock, R. W., McGrew, K. S., & Mather, N. (2001b). *Woodcock Johnson III Tests of Cognitive Ability, WJ III COG.* Itasca, IL: Riverside.

Woods, M. L., & Moe, A. J. (1998). *Analytic reading inventory.* New York: Macmillan.

Woodcock, R. W., & Pines, C. (1998). *Woodcock reading mastery tests–revised, WRMT-R.* Circle pines, MN: American Guidance Service.

Wright, P. W., & Wright, P. D. (2007). *Wrightslaw: Special education law* (2nd ed.). Hartfield, VA: Harbor House Law Press.

Yopp, H. K. (1992). Developing phonemic awareness in young children. *The Reading Teacher, 45,* 696–703.

Yuill, N. M., & Oakhill, J. V. (1991). *Children's problems in text comprehension: An experimental investigation.* Cambridge, UK: Cambridge University Press.

Ziegler, J., & Goswami, U. (2005). Reading acquisition, developmental dyslexia, and skilled reading across languages: A psycholinguistic grain size theory. *Psychological Bulletin, 13*(1), 3–29.

Index